MEDICAL *and* PSYCHOSOCIAL CARE
of the CANCER SURVIVOR

Edited by Kenneth D. Miller, MD

❝ Dr. Miller's book is the most encyclopedic approach to cancer survivorship to date. He and his co-authors tackle all of the major issues of survivorship from the psychological, to the physical and all the ramifications of trying to move one's life forward after a cancer diagnosis and the treatment that accompanies it. The thoroughness of the approach, and the manner in which the topics are tied together sheds light on the issues a cancer survivor —the whole individual—must deal with. This is a must-have book for those interested in this ever more important area of medicine. ❞

LAWRENCE SHULMAN, MD
Chief Medical Officer
Dana-Farber Cancer Institute
Boston, MA

❝ Dr. Miller has created essential reading for any professional who cares for cancer survivors. His unique perspective as a seasoned oncologist and committed husband to a cancer survivor has resulted in a no-nonsense cancer survivorship guide for physicians, nurses, and mental health professionals alike from a variety of perspectives. Essential material on psychosocial topics, medical issues, and epidemiology is presented clearly and thoroughly. This healing hero knows the science and the caring. ❞

MATTHEW LOSCALZO, MSW
Executive Director, Department of
Supportive Care Medicine
Professor, Department of Population Sciences
City of Hope
Duarte, CA

❝ With over 11 million cancer survivors nationally, Dr. Miller's book is a most welcome and needed resource for healthcare professionals, the generalist and specialist alike. This gem of a book is as comprehensive as it is practical and offers current information about the long-term and late effects of cancer and its treatment—from medical problems and psychological issues to sexual health. Most importantly, the authors give us the very important message that cancer survivorship is more than surviving—it is a distinct period of life with a unique set of healthcare challenges. This book will help us assure that survivors achieve the highest quality of life possible. ❞

MARY MCCABE, RN
Director, Cancer Survivorship Program
Memorial-Sloan Kettering Hospital
New York, NY

❝ Dr. Miller's Medical and Psychosocial Care of the Cancer Survivor *is a landmark roadmap for clinicians who care for cancer survivors and researchers. The book is written by top experts in the field and presents the state of the art and science of survivorship. It is an excellent book which reviews the medical needs of cancer survivors while sensitively discussing their psychosocial needs. I highly recommend it.* ❞

RICHARD EDELSON, MD
Director, Yale Cancer Center
Professor of Oncology
New Haven, CT

MEDICAL *and* PSYCHOSOCIAL CARE *of the* CANCER SURVIVOR

Edited by

Kenneth D. Miller, MD

Director
Lance Armstrong Survivorship Program
Dana-Farber Cancer Institute

Assistant Professor
Harvard Medical School
Boston, MA

JONES AND BARTLETT PUBLISHERS
Sudbury, Massachusetts
BOSTON   TORONTO   LONDON   SINGAPORE

World Headquarters
Jones and Bartlett Publishers
40 Tall Pine Drive
Sudbury, MA 01776
978-443-5000
info@jbpub.com
www.jbpub.com

Jones and Bartlett Publishers
Canada
6339 Ormindale Way
Mississauga, Ontario L5V 1J2
Canada

Jones and Bartlett Publishers
International
Barb House, Barb Mews
London W6 7PA
United Kingdom

Jones and Bartlett's books and products are available through most bookstores and online booksellers. To contact Jones and Bartlett Publishers directly, call 800-832-0034, fax 978-443-8000, or visit our website www.jbpub.com.

Substantial discounts on bulk quantities of Jones and Bartlett's publications are available to corporations, professional associations, and other qualified organizations. For details and specific discount information, contact the special sales department at Jones and Bartlett via the above contact information or send an email to specialsales@jbpub.com.

The authors, editor, and publisher have made every effort to provide accurate information. However, they are not responsible for errors, omissions, or for any outcomes related to the use of the contents of this book and take no responsibility for the use of the products and procedures described. Treatments and side effects described in this book may not be applicable to all people; likewise, some people may require a dose or experience a side effect that is not described herein. Drugs and medical devices are discussed that may have limited availability controlled by the Food and Drug Administration (FDA) for use only in a research study or clinical trial. Research, clinical practice, and government regulations often change the accepted standard in this field. When consideration is being given to use of any drug in the clinical setting, the healthcare provider or reader is responsible for determining FDA status of the drug, reading the package insert, and reviewing prescribing information for the most up-to-date recommendations on dose, precautions, and contraindications, and determining the appropriate usage for the product. This is especially important in the case of drugs that are new or seldom used.

Production Credits
Executive Publisher: Christopher Davis
Production Director: Amy Rose
Sr. Editorial Assistant: Jessica Acox
Production Editor: Daniel Stone
V.P., Manufacturing and Inventory Control:
    Therese Connell

Composition: Publishers' Design and Production
    Services, Inc.
Printing and Binding: Malloy, Inc.
Cover Printing: Malloy, Inc.

Cover Credits
Front Cover
Top Left: © absolut/ShutterStock, Inc.; Top Right: © Graca Victoria/ShutterStock, Inc.; Center: © Yuri Acurs/ShutterStock, Inc.; Bottom Right: © Mandy Godbehear/ShutterStock, Inc.; Bottom Left: © Studio 1One/ShutterStock, Inc.

Back Cover
Top Left: © Yuri Acurs/ShutterStock, Inc.; Center: © Studio 1One/ShutterStock, Inc.; Top Right: © Monkey Business Images/ShutterStock, Inc.

Library of Congress Cataloging-in-Publication Data
Medical and psychosocial care of the cancer survivor / edited by Kenneth D. Miller.
    p. ; cm.
  Includes bibliographical references and index.
  ISBN-13: 978-0-7637-5770-0 / ISBN-10: 0-7637-5770-5
  1. Cancer—Psychological aspects. 2. Cancer—Patients—Rehabilitation. 3. Cancer—Treatment.
I. Miller, Kenneth D., 1956–
  [DNLM: 1. Neoplasms. 2. Survivors. 3. Neoplasms—therapy. QZ 200 M48835 2009]
  RC262.M389 2009
  362.196'994—dc22
                                                                            2009014738
6048

Printed in the United States of America
13 12 11 10 09   10 9 8 7 6 5 4 3 2 1

Contents

Contributors

Editor

Kenneth D. Miller, MD
Director
Lance Armstrong Survivorship Program
Dana-Farber Cancer Institute
Assistant Professor
Harvard Medical School
Boston, MA

Contributing Authors

Ron Afshari Adelman, MD, MPH, FACS
Associate Professor of Ophthalmology
Yale University School of Medicine
New Haven, CT

Joachim Baehring, MD
Associate Professor of Neurology, Medicine, and Neurosurgery
Yale University School of Medicine
New Haven, CT

Natan Bar-Chama, MD
Associate Professor of Urology
Department of Urology
Mount Sinai School of Medicine
New York, NY

Laura A. Bayer, PhD
Staff Psychologist
Clinical Health Psychology Section, VA Connecticut Healthcare
   System
Assistant Clinical Professor of Psychiatry
Yale University School of Medicine
New Haven, CT

Dalliah Black, MD, FACS
Breast Surgical Oncologist
The Hoffberger Breast Center
Mercy Medical Center
Baltimore, MD

Rachel Blitzblau, MD, PhD
Resident
Department of Therapeutic Radiology
Yale University School of Medicine
New Haven, CT

Jason G. Bromer, MD
Instructor
Yale University School of Medicine
New Haven, CT

Michael A. Diefenbach, PhD
Associate Professor
Departments of Urology and Oncological Sciences
Mount Sinai School of Medicine
New York, NY

Debra L. Friedman, MD
Associate Professor of Pediatrics
E. Bronson Ingram Chair in Pediatric Oncology
Leader, Cancer Control and Prevention Program
Vanderbilt Ingram Cancer Center
Nashville, TN

Stephanie M. George, MPH, MA
Predoctoral Fellow
Nutritional Epidemiology Branch, National Cancer Institute
Yale School of Public Health
New Haven, CT

Sahar Ghassemi, MD
Instructor
Section of Digestive Diseases
Yale University
New Haven, CT

Mitch Golant, PhD
Senior VP Research and Training
The Wellness Community
Washington, DC

Natalie V. Haskins, MAT
Director
Public Education and Awareness
The Wellness Community
Washington, DC

Elizabeth H. Holt, MD, PhD
Assistant Professor of Medicine
Section of Endocrinology
Yale University School of Medicine
New Haven, CT

Melinda L. Irwin, PhD, MPH
Associate Professor of Epidemiology and Public Health
Yale University School of Medicine
New Haven, CT

Paul Jacobsen, PhD
Director
Psychosocial and Palliative Care Program
H. Lee Moffitt Cancer Center and Research Institute
Professor of Psychology and Oncology
University of South Florida
Tampa, FL

Heather S.L. Jim, PhD
Assistant Professor
Health Outcomes and Behavior Program
H. Lee Moffitt Cancer Center and Research Institute
Tampa, FL

Robert D. Kerns, PhD
National Program Director for Pain Management
VA Central Office
Director
Pain Research, Informatics, Medical Comorbities and Education (PRIME) Center
VA Connecticut
Professor of Psychiatry, Neurology, and Psychology
Yale University School of Medicine
New Haven, CT

Rex L. Mahnensmith, MD
Professor of Internal Medicine
Clinical Director of Nephrology
Medical Director of Dialysis
Yale University School of Medicine
New Haven, CT

Vaughn L. Mankey, MD
Assistant Director of Medical Student Education in Psychiatry
Marjorie E. Korff PACT Program (Parenting at a Challenging Time)
Child/Adolescent and Adult Staff Psychiatrist
Massachusetts General Hospital
Harvard Medical School
Boston, MA

Peter W. Marks, MD, PhD
Associate Professor of Medicine
Yale University School of Medicine
New Haven, CT

Ellen T. Matloff, MS
Research Scientist
Department of Genetics
Director, Cancer Genetic Counseling
Yale University Cancer Center/Yale University School of
   Medicine
New Haven, CT

Susan T. Mayne, PhD
Professor of Epidemiology
Yale University School of Public Health
Associate Director
Yale Cancer Center
New Haven, CT

Elias Michaelides, MD
Assistant Professor
Departments of Surgery and Pediatrics
Yale University School of Medicine
New Haven, CT

Cara Miller, BS
Graduate Fellow
Department of Clinical Psychology
Gallaudet University
Washington, DC

Andrea K. Ng, MD, MPH
Associate Professor of Radiation Oncology
Brigham and Women's Hospital
Dana-Farber Cancer Institute
Harvard Medical School
Boston, MA

Elias Obedid, MD, MPH
Medical Director
Hospital of Saint Raphael
Assistant Clinical Professor
Yale University School of Medicine
New Haven, CT

Paula K. Rauch, MD
Director
Marjorie E. Korff PACT Program (Parenting At a Challenging
    Time)
Chief
Child Psychiatry Consultation Service to Pediatrics
Massachusetts General Hospital
and
Associate Professor of Psychiatry
Harvard Medical School
Boston, MA

Kenneth B. Roberts, MD
Associate Professor
Department of Therapeutic Radiology
Yale University School of Medicine
New Haven, CT

Lynda E. Rosenfeld, MD
Associate Professor of Medicine and Pediatrics
Yale University School of Medicine
Attending Physician
Yale-New Haven Hospital
New Haven, CT

Leslie R. Schover, PhD
Professor of Behavioral Science
Department of Behavioral Science
Division of Cancer Prevention
The University of Texas M. D. Anderson Cancer Center
Houston, TX

Emre Seli, MD
Assistant Professor
Associate Director for Research, Division of Reproductive
    Endocrinology and Infertility
Director, Oocyte Donation and Gestational Surrogacy Program
Department of Obstetrics, Gynecology, and Reproductive
    Sciences
Yale University School of Medicine
New Haven, CT

Rajeev K. Seth, MD
Vitreo-Retinal Surgical Fellow
Department of Ophthalmology
Yale University School of Medicine
New Haven, CT

Antoine G. Sreih, MD
Rheumatology Section
Yale University School of Medicine
New Haven, CT

Lynn Tanoue, MD
Professor of Medicine
Section of Pulmonary and Critical Care Medicine
Yale University School of Medicine
Medical Director, Yale Cancer Center Thoracic Oncology Program
New Haven, CT

Megan Taylor-Ford
Manager
Patient Education & Outreach
The Wellness Community
Washington, DC

Lois B. Travis, MD, ScD
Director
Rubin Center for Cancer Survivorship
Professor
Department of Radiation Oncology
James P. Wilmot Cancer Center
University of Rochester Medical Center
Rochester, NY

Gina A. Turner, PhD
Post Doctoral Fellow
Department of Oncological Sciences
Mount Sinai School of Medicine
New York, NY

Guido Wollmann, MD
Associate Research Scientist
Department of Neurosurgery
Yale University School of Medicine
New Haven, CT

Preface

"When cancer treatment has helped to add years of life for many cancer survivors our next obligation is to help survivors enjoy the best possible quality of life during those years."

Many of us remember where we were when we learned that President Kennedy was shot. And most of us remember Where we were when we heard about the World Trade Center attacks on September 11th, 2001. Similarly, people vividly recall the moments leading up to and the moment when they were told that they, a friend, or loved one has cancer. Some describe it as raw terror and others as "ice water poured through my veins." The day of diagnosis is essentially as "unforgettable" as are the days that follow when treatment starts and then finishes. Thankfully, a growing majority of cancer survivors live with and beyond cancer and spend far more time with a history of cancer than during the time of diagnosis and treatment. Natalie Spingarn writes about them: "The new population of survivors hanging in there can be found everywhere . . . in offices and factories, on bicycles and cruise ships, on tennis courts and beaches, and in bowling alleys. You see them in all ages, shapes, sizes, and colors, usually unremarkable in their appearance, sometimes remarkable for the way they learn to live with disabilities."*

For cancer survivors there are "seasons of survivorship." Dr. Fitzhugh Mullen described three seasons of survival in the *New England Journal of Medicine*. Acute survivorship includes the time of diagnosis, testing, and treatment. Extended survivorship is a period of surveillance for recurrence. Finally, permanent survivorship begins with a

---

Source: Spingarn, Natalie. *The New Cancer Survivors. Living with Grace, Fighting with Spirit.* Johns Hopkins University Press, 1999.

renewed sense of confidence in one's health and continues for what we hope will be many years of life. Twenty years after Dr. Mullen defined these seasons it is helpful to reexamine this concept in light of the many changes that have occurred in regards to diagnosis, treatment, and prognosis. Acute survivorship is still a period of intense activity with diagnosis and treatment. The next season we might refer to as transitional survivorship when treatment ends then begins extended survivorship. Next, survivors in the extended season of survivorship are a heterogeneous group—some are living with cancer and don't require additional treatment, some are in a "maintained remission" and require ongoing treatment with a hormonal therapy of targeted agent such as Imitinib. Finally others are "living with cancer," and living well for many years. In many established clinical practices the growing majority of the cancer survivors are "permanent survivors." In permanent survivorship, however, great heterogeneity is seen because other cancer survivors are cancer free but not "free of cancer" meaning that they have some late or long-term consequences of their cancer diagnosis or treatment. Others go on to develop a second cancer that may or may not be related to their primary diagnosis, and finally others develop a cancer that is secondary to their initial treatment. Cancer survivors are very hesitant to refer to themselves as cured, but, thankfully many go on to lead long and healthy lives.

Cancer survivorship care is deeply embedded in the "normal" care that we offer to cancer survivors, and many clinicians when asked about survivorship rightfully say, "I do that already" and they do. Good cancer survivorship care need not involve a dedicated cancer survivorship program, but, ideally this can be expectantly designed and delivered within many different care settings to meet the needs of cancer survivors in each of the seasons of survivorship. These needs may be very few or very great, may be medical, psychosocial, legal, spiritual, and financial to name a few, and the type and intensity of needs will tend to change over time.

This manual was created to enhance the readers' knowledge about the psychosocial, medical, and epidemiologic issues in the survivorship field, for survivors as a group, and as individuals. Reading this book will give you the most current information on multiple topics in cancer survivorship, as well as state of the art information on delivering survivorship care. We hope that this manual will increase your breadth of knowledge and increase your confidence in caring for cancer survivors during their seasons of survivorship. Surviving cancer is the first goal and then healthy cancer survivorship is the next.

Kenneth D. Miller, MD

Acknowledgments

I have been married for almost 30 years, a medical oncologist for 20, and the husband of a cancer survivor for about 10. Joan, I want to thank you for teaching me what cancer survivorship really is and for your strength, determination, and raw courage that helped you to be here today with our three daughters and with me. In the same manner I also want to thank Cara, Julie, and Kim, who like me, are also cancer survivors, or "cosurvivors" as some might say. The three of you are wonderful, bright, caring young women and we are incredibly proud of you.

My sincere thanks to Jeffrey Keith who is an almost 30-year survivor of osteosarcoma.

Jeff was the first man to run across the entire United States on a prosthetic leg, and 3 years ago provided the inspiration and the perspiration to spark the development of the first adult cancer survivorship program in Connecticut. Jeff, the Connecticut Challenge Cancer Survivorship Program at Yale is a wonderful testimony to your efforts and those of John Ragland, Bob Mazzone, and hundreds of bicycle riders who are equally passionate about this cause. Similarly, thank you to my colleagues at Yale including Drs. Rick Edelson and Ed Chu and to those who crafted the clinic program along with me including Maura Harrigan, Scott Capposa, Lina Chase, and Tom Quinn.

Special thanks to those who contributed their knowledge and expertise by writing the chapters in this book. Our goal collectively is to spread as much of our knowledge as possible to clinicians who are providing care for cancer survivors. Similarly, thank you to our editor Chris Davis and production editor Daniel Stone at Jones and Bartlett for making this book both possible and now a reality.

Kenneth D. Miller, MD

PART

1

Introduction

chapter

1

Challenges in Cancer Surviorshp

Kenneth D. Miller, MD

A person becomes a cancer survivor at the moment of a cancer diagnosis and remains one for as long as he or she lives. This definition, developed by the National Coalition for Cancer Survivorship in 1984 and later adopted by the National Cancer Institute, now applies to over 12 million Americans and their families and caregivers as well. Many embrace this definition, while others are uncomfortable with it. Some people believe that the term cancer survivor should be reserved for people who are in a long-term remission or are cured and that accepting this title early risks being overly confident of one's health. Others do not adopt the term survivor because historically it has been linked with the holocaust or with natural disasters. Other titles have been used for cancer survivors, including cancer veterans, victors, and heroes.

The term "cancer survivorship" is perhaps better received because it describes a process rather than a person. The process of survivorship starts at the time of diagnosis and then changes over time. The significance of the term "survivorship" is that it establishes some degree of connection between the issues and decisions that individuals with cancer face at the time of diagnosis with the issues and decisions they may face 5, 10, and 20 years later. For example, difficult treatment decisions are made for children with leukemia and have implications throughout that child's adolescence and adulthood. One of the goals of therapy is cure, but there is growing awareness of the "price of success," the short but also the long-term sequelae of therapy. One trend in cancer therapy has been increasing dose intensity and dose density, but at the same time there have been efforts to reduce the toxicities of therapy without compromising the efficacy. The use of prophylactic cranial irradiation is no longer automatic in the treatment of childhood leukemia, the total dose of anthracyclines used in the treatment of women with breast cancer has been reduced, and fertility preservation is also considered.

People diagnosed with cancer come in all ages, shapes, colors, ethnicities, and religions, and they have different diagnoses and treatment regimens and outcomes. It is difficult to define a specific path of cancer survivorship. For cancer survivors there may be phases of the experiences that are related to the cancer, to normal aging, and some to the interaction of both. Medically, phases include:

1. The period prior to diagnosis, when symptoms may be developing but are occult
2. The time of diagnosis and the trauma associated with it
3. A treatment phase of varying duration and intensity
4. A post-treatment transition from active treatment to observation
5. A longer period of observation during which the frequency of testing and medical care may decrease
6. For some, a long period of non-cancer-related life.

Each of these phases involves a complex combination and interaction of physical, emotional, and social challenges and changes. The phases have been referred to as the "seasons of survivorship." In 1990, Dr. Fitzhugh Mullen wrote about this in the *New England Journal of Medicine*.

The journey that cancer survivors make is individual, intense, and life changing and an important one for clinicians to understand from a medical, psychosocial, and epidemiologic perspective. Medical treatment for some cancers may be relatively brief and "minor," such as a wide lumpectomy for a minute focus of ductal carcinoma in situ, not followed by radiation, chemotherapy, or hormonal therapy in an 85-year-old woman. Alternatively, treatment can be long and intensive. A

45-year-old woman might undergo neoadjuvant chemotherapy for treatment of breast cancer followed by surgery, radiation therapy, and then hormonal therapy. Yet another patient may be treated for acute leukemia before undergoing an allogeneic bone marrow transplant.

Providing medical care for cancer survivors is complex by virtue of the diversity of sex, age, diagnoses, and treatments. *Medical and Psychosocial Care of the Cancer Survivor* provides information on the common medical issues faced by cancer survivors as well as some of the uncommon ones. Many cancer survivors do not experience long-term consequences of treatment, but on the other hand, there are survivors of Hodgkin disease who after radiation and chemotherapy are at risk of a myriad of problems, including damage to coronary, valvular, and conduction systems as well as pericardial types of heart disease, pulmonary fibrosis, hypothyroidism, breast cancer, and secondary leukemia.

An understanding of the psychosocial issues of cancer survivorship is also important for clinicians. The fear of recurrence is a major issue and may be inversely proportional to the actual risk. A woman who has a small, noninvasive breast cancer may feel far more at risk of recurrence than a similar woman who has a large invasive cancer with multiple positive lymph nodes. Multiple other issues include depression, anxiety, change in family structure and dynamics, and problems related to sexuality and intimacy. Cancer survivorship affects children of cancer survivors, other family members, and caregivers in ways that are not well understood, but their experiences are important both to the patient and also later during their own lifetime. Some problems that may follow a cancer diagnosis include exacerbation of already existing financial or marital distress and divorce. Children of cancer survivors may also manifest their own stress reactions in expected and unexpected ways. A cancer diagnosis has a "ripple effect" on an entire community in positive as well as negative ways.

Cancer survivorship is not just a personal but also a public health issue. If every oncologist in practice were to continue to frequently see the growing number of new patients each year who fortunately are living to be long-term survivors, they would eventually have less time to see patients who present with a new cancer diagnosis. The healthcare system needs to gradually adopt a strategy to transition some of their care back to primary care providers who also are adept at providing care for their routine healthcare needs and the special issues related to aging. In this regard, however, it should be noted that 15% to 20% of the patients who are diagnosed with cancer any year are experiencing this as a second or greater malignancy. Screening for second malignancies needs to be a priority of a survivor's care based on normal cancer screening guidelines but also reflecting the special needs of cancer survivors, including genetic risks, increased risks of certain cancers related to the primary tumor, as well as the risk of second malignancies related to their cancer therapy.

Cancer survivorship may also be a "teachable moment," meaning that cancer survivors can change health-related behaviors to reduce their risk of developing another cancer or cardiac disease. Smoking cessation, better nutrition, and increased physical activity are important goals for everyone but potentially even more so for cancer survivors. In addition, ongoing screening for recurrence but also for the development of other common cancer is a priority and includes breast, colon, prostate, and cervical cancer screening. Hence, clinicians have an opportunity to promote good health.

Finally, there can be post-traumatic stress after cancer but also post-traumatic growth for cancer survivors. Cancer survivors often point to a new sense of purpose in life and a greater appreciation for living. The expression "taking time to smell the roses" can be considered a cliché but is a true experience for many cancer survivors. Cancer survivors can also have an improved sense of self-esteem, with a greater confidence in themselves and in their ability to meet this and other challenges.

Medical and Psychosocial Care of the Cancer Survivor is written for oncologists, primary care providers, oncology nurses, advanced practice nurses, social workers, psychologists, and other healthcare professionals. The three major areas presented in the book include:

1. Psychosocial issues in cancer survivorship, which focuses on the emotional journey of cancer survivors including the patients, their family, and caregivers. This portion of the book is written by experts in psycho-oncology, many of whom focus on the cancer survivors' family system and on psychosocial changes over time, post-traumatic stress, and post-traumatic growth.
2. Medical issues in cancer survivorship, which focuses on the most common problems faced by survivors after the experience of cancer and its treatment. This section has been designed to focus on the

most important medical issues. For example, rather than provide an exhaustive description of every type of cardiac condition, the book provides an in-depth description of the most common types of heart disease seen in cancer survivors.

3. Epidemiologic issues in cancer survivorship, which focuses on the risk of second malignancies in general and those secondary to chemotherapy or to radiation therapy. In addition, this section of the book focuses on the role of nutrition and exercise in secondary risk reduction.

Fortunately, there is a growing number of cancer survivors. The need to respond effectively to the problems and challenges they face will continue to be a growing challenge to healthcare providers.

chapter

2

Cancer Survivorship Today

Kenneth D. Miller, MD

ABSTRACT

Presently, it is estimated that there are 12 million cancer survivors in the United States and fortunately this number is continuing to increase as the result of earlier diagnosis and better treatment. Most cancer survivors recover well after their diagnosis and treatment but others are "cancer-free but not free of cancer" and continue to have medical, psychosocial, and other consequences of this experience. Preventing, recognizing, and treating these problems is essential to help cancer survivors enjoy the best possible quality of life.

Many lessons have been learned from and about cancer survivors. One of them is that cancer is a "teachable moment." More specifically, following cancer, survivors may be able to make changes in diet, exercise, smoking, and other behaviors which can result in life long health improvement.

INTRODUCTION

There has been a dramatic increase in the number of cancer survivors (Figure 2.1). This change reflects the broader definition of who is labeled a survivor but even more the improved likelihood that people diagnosed with cancer can go on to live free of cancer or with cancer as a chronic

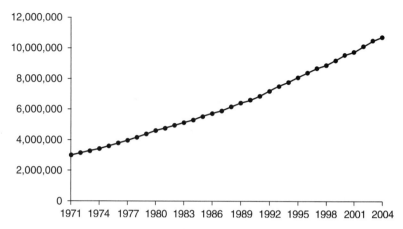

FIGURE 2.1   Estimated number of cancer survivors in the United States from 1971 to 2004.

Source: Data obtained from Ries LAG, Melbert D, Krapcho M, et al, eds. *SEER Cancer Statistics Review, 1975–2004*, National Cancer Institute Web site. http://seer.cancer.gov/csr/1975_2004. Published November 2006. Updated November 15, 2007. Accessed November 18, 2008.

disease. Earlier detection, newer and more effective therapies, and better supportive care have all contributed.

More individuals can expect to be living long term following a cancer diagnosis (Figure 2.2). Sixty-five percent of adults diagnosed today will be alive 5 years from now, and 75% of children treated for cancer will be alive 10 years from now.[1,2] Currently in the prevalent cancer survivor population, 14% of survivors were diagnosed 20 or more years ago.[3] The largest constituent of all cancer survivors, which represents 3.6% of the US population, is women breast cancer survivors followed by prostate and colorectal cancer survivors.[1,4] Together these groups account for 50% of the prevalent population of survivors in this country (Figure 2.3). Reviewing these data in detail reveals some interesting perspectives. For example, lung cancer is very prevalent, but unfortunately there is a relatively smaller population of long-term survivors. Another large group, 19% of the prevalent cancer survivor population, has been treated for colorectal cancer.[2,5] However, compared to breast cancer survivors, lung and colorectal cancer survivors are not typically vocal advocacy groups.

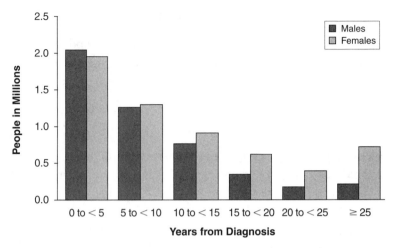

FIGURE 2.2   Estimated number of persons alive in the United States diagnosed with cancer as of January 1, 2004, by time from diagnosis and gender.

Source: Data obtained from Ries LAG, Melbert D, Krapcho M, et al, eds. *SEER Cancer Statistics Review, 1975–2004.* National Cancer Institute Web site. http://seer.cancer.gov/csr/1975_2004. Published November 2006. Updated November 15, 2007. Accessed November 18, 2008.

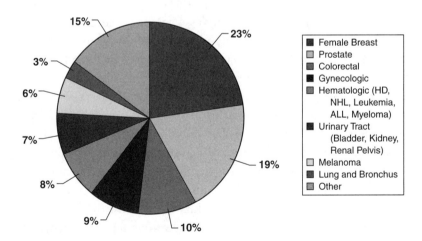

FIGURE 2.3   Estimated number of persons alive in the United States diagnosed with cancer as of January 1, 2004, by site (N = 10.8 million).

Source: Data obtained from Ries LAG, Melbert D, Krapcho M, et al, eds. *SEER Cancer Statistics Review, 1975–2004.* National Cancer Institute Web site. http://seer.cancer.gov/csr/1975_2004/, Published November 2006. Updated November 15, 2007. Accessed November 18, 2008.

SUCCESS AT A PRICE

Cancer survivorship is a process that extends over time and is a different journey for each individual and for his or her family members and caregivers. In general the impact of cancer and its treatment is:

Physical/Medical (e.g., second cancers, cardiac dysfunction, pain, lymphedema, sexual impairment)

Psychological (e.g., depression, anxiety, uncertainty, isolation, altered body image) and **social** (e.g., changes in interpersonal relationships, concerns regarding health or life insurance, job lock/loss, return to school, financial burden)

Existential and Spiritual (e.g., sense of purpose or meaning, appreciation of life)

The medical impact of cancer on an individual is related to many factors, including the cancer survivor's age and comorbidities, the specific diagnosis, location of the tumor, type of treatment (ie, surgery, radiation, or chemotherapy), the intensity of the treatment, and the effect of time and age after cancer treatment. Studies demonstrate that cancer survivors are more likely to have some difficulty with activities of daily living (Figure 2.4).[6] Other conditions associated with specific organ systems can also be seen. For example, in Chapter 19 of this book, Dr. Lynda Rosenfeld writes, "Cardiac complications of such treatment are a relatively infrequent, but important cause of morbidity and mortality in these patients, and some cancer survivors face a higher risk of death from cardiovascular causes than from recurrent cancer." Pulmonary toxicities may be common as well; as noted in this book, "up to 20% of patients who had chemotherapy will have some long-term pulmonary complications, and up to 50% of patients with thoracic radiation also have long-term complications."[7–11] During previous decades, when people diagnosed with cancer were not likely to live beyond the diagnosis, these toxicities may not have been relevant, recognized, or treated. Now, however, with a large and growing number of cancer survivors, short- and long-term sequelae of treatment have been identified in essentially all organ systems. It might be anticipated also that because cancer survivors are living longer, new problems may be identified that represent the interaction of time, age, and previous treatment. In addition, the in-

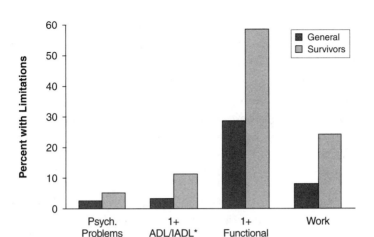

FIGURE 2.4 Percent with limitations: Survivors versus general population.

*ADL - Activities of Daily Living; IADL - Instrumental Activities of Daily Living.

Source: Data obtained from Hewitt M, Rowland JH, Yancik R. Cancer survivors in the United States: age, health, and disability. *J Gerontol.* 2003;58(1):82.

cidence of toxicity with newer agents including monoclonal antibodies, small-molecule inhibitors, and other new agents is still unknown.

The risk of a second or subsequent malignancy is also becoming more relevant because of the side effects of high-dose therapy and because cancer survivors are living longer, and with age comes an increased risk of cancer. In Chapter 15 of this book, Ng and Travis write, "The number of patients who develop second or higher order cancers is increasing, with these diagnoses now comprising about 1 of every 6 (16%) cancer incidents reported to the National Cancer Institute's Surveillance, Epidemiology, and End Results Program in 2004.[3] Moreover, solid tumors are an important cause of mortality among a number of groups of long-term survivors, in particular, patients with Hodgkin disease."[12]

Similarly, *the psychosocial impact on cancer survivors* is related to an individual's premorbid emotional life, social relationships, and support as well as factors related to the cancer and its treatment, including the intensity and duration of the treatment. The experience of a woman who receives outpatient adjuvant therapy for colon cancer is very different from that of a man who undergoes a prostatectomy or of a 35-year-old hospitalized for 6 weeks for treatment of acute leukemia. Similarly, the short- and long-term psychosocial "fallout" for these individuals may be very different. For example, in Chapter 6 of this book, Dr. Leslie Schover writes on the topic of sexuality, "Sexual problems are observed in at least 50% of survivors of breast cancer and gynecological cancer, as well as up to 90% of men treated for prostate cancer.[13] After treatment for colorectal cancer, 30% to 70% of patients have impaired sex lives, depending on the surgical procedure, their gender, and their age."[14]

In Chapter 12 of this book, Dr. Mitch Golant and Natalie Haskins describe some of the important emotional sequelae of the cancer experience:

> For many cancer patients, the most significant psychosocial stressors are unwanted aloneness, loss of control, and loss of hope. Unwanted aloneness occurs at the time of diagnosis—just imagine what it feels like when a patient hears the words from the doctor, "You have cancer." In effect, not only do patients feel different from others in their social network, but this experience also may create shifts in intimacy between them and the family caregiver. Loss of control is often reflected in feelings of helplessness, especially when patients realize that cancer is in their bodies and are unsure of the right course of treatment when faced with conflicting treatment options. Loss of hope is associated with the ups and downs of treatment and the side effects from treatment (fatigue, pain, and nausea), and is especially likely when one receives bad news.

The existential issues in cancer survivorship are perhaps the least studied but may be quite profound. Cancer survivors often report great personal growth after the cancer experience. In Chapter 5 of this book, Drs. Jim and Jacobsen write, "Evidence suggests that the fear, uncertainty, and loss wrought by cancer often spur a search for deeper meaning and a fresh perspective on old problems. As a result, survivors frequently report that life after diagnosis is characterized by a richness and depth that was previously lacking."

WHY IS THE CONCEPT OF CANCER SURVIVORSHIP IMPORTANT?

In the past, defining a survivor as a person who is disease free for 5 years focused interest and concern about the impact of cancer and treatment beginning after 5 years. In contrast, the redefinition of cancer survivors to include people from the moment of diagnosis emphasizes the need to address quality-of-life concerns at the time of diagnosis and to not wait 5 years to realize that survivors are dealing with long-term sequelae of therapy. Pediatric oncology has been at the forefront of this movement to view diagnosis and treatment as just a small part of the survivorship trajectory and to incorporate this perspective into treatment planning.

Changes in cancer treatment patterns reflect evidence-based progress but also an awareness that treatment choices have these long-term consequences. Some examples include:

▷ Neoadjuvant chemotherapy and radiation therapy allow for limb-sparing surgery in the treatment of adults with sarcoma
▷ Greater interest in the use of non-anthracycline-containing adjuvant chemotherapy in breast cancer to reduce the risk of cardiomyopathy and leukemogenesis
▷ Sperm banking or ovum preservation prior to initiation of chemotherapy

LESSONS LEARNED FROM CANCER SURVIVORS

Working with cancer survivors has taught clinicians and researchers many lessons. Dr. Julia Rowland, Director of the Office of Cancer Survivorship at the National Cancer Institute, shared the following at a recent address at the Yale Cancer Center:[15]

Lesson #1: Being cancer free does not mean being free of cancer.

Lesson #2: Transitioning to recovery is stressful.

Lesson #3: Despite risk, survivors manifest remarkable *resilience* with respect to the cancer experience and even the potential to *find benefit* from the experience.

Lesson #4: A number of key factors are associated with optimal adaptation.

Lesson #5: Cancer for many may provide a "teachable moment."

"Being cancer free does not mean being free of cancer."

Symptoms can persist after cancer treatment. Cancer survivors often say, "I am cancer free but I do not feel free of my cancer." Most of the acute symptoms that patients experience resolve, including postoperative pain or chemotherapy-associated nausea, vomiting, and hair loss. In contrast, however, for some cancer survivors the effects of cancer and its treatment are lingering and can go on for weeks, months, or years afterward. Sometimes symptoms are noted during or soon after treatment is completed, but some develop after a long latency period. Some of these complaints include chronic postoperative pain syndromes or neuropathy following chemotherapy, chronic fatigue, cognitive dysfunction (or "chemobrain"), or arthralgias and myalgias referred to as postchemotherapy rheumatism.

Aside from persistent symptoms, cancer survivors are at increased risk of disease recurrence, second primary tumors, cardiovascular disease, obesity/diabetes, and osteoporosis.

Some survivors have very few sequelae of therapy, while others have multiple problems. Stroke, cardiovascular disease, and other kinds of major life-threatening consequences need to be monitored because early intervention has the potential to make a difference.

"Transitioning to recovery is stressful."

Patients sometimes are seeing their oncologist or oncology nurse once a week for months, and then when treatment has ended, they are asked to return in 3 months. For many patients, this is a time of celebration but can be mixed with stress associated with fear that the cancer will return, concern about ongoing monitoring, loss of a supportive environment, diminished sense of well-being due to treatment effects, and social demands. These problems are often referred to as "reentry" problems.

Clinicians do not always do a good job of saying what is next and helping people prepare for the transition to the next seasons of survivorship. It is very important to acknowledge that these transitions are difficult and to create a follow-up care plan.

"People are remarkably resilient."

Remarkably, the majority of cancer survivors get through what is often an incredibly difficult time in their lives and often report an increased sense of mastery and self-esteem, and an enhanced appreciation of life.

This is a benefit as people make sense out of adversity and an incredible deepening of life experiences that many people report as a consequence of surviving cancer.

"A number of key factors are associated with optimal adaptation."

Dr. Rowland and other experts report that a number of key factors are associated with optimal adaptation. They find the following to be true:

▷ Accessing state-of-the-art care is important.
▷ Being an active participant in one's care leads to a better outcome. People who are actively involved in their care, participating in whatever treatments they are having and doing what they can for themselves, may do better during and after treatment.
▷ Being physically active may be important.
▷ Having and using a social support network predicts an improved outcome. Social support is a buffer to adverse health outcomes, so having it and building it is very important. In fact, just believing there is a network available to you is very important.
▷ Having a sense of purpose or meaning in one's life is helpful. Some studies suggest that this is a religious affiliation, while other studies indicate that this sense of purpose is built around the tasks that a person performs.

Provocative research suggests that learning to express oneself is important as well. This process enables people to find meaning and make sense of what is happening.

"Cancer may provide a teachable moment."[16]

People come into this illness often unaware that they are at risk. Cancer survivors then often want to try to regain a sense of mastery and reduce their risk, so they change their diet, take vitamins and herbals, and try tai chi, meditation, and yoga.

Lifestyle interventions can have profound effects on issues like depression or fatigue, changes in body composition and body image, functional status, and comorbid conditions. Wendy Demark-Wahnefried summarizes the possible impact of these lifestyle changes in Table 2.1.

TABLE 2.1 ∾ Potential Role of Lifestyle Modification

	Diet	Exercise	Smoking Cessation
Depression	✓	✓✓	
Fatigue	✓	✓✓	
Adverse Body Composition	✓	✓✓✓	✓
Functional Decline	✓	✓✓✓	✓✓
Comorbidity	✓✓✓	✓✓✓	✓✓✓

Source: Demark-Wahnefried[16]

CONCLUSION

Perhaps the most frightening words that individuals can hear are that they or a loved one has cancer. Fortunately, for an increasingly large percentage of these individuals, cancer is a treatable disease with an improved chance for the person to live cancer free or with cancer as a chronic disease. The definition of a cancer survivor now includes the time from the moment of diagnosis to the remainder of that person's life; this definition applies to family members and caregivers as well. The term cancer survivor has added hope while the concept of cancer survivor has led to an increased emphasis on improving our understanding of the impact of treatment on an individual's future health and the effect of different treatment decisions. It is hoped that improved understanding of the seasons of survivorship will lead to improvements in not only survival free of cancer but also on quality of life.

REFERENCES

1. Hewitt M, Greenfield S, Stovall E. From cancer patient to cancer survivor: lost in transition. Washington, DC: Institute of Medicine and National Research Council of the National Academies; 2006.
2. Hewitt M, Weiner SL, Simone JV. Childhood cancer survivors: improving care and quality of life. Washington, DC: The National Academies Press; 2003.

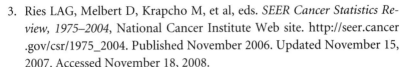

3. Ries LAG, Melbert D, Krapcho M, et al, eds. *SEER Cancer Statistics Review, 1975–2004*, National Cancer Institute Web site. http://seer.cancer.gov/csr/1975_2004. Published November 2006. Updated November 15, 2007. Accessed November 18, 2008.

4. President's Cancer Panel. Living beyond cancer: finding a new balance. Bethesda, MD: National Cancer Institute; 2004.

5. Lance Armstrong Foundation. Centers for Disease Control and Prevention. A national action plan for cancer survivorship: advancing public health strategies. Atlanta, GA: U.S. Department of Health and Human Services, Centers for Disease Control and Prevention; 2004.

6. Hewitt M, Rowland JH, Yancik R. Cancer survivors in the United States: age, health, and disability. *J Gerontol.* 2003;58(1):82.

7. Putterman C, Polliack A. Late cardiovascular and pulmonary complications of therapy in Hodgkin's disease: report of three unusual cases, with a review of relevant literature. *Leuk Lymphoma.* 1992;7(1–2):109–115.

8. Brice P, Tredaniel J, Monsuez JJ, et al. Cardiopulmonary toxicity after three courses of ABVD and mediastinal irradiation in favorable Hodgkin's disease. *Ann Oncol.* 1991;2(suppl 2):73–76.

9. Hohl RJ, Schilsky RL. Nonmalignant complications of therapy for Hodgkin's disease. *Hematol Oncol Clin North Am.* 1989;3(2):331–343.

10. Moreno M, Aristu J, Ramos LI, et al. Predictive factors for radiation-induced pulmonary toxicity after three-dimensional conformal chemoradiation in locally advanced non-small-cell lung cancer. *Clin Transl Oncol.* 2007;9(9):596–602.

11. Sleijfer S. Bleomycin-induced pneumonitis. *Chest.* 2001;120:617–624.

12. Dores G, Schonfeld S, Chen J, et al. Long-term cause-specific mortality among 41,146 one-year survivors of Hodgkin lymphoma (HL). *Proc Am Soc Clin Oncol.* 2005;23:562.

13. Schover LR. Reproductive complications and sexual dysfunction in the cancer patient. In: Chang AE, Ganz PA, Hayes DF, et al, eds. *Oncology: An Evidence-Based Approach.* New York: Springer-Verlag; 2005:1580–1600.

14. Schover LR, Fouladi RT, Warneke CL, et al. Defining sexual outcomes after treatment for localized prostate cancer. *Cancer.* 2002;(95):1773–1785.

15. Rowland J. What cancer survivors are telling us. New Haven, CT: Defining Excellence in Cancer Survivorship, Yale Cancer Center; January 14–15, 2008.

16. Demark-Wahnefried W, Aziz NM, Rowland JH, et al. Riding the crest of the teachable moment: promoting long-term health after the diagnosis of cancer. *J Clin Oncol.* 2005;23:5458–5460.

PART

2

Psychological Issues

3

Symptom Burden in Cancer Survivorship: Managing Mood, Pain, Fatigue, and Sleep Disturbances

Robert D. Kerns, PhD

&

Laura A. Bayer, PhD

ABSTRACT

Cancer survivors generally regain "normal" quality of life following their treatment. Symptom burden among survivors tends to be disease-specific symptoms associated with physiological functioning such as fatigue or pain. Recurrence is associated with diminished quality of life for some cancer populations. There are effective treatments for the most common symptoms: mood disturbance, pain, fatigue, and depression. Early intervention of symptoms and discussion of survivorship issues need to be incorporated into initial treatment planning.

INTRODUCTION

Achieving optimal adaptation to cancer is a highly complex and variable phenomenon. The following vignette illustrates the complexity of a patient's illness experiences. Cancer can have an impact at multiple levels, including not only one's physical health and vitality, but also one's sense of identity and mortality. It can also impact one's roles and responsibilities related to extended networks of family, friends, and coworkers. This vignette comes from a doctoral student of ours from South Africa who recently sent us the following email message.

> Life has been a bit challenging. . . . A few months ago I had a cancer scare while I was pregnant. Exposure to radiation during my pregnancy resulted in a miscarriage at a relatively late stage. Thank God, I am pregnant again, but this has been a complicated pregnancy. . . . I am still bedridden in South Africa but have periods where I am better than before. The great news is that the baby is doing well and that I will be fine, at the latest, following the birth. I am grateful for my excitement about having another child, the tremendous family support, my sense of humor and resilience, which have kept me going during this challenging time.

CANCER SURVIVORS GO ON TO RESUME NORMAL LIVES

The vignette also speaks to the resilience that cancer survivors experience. While cancer can have complex impacts across different domains of one's life, resilience is a predominant theme in patients' experience of their illness. Recent longitudinal studies of cancer survivorship suggest that most are able to reclaim their quality of life.[1] Studies of breast cancer patients indicate that they regain activity and overall quality of life shortly after treatment ends—within the first year[2]—and that as time progresses, the influence of cancer continues to wane. Recurrence and subsequent treatment place additional demands, and survivors with recurrence score worse on a variety of quality-of-life domains.[1,3–4]

Other follow-up studies indicate that survivors generally return to work and resume other roles and activities. Taskila-Abrandt and colleagues found that overall cancer survivors were 9% less likely to be employed than the general public; however, that varied significantly by cancer type.[5] There were no decreases in employment rates for colon and prostate cancer survivors, while lung cancer survivors were 37% less likely to be employed compared to the general population.

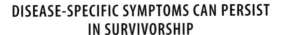

DISEASE-SPECIFIC SYMPTOMS CAN PERSIST IN SURVIVORSHIP

When symptoms do persist in survivorship, they tend to be disease-specific and related to treatment, for example, lymphedema or sexuality issues.[6,7] Symptom burden will differ according both to the type of cancer and to the type of treatments involved. Fatigue, sleep disturbance, and pain are common persistent symptoms, even into long-term survivorship.[1,8]

The relationships among chronic pain, sleep disturbance, fatigue, and mood disturbance are complex and intertwined.[9] For example, depression is often associated with sleep disturbance and fatigue. Chronic pain is known to contribute to depression, fatigue, and sleep disturbances. While the interconnection of these relationships can lead to the persistence of these symptoms, each of them also responds well to behavioral strategies such as increased activity and cognitive-behavioral therapy.

MOOD DISTURBANCES

Patients typically experience anxiety and depression following their initial diagnosis. While these emotions can be intense, they tend to be short-lived.[2] Deshields and colleagues found that mood and quality of life improved significantly within the first weeks of completing treatment. For those who continue to have difficulty, psychological issues in survivorship include fear of recurrence, sexuality issues, and difficulty transitioning to survivor status and reentering into work.[8]

Identification and appropriate treatment of depression and other mood disturbances are important to overall recovery. Depression at diagnosis was the single most important predictor of distress at 6 and 12 months following treatment of lung and gastrointestinal cancers.[10–12] Depression is associated and intertwined with pain, fatigue, and overall symptom burden. Depression affects decision making and is reliably associated with poorer clinical outcomes. Patients who are younger, socially isolated, or who have a history of depression and anxiety are at greater risk of depression.

Depression, anxiety, and other forms of psychological distress most often are responsive to treatment. Effective treatments include support groups, cognitive-behavioral therapy, and psychotropic medications. Professionally led support groups are associated with improved psychological functioning in randomized clinical trials.[13] Support groups are proven to be beneficial regardless of cancer type, particularly groups that meet for 12 weeks or longer. In addition to support groups, individual cognitive-behavioral therapy is an effective time-limited treatment for survivorship issues.

While cancer treatment and survivorship are stressful experiences and are often associated with short-term emotional distress, many survivors report unanticipated positive benefits. These may include a sense of purposefulness, hopefulness, and renewed spirituality.[1,8]

FATIGUE AND SLEEP DISTURBANCES

Fatigue and sleep disturbances are some of the most commonly reported symptoms in survivorship across cancer type.[9] Among breast cancer survivors, one-third continue to experience significant fatigue more than a year following treatment.[14] Over time, fatigue complaints decrease. Neyt and Albrecht found that long-term breast cancer survivors (5 years or more) reported significantly less fatigue than more recent survivors. Fatigue has a negative impact on mood, social relationships, daily activities, and overall quality of life. Similar to depression, survivors who are single and low-income are more likely to be fatigued. It is likely that these demographic factors are markers of chronic stress and/or fewer social resources that can serve to buffer or moderate negative effects of stress.[15,16]

The etiology of cancer-related fatigue remains unclear. The most likely contributor is activation of the immune system in response to the tumor or cancer treatments. While the etiology and mechanisms of fatigue continue to be explored, increased activity and other behavioral interventions are known to be effective interventions. Low activity levels at the end of cancer treatment are predictive of fatigue 6 months later.[16] Exercise and cognitive-behavioral therapy are both effective in reducing fatigue and insomnia among breast cancer survivors.[17–19] In a manner similar to chronic pain, fatigue and sleep disturbances are well suited to a biopsychosocial model of treatment that can address expectations and depressive symptoms as well as activity levels and sleep hygiene.

PAIN

While there has been much focus over the past 20 years in addressing pain during cancer treatment and as part of palliative care, relatively little is known about the prevalence of chronic pain in survivorship. Often the treatments that are used to optimize survival (ie, surgery, radiation therapy, and chemotherapy) are associated with recurrent or persistent pain issues. Chronic pain occurs in 50% of patients undergoing thoracotomy and 25% for breast surgery.[20–21] For head and neck cancer, approximately 40% of survivors at 1 year report pain, and it persists for 15% of long-term survivors at 5 years post-treatment.[20]

It is necessary to intervene early in controlling moderate to severe pain during initial treatment to prevent chronic pain in survivorship. In an 18-month follow-up study of survivors who had thoracotomies, 52% reported chronic pain, and postsurgical pain was the only significant predictor of continuing pain.[22] Other treatment factors associated with chronic pain include prior history of chronic pain and type of treatment (ie, radiation and chemotherapy). Psychological predictors include passive coping, anxiety, and secondary gain issues associated with worker's compensation claims.

Effective treatment of chronic pain in survivorship involves an interdisciplinary and multidimensional approach informed by a biopsychosocial model. Survivors need an ongoing mechanism-based approach to management of chronic pain and acute exacerbations, and possibly a referral to a specialty pain clinic. Psychological aspects of care include providing emotional support that acknowledges that pain is a problem that needs to be addressed. Survivors need to be encouraged to adopt an active coping style, enhancing their sense of control. Referrals for cognitive-behavioral therapy should be considered for those who display maladaptive coping to chronic pain. This includes being passive-dependent, having limited insight into self-defeating behaviors, and catastrophizing about their pain condition.

SUMMARY AND RECOMMENDATIONS

As we begin to approach cancer as a chronic illness, the importance of addressing survivorship issues as early as initial diagnosis becomes more apparent. Issues to address include acknowledging likelihood of cancer survival and planning for recovery and optimal adaptation. In addition, the risk of persistent symptoms and the potential burden of long-term symptoms need to be addressed.

The Institute of Medicine's 2005 report, "From Cancer Patient to Cancer Survivor: Lost in Transition," recommends that as patients complete their primary cancer treatment, a "Survivorship Care Plan" be created.[23] They recommend that it include the following information:

▷ Cancer type, treatments received, and their potential consequences
▷ Specific information about the timing and content of recommended follow-up
▷ Recommendations regarding preventive practices and how to maintain health and well-being
▷ The availability of psychosocial services in the community

RESOURCES

Facing Forward: Life After Cancer Treatment—a patient booklet available online from the National Cancer Institute, at http://www.cancer.gov/cancer topics/life-after-treatment. The booklet discusses symptom management and the transition after treatment.

"Cancer-Related Fatigue"—an excerpt from *NCCN Clinical Practice Guidelines in Oncology* (2007), available from the National Cancer Control Network at http://www.nccn.org/JNCCN/toc/2007nov.asp#fatigue

"Distress Management"—an excerpt from *NCCN Clinical Practice Guidelines in Oncology* (2007), available from the National Cancer Control Network at http://www.nccn.org/professionals/physician_gls/PDF/distress.pdf

REFERENCES

1. Helgeson VS, Tomich PL. Surviving cancer: a comparison of 5-year disease-free breast cancer survivors with healthy women. *Psycho-Oncol.* 2004; 14:307–317.
2. Deshields TL, Tibbs T, Fan M, Bayer L, Taylor ME, Fisher EB. Ending treatment: the course of emotional adjustment and quality of life among breast cancer survivors immediately following radiation therapy. *Support Care Cancer.* 2005;13:1018–1026.
3. Northouse LL, Mood D, Kershaw T, et al. 2002. Quality of life of women with recurrent breast cancer and their family members. *J Clin Oncol.* 2002; 20:4050–4064.

4. Oh S, Heflin L, Meyerowitz BE, Desmond KA, Rowland JH, Ganz PA. Quality of life of breast cancer survivors after a recurrence: a follow-up study. *Breast Cancer Res Treatment*. 2004;87:45–57.

5. Taskila-Abrandt T, Pukkala E, Martikainen R, et al. Employment status on Finnish cancer patients in 1997. *Psycho-Oncology*. 2005;14:221–226.

6. Ganz PA, Desmond KA, Leedham B, Rowland JH, Meyerowitz BE, Belin TR. Quality of life in long-term, disease-free survivors of breast cancer: a follow-up study. *J Natl Cancer Inst*. 2002;94:39–49.

7. Kleinberg L, Wallner K, Roy J, et al. Treatment-related symptoms during the first year following transperineal 125I prostate implantation. *Int J Radiat Oncol Biol Phys*. 1994;28:985–990.

8. Dow KH, Ferrell BR, Leigh S, Ly J, Gulasekaram P. An evaluation of the quality of life among long-term survivors of breast cancer. *Breast Cancer Res Treatment*. 1999;39:261–273.

9. Fossa SD, Dahl AA, Loge JH. Fatigue, anxiety, and depression in long-term survivors of testicular cancer. *J Clin Oncol*. 2003;21:1249–1254.

10. Akechi T, Okuyama T, Akizuki N, et al. Course of psychological distress and its predictors in advanced non-small cell lung cancer patients. *Psycho-Oncol*. 2006;15:463–473.

11. Nordin K, Glimelius B. Predicting delayed anxiety and depression in patients with gastrointestinal cancer. *Br J Cancer*. 1999;79:525–529.

12. Uchitomi Y, Mikami I, Magai K, et al. Depression and psychological distress in patients during the year after curative resection on non-small lung cancer. *J Clin Oncol*. 2003;21:69–77.

13. Gottlieb BH, Wachala ED. Cancer support groups: a critical review of empirical studies. *Psycho-Oncol*. 2007;16:379–400.

14. Bower JE, Ganz PA, Desmond KA, Rowland JH, Meyerowitz BE, Belin TR. Fatigue in breast cancer survivors: occurrence, correlates, and impact on quality of life. *J Clin Oncol*. 2000;18:743–753.

15. Bower JE, Ganz PA, Aziz N, Fahey JL. Fatigue and proinflammatory cytokine activity in breast cancer survivors. *Psychosom Med*. 2002;64:604–611.

16. Donovan KA, Small BJ, Andrykowski MA, Munster P, Jacobsen PB. Utility of a cognitive-behavioral model to predict fatigue following breast cancer treatment. *Health Psychol*. 2007;26:464–472.

17. Courneya KS, Friedenreich CM, Sela RA, Quinney HA, Rhodes RE, Handman M. The group psychotherapy and home-based exercise (Group-Hope) trial in cancer survivors: physical fitness and quality of life outcomes. *Psycho-Oncol*. 2003;12:357–374.

18. Davidson JR, Waisberg JL, Brundage MD, MacLean AW. Nonpharma-cological group treatment of insomnia: a preliminary study with cancer survivors. *Psycho-Oncol.* 2001;10:389–397.

19. McNeely ML, Campbell KL, Rowe BH, Klassen TP, Mackey JR, Courneya KS. Effects of exercise on breast cancer patients and survivors: a system-atic review and meta-analysis. *CMAJ.* 2006;175:34–41.

20. Burton AW, Fanciullo GJ, Deasley RD, Fisch MJ. Chronic pain in the cancer survivor: a new frontier. *Pain Med.* 2007;8:189–198.

21. Tasmuth T, von Smitten K, Hietanen P, Kataja M, Kalso E. Pain and other symptoms after different treatment modalities of breast cancer. *Ann Oncol.* 1995;6:453–459.

22. Katz J, Jackson M, Kavanagh BP, Sandler AN. Acute pain after thoracic surgery predicts long-term post-thoracotomy pain. *Clin J Pain.* 1996;12:50–55.

23. Hewitt M, Greenfield S, Stovall E, eds. Committee on cancer survivorship: improving care and quality of life. In: *From Cancer Patient to Cancer Sur-vivor: Lost in Transition.* Washington, DC: The National Academies Press; 2005.

4

Post-Traumatic Stress in Cancer Survivors

Mitch Golant, PhD

&

Megan Taylor-Ford

ABSTRACT

Research has shown that professionally facilitated support groups reduce emotional distress and post-traumatic stress symptoms for people with cancer. A primary component of The Wellness Community (TWC) model and many community cancer support organizations is support groups. It is vital for TWC, as an evidence-based organization with support groups in 24 cities worldwide as well as on the Web through The Wellness Community Online, to incorporate a theoretical framework that explains how change occurs for people with cancer who participate in our support programs. Likewise, it is important to understand and validate the effectiveness of support groups for people with cancer in a community setting where nearly 85% of patients are treated. Therefore, TWC engaged in several research studies evaluating the relationship between social support, reductions in post-traumatic stress symptoms, and distress. Following this, the Social-Cognitive Processing model of emotional adjustment to cancer was applied to the research findings to better understand how support groups help mitigate distress and reduce post-traumatic stress associated with the illness, and to determine how these groups add value to community-based support organizations. It is theorized that professionally facilitated support groups play a crucial role in providing a safe environment for people affected by cancer to express emotions with others, thereby reducing distress and post-traumatic stress.

INTRODUCTION

The purpose of this chapter is to present a clinical discussion pertaining to the psychosocial issues facing oncology's survivorship movement. More specifically, this chapter discusses the post-traumatic stress that people affected by cancer experience and TWC's theoretical model for decreasing distress. The chapter is divided into 3 sections. The first section provides background information on TWC. The second section discusses TWC's findings on distress and the role of support in decreasing post-traumatic stress. Thirdly, this chapter outlines a social-cognitive processing model developed by Steve Lepore, which TWC has adopted to more fully understand and explain the findings of our research. We would like to thank, in particular, Diana Jeffery, PhD, at the National Cancer Institute's (NCI) Office of Cancer Survivorship. She has been supportive in helping TWC consider and adopt this theoretical model. It is vital for TWC, as an evidence-based organization, to have a theoretical framework that explains how change occurs for people with cancer who participate in our support programs.

ABOUT THE WELLNESS COMMUNITY

The Wellness Community is an international nonprofit organization dedicated to providing free support, education, and hope to people with cancer and their loved ones. It is our goal that through participation in professionally led support groups, educational workshops, nutrition and exercise programs, and mind–body classes, people affected by cancer learn vital skills that enable them to regain control, reduce isolation, and restore hope regardless of the stage of their disease. Most importantly, TWC provides a homelike setting for people fighting cancer in which they connect with and learn from each other. At TWC, all programs are free of charge and are led by licensed healthcare professionals. Furthermore, all core programs and training curricula at TWC are

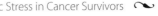

consistent throughout the country, allowing for streamlined, system-wide adoption of national programs and initiatives.

The vision of TWC is to establish TWC's model as the gold standard of psychosocial support for people affected by cancer. This vision is reinforced by TWC's eloquent yet simple program philosophy entitled the Patient Active Concept. The Patient Active Concept states, "People with cancer who participate in their fight for recovery from cancer will improve the quality of their lives and may enhance the possibility of their recovery." People who see themselves as *patient active* consider themselves part of the fight for recovery along with their physicians and healthcare team.

The Wellness Community has developed 10 core principles that underlie the programs and services we deliver. These 10 core principles follow.

Focused on the Patient Active Concept

Community-Based

Free of Charge

Inclusive of All Cancers and Families

Adjunctive to Conventional Medical Treatment

Evidence-Based

Committed to Quality Assurance

Professionally-Facilitated Programs

Collaborative

Signature Cancer Educational Programs

The Wellness Community is proud to offer patient and professional education programs across the United States. These programs often include a patient education booklet, professionally led educational workshop, online content, and interactive educational components such as podcasts and continuing education courses for professionals.

The Wellness Community also has a very large presence on the Internet in The Wellness Community Online (TWC Online www.the wellnesscommunity.org). Launched in 2002, TWC Online served 243 000 unique visitors in 2006. It currently offers online support groups including tumor-specific groups, mixed diagnosis groups, caregiver groups, teen groups, parents of teen groups, Spanish language groups, and bereavement groups.

In 2006, TWC held 13 486 support groups, including nearly 9000 patient groups and over 4400 caregiver groups at our brick-and-mortar facilities and online. There were over 70 000 visits to these groups. Additionally, TWC provided 2343 educational workshops at facilities across the United States and 6354 exercise and stress management classes.

CANCER AS A CHRONIC DISEASE

Consider the hopeful statistic that there are approximately 12 million cancer survivors alive today.[1] Encouraged by earlier detection and better treatments, cancer is becoming a chronic illness with which many people will live for years. Patients diagnosed with cancer may go through treatment, some may experience recurrence, and others may experience a second course of treatment or even a third. Through this lengthy and ever-extending pattern of diagnosis/recurrence and treatment, it is evident that the concept of survivorship is becoming an integral part of our model of cancer care. As we face this reality of longer survival periods and increased numbers of cancer survivors, it is imperative to recognize that our very notion of cancer survivorship is changing as well. Therefore, when considering a comprehensive model of care, it is essential to visualize the wide spectrum of needs cancer survivors and caregivers will encounter during the cancer continuum, including the need for support.

When considering cancer as a chronic illness, it behooves us to look at an integrative model that includes 3 primary types of care: tertiary care, community cancer care, and community-based support (Figure 4.1).

In this model, tertiary care refers to NCI-designated comprehensive cancer centers. These centers offer a full spectrum of cancer-related services including psychosocial support services that may consist of support groups, individual counseling, and educational workshops. While impressive and effective in their goal to treat the whole cancer experience from the tumor to the emotional side effects, tertiary care facilities reach only a small portion of cancer patients and never provide services to the vast majority. Indeed, most cancer care in the United States occurs in community cancer care centers. Unlike tertiary facilities, com-

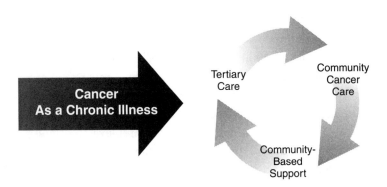

FIGURE 4.1   Cancer as a chronic illness.

munity centers do not necessarily provide support services, often due to resource restrictions such as lack of space, funding, staffing, and clinical expertise. Consequently, a gap exists for patients in these communities, creating a great need for community-based support organizations such as TWC.

This need will continue to grow as the profile of cancer evolves from a fatal disorder toward a chronic condition. For example, community cancer care centers provide care to nearly 85% of cancer survivors. Many of these survivors are returning to work after treatment sooner than they would have in the past, or they are continuing to work while undergoing treatment. With such a comparatively active and "healthy" patient population and with outside pressures such as work or family obligations, it is unlikely—even if they were available—that a patient will return after treatment to receive support services. Some patients may actively avoid returning to the medical center or hospital because it brings up negative memories of treatment or they cannot afford such services. Thus, there is a growing need for community-based support.

THE WELLNESS COMMUNITY'S RESEARCH ON DISTRESS: MAKING THE CASE FOR A THEORETICAL MODEL

A primary component of The Wellness Community model is face-to-face support groups. It is important to TWC to validate the effectiveness of support groups for people with cancer. Therefore, TWC engaged in several research studies evaluating the relationship between social support and distress. Across all the studies that follow, the general hypothesis was that support, and specifically support received and given in a support group setting, reduces distress in cancer survivors.

The Wellness Community felt strongly that a theoretical model of change was needed to explain how the support services offered at TWC translate into improvements in quality of life for people with cancer. In particular, TWC felt a responsibility to find or develop a model that could explain the positive impact of individual and group support that was at the very foundation of its organization.

Although only 6% to 10% of cancer patients are fully diagnosed with post-traumatic stress disorder, distress is a prevalent reaction to cancer.[2] Therefore, TWC sought to investigate whether a relationship existed between the reduction of this distress and other traumalike symptoms related to the diagnosis/treatment of cancer and social support. The Wellness Community engaged in 4 research studies to establish this relationship.

Study 1: Support Groups Buffer Intrusion (2001)

The Impact of Event Scale developed by Mardi Horowitz, Nancy Wilner, and William Alvarez found that the most commonly reported responses to traumatic events were intrusive thoughts and avoidance.[3] Applying this finding, TWC considered the cancer experience a key source of intrusive thoughts and avoidance (referred to as traumalike symptoms). For the person living through cancer, intrusion may be experienced as nightmares about death, anxious thoughts as an anniversary of diagnosis approaches, overwhelming fear of recurrence, and so forth. In their efforts to deal with these intrusive thoughts, people affected by cancer may use avoidance tactics such as going out of their way to prevent driving by the hospital because it brings up negative memories of treatment, skipping treatments because it is a reminder of the illness, or ignoring friends' expressions of support in an effort not to talk about the cancer. Using the Impact of Event Scale, the Support Groups Buffer Intrusion correlational study sought to measure the impact of intrusion and avoidance caused by cancer.

The Support Groups Buffer Intrusion study found that compared to cancer patients who were not in a support group, those who participated in a support group at the time of a recurrence experienced fewer

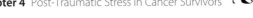

intrusive thoughts. Furthermore, those individuals in a support group expressed:

▷ Feeling supported by the group
▷ Ease in verbalizing their true feelings
▷ Increased control over treatment decisions
▷ Less loneliness

All of these experiences appeared to act as a buffer to intrusion. These initial findings encouraged TWC to think that the services provided in support groups may have some positive effect on people affected by cancer.[4]

Study 2: Mood Disturbance in Community Cancer Support Groups: The Role of Emotional Suppression and Fighting Spirit (2003)

In this second correlational study, TWC found that community support groups that encouraged preparing for the worst while hoping for the best reduced patients' overall distress. The significance of this finding was that in embracing a realistic assessment of their cancer experience and not just thinking "positive," patients were better able to cope with the illness.[5]

Study 3: Effectiveness of Electronic Support Groups for Women with Breast Carcinoma: A Pilot Study of Effectiveness (2003)

In this study, TWC found that women with breast cancer in professionally facilitated online support groups experienced significant increases in post-traumatic growth in 3 areas: seeing new possibilities, zest for life, and spirituality. These women also experienced decreases in depression. This study was significant because it suggested that even support received in a nontraditional setting such as in an online support group was associated with reductions in depression and also the ability to "see the silver lining" in the traumatic experience.[6]

Study 4: Do Cancer Support Groups Reduce Physiological Stress? A Randomized Clinical Trial (2007)

In this randomized clinical trial, TWC found that women in TWC support groups, when compared to those in supportive-expressive therapy, showed significant reductions in post-traumatic stress symptoms, as well as significant increases in making changes, developing a new attitude toward their illness, better access to cancer-related information/resources, and better partnering with their physicians.

Together, these 4 research studies make a strong case for the positive impact that support groups have on reducing traumatic stressors such as intrusive thoughts and avoidance, and improving quality of life among people affected by cancer. Furthermore, they illuminate the next question that TWC faced: Why are support groups improving quality of life for their members? To answer this question, TWC turned to a theoretical model: the social-cognitive processing model.[7]

SOCIAL-COGNITIVE PROCESSING MODEL

After a thorough examination of the previous findings, TWC sought a model in the literature to explain the positive results that emerged from their studies that also complemented the Patient Active Concept. We found that the social-cognitive processing model of emotional adjustment to cancer, as outlined by Stephen Lepore, PhD, in *Psychosocial Interventions for Cancer*, best explained our research findings.[8] Illuminating the process of adjusting to a cancer diagnosis and comparing people with positive support interactions (social support) with those who have negative support interactions (social constraint), the social-cognitive processing model sheds light on the value of support groups in community-based support organizations.

Process of Adjusting to a Cancer Diagnosis

Distress, defined as an unpleasant emotional experience that can impact cognitive, behavioral, social, emotional, and spiritual functioning, is a common reaction among people with cancer.[9] Distress may interfere with one's ability to cope effectively with the physical symptoms of the illness and may impact the likelihood of a patient receiving treatment. Cancer is a multiple traumatic event experienced over a lifetime and is defined by numerous unpleasant experiences such as diagnosis, treatment, side effects, fear of recurrence, and fear of dying. Emotional distress is the most underreported yet most common side effect of cancer, highlighting a need within the clinical community to pay close attention to this devastating component of the cancer journey.[9]

Symptoms of distress include a wide spectrum of feelings ranging from sadness, fear, anger, and unhappiness to severe depression, panic, and debilitating anxiety. Thus it is crucial for practitioners to monitor the severity of symptoms. Furthermore, it is important to recognize that there are both reliable and unreliable symptoms of distress. Reliable symptoms may include persistent depression or angry mood, sadness, fearfulness, overwhelming anxiety, or lack of pleasure in activities. These are normal symptoms of distress that are most often directly related to a traumatic experience such as a cancer diagnosis. Other symptoms such as fatigue, insomnia, eating disturbances, and decreased libido can also be symptoms of distress, but they may be unreliable because they are also potential side effects of treatment. Regardless, whether reliable or unreliable, all of these symptoms diminish quality of life.

The cognitive-processing theory suggests that distress is related to an overwhelming and disturbing incongruity between an individual's worldview and the meaning or experience of a traumatic event.[10] Cancer radically changes individuals' worldviews, causing many people to question their core assumptions about life, their relationships, and themselves.[11] For example, a diagnosis may deliver a striking blow to a previously held belief that one is healthy and will have a long life. Cancer challenges us to recognize our own mortality.

Theoretically, diminishing distress may be achieved by reconciling one's previously held worldview with the cancer diagnosis through cognitive integration (e.g., confrontation, contemplation, and reevaluation).[11–16] Moreover, there are 2 categories of cognitive integration: assimilation and accommodation. Assimilation is a reappraising of the traumatic events in order to make them fit one's worldview or preconceptions of life. For example, when diagnosed with cancer, individuals may feel that their bodies are out of control. By adopting an understanding that they may not be able to control the actual tumor but that they *can* control their diet, exercise, and treatment decisions, individuals are able to assimilate the traumatic cancer reality into their worldview or mental schema. Accommodation is adjusting mental models to fit the traumatic situation. For example, initially cancer patients may hope to become cancer free, but over time, because this goal may not be met, the individuals may, through accommodation, change their worldview to see cancer as a chronic illness—something that they may never get rid of but, instead, can live with. Assimilation and accommodation facilitate discovery of meaning in a traumatic event.[8]

Additionally, cognitive integration may vacillate between 2 coping mechanisms, intrusion and avoidance. Intrusion may include overwhelming and invasive thoughts that interrupt normal thought processes. Adaptively, avoidance becomes a coping strategy to manage the intrusive thought (e.g., avoiding driving by the hospital, not thinking about the treatments, or not discussing the disease). Intrusive thoughts represent an attempt to integrate the traumatic experience in order to achieve a sense of completion, resolution, and/or understanding. Thus, intrusion and avoidance represent not only emotional distress but also incomplete cognitive processing.[12]

The Role of Social Interactions in Cognitive Processing

The social-cognitive processing model theorizes that social interactions play a crucial role in the success or failure of cognitive integration and completion. Social support can be defined as positive, affirmative, and empathetic social interactions.[8] Supportive interactions include talking about the traumatic event and, as a result, lead to cognitive processing and integration. Support assists in cognitive processing by validating the individual's feelings,[17] identifying novel solutions to the stressful experience,[18] and providing information on better coping skills.[19] In contrast, social constraints on disclosure are unsupportive social interactions that discourage talking about a stressful event.[8] For example, caregivers or family members may want to be supportive but may not know what to say. They may say, "Don't worry, it will all be okay," although battling cancer often brings many challenges. Additionally, family members may feel threatened and distance themselves from their loved one with cancer. These situations discourage emotional expression. In effect, constraint on disclosure leads to emotional suppression, which may prevent effective cognitive processing of the trauma associated with cancer and thereby prolong psychological distress.[8]

The Importance of Support Groups

In essence, if families or friends are unable to provide the much-needed emotional support for people with cancer as they go through the continuum of diagnosis, treatment, and side effects of treatment, then professionally facilitated support groups play a crucial role, providing a safe environment for individuals to express emotions with others who share their experiences. Support groups encourage confronting, contemplating, and reevaluating traumatic events, and may counteract social constraint encountered in other relationships, thereby facilitating emotional assimilation and accommodation. Effective support groups also create a forum for safe expression of emotions. One can extend these safe environments for emotional expression to many different situations, including individual therapy, psychoeducational programs, online support groups, and face-to-face support groups. In conclusion, community-based support programs like TWC offer survivors a place where they can join together with other survivors in order to reduce the distress associated with battling the disease.

REFERENCES

1. Cancer survivorship research. National Cancer Institute Office of Cancer Survivorship Web site. http://www.cancercontrol.cancer.gov/ocs/prevalence/prevalence.html. Accessed November 13, 2008.
2. Green BL, Rowland JH, Krupnick JL, et al. Prevalence of posttraumatic stress disorder (PTSD) in women with breast cancer. *Psychosom.* 1998;32:102–111.
3. Horowitz M, Wilner N, Alvarez W. Impact of event scale: a measure of subjective stress. *Psychosom Med.* 1979;41:209–218.
4. Golant M, Giese-Davis J, Benjamin H, et al. Gender difference, group support's buffering effect on intrusion symptoms after cancer diagnosis. In: Society of Behavioral Medicine 22nd Annual Meeting; March 21–24, 2001; Seattle, WA.
5. Cordova M, Giese-Davis J, Golant M, et al. Mood disturbance in community cancer support groups: the role of emotional suppression and fighting spirit. *J Psychosom Res.* 2003;55:461–467.
6. Lieberman M, Golant M, Giese-Davis J, et al. Electronic support groups for breast carcinoma: a clinical trial of effectiveness. *Cancer.* 2003;97(4): 920–925.
7. Giese-Davis J, Kronenwetter C, Golant M, et al. Cancer support groups: different models, different participant experiences. *Group Dynamics: Theory, Research and Practice.* In press.
8. Lepore, SJ. A social-cognitive processing model of emotional adjustment to cancer. In: Baum A, Anderson B, eds. *Psychosocial Interventions for Cancer.* Washington, DC: APA; 2001:99–118.

9. Jacobsen PB, Donovan KA, Trask PC, et al. Screening for psychological distress in ambulatory cancer patients. *Cancer*. 2005;103(7):1494–1502.
10. Epstine S. The self-concept, the traumatic neurosis and the structure of personality. In: Ozer D, Healy JN, Stewart AJ, eds. *Perspectives on Personality*. Greenwich, CT: JAI Press; 1991:80–95.
11. Janoff-Bulman R. *Shattered Assumptions: Toward a New Psychology of Trauma*. New York: Free Press; 1992.
12. Horowitz M. *Stress Response Syndromes*. 2nd ed. New York: Jason Aronson; 1986.
13. McCann IL, Pearlman LA. *Psychological Trauma and the Adult Survivor: Theory, Therapy, and Transformation*. New York: Brunner/Mazel; 1990.
14. Parkes CM. Psycho-social transitions: a field study. *Soc Sci Med*. 1971;5:101–115.
15. Rachman S. Emotional processing. *Behav Res Ther*. 1980;18:51–60.
16. van der Kolk BA, van der Hart O. The intrusive past: the flexibility of memory and the engraving of trauma. *Am Imago*. 1991;48:425–454.
17. Silver RL, Wortman CB. Coping with undesirable life events. In: Garber J, Seligman MEP, eds. *Human Helplessness: Theory and Applications*. New York: Academic Press; 1980:279–340.
18. Silver RC, Boon C, Stones MH. Searching for meaning in misfortune: making sense of incest. *J Soc Issues*. 1983;39:81–102.
19. Lepore SJ. Cynicism, social support, and cardiovascular reactivity. *Health Psychol*. 1995;14:210–216.

5

Finding Benefits in the Cancer Experience: Post-Traumatic Growth

Heather S. L. Jim, PhD

&

Paul Jacobsen, PhD

"The truth is that cancer is the best thing that ever happened to me. I don't know why I got the illness, but it did wonders for me, and I wouldn't want to walk away from it. Why would I want to change, even for a day, the most important and shaping event of my life?"[1]

—Lance Armstrong

ABSTRACT

Cancer is often considered a dread disease, yet the opening quote illustrates that survivors do not always view cancer negatively. Most survivors are able to point to benefits in one or more areas of life as the result of cancer.[2] These benefits are not mutually exclusive of the many difficulties survivors and their families endure. Evidence suggests that the fear, uncertainty, and loss wrought by cancer often spur a search for deeper meaning and a fresh perspective on old problems. As a result, survivors frequently report that life after diagnosis is characterized by a richness and depth that was previously lacking.

INTRODUCTION

This chapter focuses on benefit-finding in individuals diagnosed with cancer. It begins with a theoretical overview of cancer as a traumatic experience, then defines and describes benefit-finding. Measurement issues are also reviewed. A discussion follows of the controversy over whether perceived benefits represent real change or motivated illusion. The chapter then examines the question of which survivors are most likely to find benefits in the cancer experience. The relationship between benefit-finding and mental health, as well as interventions to enhance benefit-finding, are also reviewed. The chapter concludes with a summary and recommendations for clinicians.

CANCER AS A TRAUMATIC EXPERIENCE

As a potentially life-threatening illness, cancer can be conceptualized as a traumatic life event.[3] Loss of physical health and well-being, functional independence, fertility, and employment are among the possible consequences. At best, many of these losses are temporary and patients rebound, albeit often with physical scars, late effects of treatment, and other reminders of their battle with cancer. At worst, these losses represent permanent changes in patients' lives.

Although post-traumatic stress disorder due to cancer diagnosis and treatment is relatively uncommon,[4] it is not unusual for patients to report some symptoms of traumatic stress, particularly at diagnosis. These symptoms commonly include intrusive thoughts about the cancer and efforts to avoid reminders of the disease.[5,6] Consequently, models of adaptation to other traumatic life events, such as car accidents and natural disasters, have been applied to cancer.[7,8] These models posit that in Western cultures, individuals typically live according to a series of assumptions that the world is just and predictable, life is meaningful and orderly, and the self is worthy and in control. In contrast, a cancer diagnosis may seem unfair, unpredictable, and entirely out of one's control. For example, following his wife's diagnosis of cancer, C.S. Lewis described God as "a door slammed in your face, and a sound of bolting and double bolting on the inside."[9] Patients may struggle with the question "Why did this happen to me?" Consequently, patients must reconcile their disease with previous assumptions about life. They must either build a new series of assumptions to accommodate the reality of their disease or change the meaning of the cancer to maintain positive assumptions about the world and themselves.[10]

THE PHENOMENON OF BENEFIT-FINDING

Benefit-finding is an effort to change the meaning of cancer to maintain previous positive assumptions. Also known as post-traumatic growth,[11] stress-related growth,[12] or meaning-making,[13] benefit-finding refers to the reinterpretation of cancer as an opportunity for personal growth. Davis and colleagues suggest that benefit-finding occurs as the result of the question "What has the experience taught me about myself and about my relationships with others in my life?"[13] Benefits may be directly attributed to the cancer itself or indirectly through attempts to cope with the disease.[14] Benefits represent something new and positive that is believed to surpass what was present before diagnosis. As Tedeschi and Calhoun note, benefit-finding "is not simply a return to baseline—it is an experience of improvement that for some persons is deeply profound."[11]

Survivors commonly report benefits in 3 specific domains of life: enhanced social resources, enhanced personal resources, and improved coping skills[15] (Table 5.1). Enhanced social resources take several forms, such as increased love for one's spouse,[16] improved relationships with family and friends,[16] and increased time invested in relationships.[17] Enhanced personal resources may include a better outlook on life[16]; greater satisfaction with religion[16]; a greater appreciation for life[18]; and increased compassion, sympathy, and sensitivity for others.[17] Finally, survivors may report better coping skills, including acceptance of things that cannot be changed, learning to take things as they come, and more effective coping with stress and problems.[19]

To illustrate these benefits, we present a case study. The survivor is a 59-year-old woman who was diagnosed with ovarian cancer in 2005. Treated initially with surgery and chemotherapy, she is now undergoing a second course of chemotherapy. She draws a distinction between her attitude before cancer compared to now. Referring to the time before her diagnosis, she says:

> I had experienced some difficult circumstances in my life and thought of myself as a victim. I believe that my depression, resentment, and negative self-talk caused my cancer. When I was diagnosed, I took

TABLE 5.1 ∾   Commonly-Reported Benefits of Cancer

Social resources
Deeper love for spouse and family
Improved relationships with family and friends
Increased time and effort invested into relationships
Personal resources
Better outlook on life
Greater satisfaction with religion
Increased compassion, sympathy, and concern for others
Coping skills
Greater acceptance of circumstances
Learning to take things as they come
More effective coping with stress

Source: Adapted from Schafer and Moos, 1992

responsibility for my negative thoughts. I concluded that if I wanted to get better, I would have to change my thoughts. One of the most important things I have done is to set aside time every day to write out positive affirmations. I envision myself healthy, I quote inspiring passages from the Bible, and I write about my gratitude for the many blessings in my life. I am so much more appreciative of life now. My relationships with my family are much better. I want people to know not to waste their lives thinking negative thoughts—not to wait until they have cancer to start appreciating life.

MEASURING BENEFIT-FINDING

Measurement of benefit-finding has been conducted using both qualitative[2,20] and quantitative[21–23] methods. Qualitative interviews typically ask survivors to describe any changes[20] or benefits[2] resulting from the cancer experience. Responses are then categorized by multiple independent raters.[2,20] Although qualitative interviews ensure adequate assessment of the domain of all possible benefits, they are time-consuming and generally lack reliability and validity information. Quantitative scales typically ask patients to rate the extent to which they have experienced specific benefits. Two commonly used quantitative scales are the Posttraumatic Growth Inventory (PTGI)[24] and Behr's Positive Contributions Scale (PCS).[19,25,26] The PTGI is composed of 5 subscales: relating to others, new possibilities, personal strength, spiritual change, and appreciation for life.[24] The PCS is composed of a single scale.[19,25] Both were developed to assess benefit-finding in other populations (ie, PTGI: trauma victims; PCS: family members of individuals with disabilities) and have been modified for use with cancer samples.

BENEFIT-FINDING: REAL CHANGE VERSUS MOTIVATED ILLUSION

An important issue in benefit-finding research is the extent to which perceived benefits indicate actual change. It has been suggested that benefit-finding may not indicate change per se but rather social desirability,[19] a general tendency to report personal growth over time,[21,27] or motivated illusion.[28,29] Motivated illusion refers to the theory that individuals need to maintain a coherent and integrated identity over time.[30] A threat to one's identity, such as a cancer diagnosis, compels individuals to seek ways to maintain or enhance self-esteem.[29] One way to do so is to engage in temporal self-comparisons or derogation of one's own past personal attributes so that one's current attributes appear to have changed favorably over time.[28] A study of undergraduates by McFarland and Alvaro found that victims of traumatic life events perceived improvement in personal attributes by derogating their pre-event attributes.[28] The degree to which the event was evaluated as threatening was positively correlated with perceived improvement. Studies comparing survivors' reports of benefits due to cancer to the reports of non-cancer control groups over a similar time period indicate that survivors report more benefits.[16,21] Similarly, Widows and colleagues found that greater perceived, but not actual, improvement in distress over time was related to post-traumatic growth in bone marrow transplant survivors.[31]

In contrast, the argument that benefit-finding reflects actual change is supported by evidence suggesting that individuals' reports of benefit-finding can be corroborated by loved ones. In a study of undergraduates, participants' perceived benefits from their most stressful experience in the past year were significantly correlated with benefits observed in the participants by their family and friends.[12] In a study of breast cancer patients, patients' reported benefits were significantly correlated with their husbands' reports of the patients' benefits. Similarly, the patients' reports of their husbands' benefits were significantly correlated with their husbands' own reported benefits. With evidence to support both sides of the debate, the issue of actual change versus motivated illusion is far from resolved.[27]

WHICH SURVIVORS ARE MOST LIKELY TO FIND BENEFITS?

Benefit-finding appears to be influenced by factors related to the survivor, to the survivor's environment, to the cancer itself, and to the survivor's coping strategies. Regarding survivor factors, those who are younger[31,33] and members of racial or ethnic minority groups[19,22] have been found to report greater benefits. Gender does not appear to be related to benefit-finding.[17,34,35] The relationship between benefit-finding and socioeconomic status is unclear, with some research demonstrating a positive relationship[20,21] and other research demonstrating a negative relationship.[19] Similarly, education has been both positively[2] and negatively[31] correlated with perceived benefits. In terms of environmental factors, social support appears to be helpful.[21,35] Regarding cancer-related factors, more severe disease[20,22] and longer time since diagnosis[2,21] have been associated with greater perceived benefits. Type of treatment received does not appear to be a predictor of benefit-finding.[20,21,36] Finally, the coping strategies of problem solving, positive reinterpretation, and involving oneself in enjoyable activities have been associated with greater perceived benefits.[2,17,31] (See Figure 5.1.)

THE RELATIONSHIP BETWEEN BENEFIT-FINDING AND MENTAL HEALTH

The relationship between benefit-finding and mental health has been the subject of much debate. Some studies have found benefit-finding associated with better mental health; for example, Carver and Antoni reported that benefit-finding in the year post-surgery was associated with less distress and depression 4 to 7 years later, controlling for initial distress and depression.[37] In addition, a meta-analysis examining benefit-finding across a variety of negative life events found that

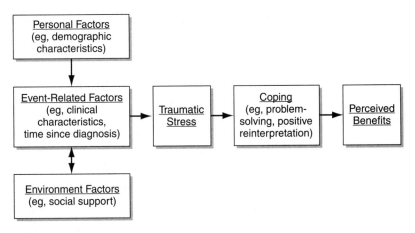

FIGURE 5.1 Model of benefit-finding in cancer survivors.

benefit-finding was related to more event-related distress but less depression.[38] Other studies have found no relationship between benefit-finding and mental health.[2,21,31] Still other studies have found a negative relationship; for example, Tomich and Helgeson found that benefit-finding at 4 months post-diagnosis predicted worse mental health at 7 months post-diagnosis for women with more advanced breast cancer.[19]

Results from a study by Lechner and colleagues may shed light on these conflicting findings.[22] They examined benefit-finding in breast cancer survivors in the year post-surgery and again 5 to 8 years later. Benefit-finding was related in a curvilinear manner to concurrent psychological adjustment at both times. Better adjustment was related to high and low benefit-finding, while poorer adjustment was related to intermediate benefit-finding. They interpreted these results to mean that some survivors fail to interpret cancer as threatening, and thus experience no impetus to find benefits. Survivors in the intermediate benefit-finding group may have been struggling with both benefit-finding and poor adjustment, while survivors who reported good adjustment and greater benefits have successfully coped with the threat of breast cancer. This interpretation is consistent with studies indicating that the perception of cancer as threatening is associated with greater perceived benefits.[2,21] Lechner and colleagues point out that if the true relationship between benefit-finding and mental health is curvilinear, studies testing linear relationships will report varying results.[22] Studies with samples with survivors falling at one end of the curve or the other will report a positive or negative relationship accordingly, while samples with a mix of survivors will report no relationship.

INTERVENTIONS TO PROMOTE BENEFIT-FINDING IN SURVIVORS

Although the relationship between benefit-finding and mental health is unclear, two types of psychosocial interventions have been tested to increase benefit-finding in cancer survivors: written emotional disclosure and cognitive-behavioral stress management. In a study of written emotional disclosure,[39] survivors were randomized to write about positive thoughts and feelings about their breast cancer, their deepest thoughts and feelings about their breast cancer, or facts of their breast cancer experience. Survivors who wrote about positive feelings reported less physician visits for medical comorbidities than survivors who wrote about facts of their cancer experience. Additionally, survivors who were high in avoidance and wrote about positive feelings reported less distress.[39]

The effects of cognitive-behavioral stress management on benefit-finding have been examined in breast cancer survivors[25] and prostate cancer survivors.[23] The intervention was the same across both studies. It consisted of 10 weekly 2-hour group sessions that included coping skills training, relaxation exercises, conflict resolution, and emotional expression. Control participants attended a half-day seminar consisting of a condensed, educational version of the intervention. In the prostate study, the experimental group showed an increase in benefit-finding at a 2-week follow-up, while the control group did not.[23] In the breast study, the intervention had a beneficial effect on benefit-finding at 6- and 12-month follow-ups.[25] This intervention also resulted in improved quality of life,[23] increased emotional well-being,[25] and positive affect.[25] These findings suggest that increases in benefit-finding are associated with increases in positive psychological outcomes. However, it is unclear whether benefit-finding contributed to these outcomes. Given the conflicting evidence between benefit-finding and mental health, it is premature to recommend interventions for benefit-finding. Further research is needed to determine whether benefit-finding does indeed contribute to improved adjustment.

SUMMARY AND RECOMMENDATIONS FOR CLINICIANS

Survivors commonly attribute benefits to the cancer experience, including enhanced social resources, enhanced personal resources, and improved coping skills. Benefits are more likely to be reported by survivors who are younger, are members of racial or ethnic minority groups, have more severe disease, or undergo more aggressive treatment regimens. Longer time since diagnosis and engaged coping strategies are also associated with greater benefits. The question of whether benefit-finding represents actual change or motivated illusion is in some ways unimportant. If survivors believe that benefit-finding strengthens fragile hope, offers a sense of meaning, and makes the destruction wreaked by cancer seem more manageable, then it is valuable. This is the intuitive appeal of benefit-finding and perhaps the reason that benefit-finding interventions have been created in the absence of solid evidence associated with psychological adjustment. Clinicians would do well to take a moderate approach to benefit-finding, neither rejecting reported benefits nor insisting on a rosy interpretation of the cancer experience. Clinicians should acknowledge benefits reported by patients but should not convey the impression that survivors should find benefits. Survivors must ultimately decide for themselves whether cancer has resulted in positive changes in their lives.

REFERENCES

1. Armstrong L, Jenkins S. *It's Not About the Bike: My Journey Back to Life*. New York: G.P. Putnam's Sons; 2000.
2. Sears SR, Stanton AL, Danoff-Burg S. The yellow brick road and the emerald city: benefit finding, positive reappraisal coping, and posttraumatic growth in women with early-stage breast cancer. *Health Psychol.* 2003; 22(5):487–497.
3. American Psychiatric Association. *Diagnostic and Statistical Manual of Mental Disorders*. 4th ed. Washington, DC: Author; 1994.
4. Shelby, RA, Golden-Kreutz DM, Andersen BL. Mismatch of posttraumatic stress disorder (PTSD) symptoms and DSM-IV symptom clusters in a cancer sample: exploratory factor analysis of the PTSD Checklist-Civilian Version. *J Trauma Stress.* 2005;18(4):347–357.
5. Butler LD, Koopman C, Classen C, Spiegel D. Traumatic stress, life events, and emotional support in women with metastatic breast cancer:

cancer-related traumatic stress symptoms associated with past and current stressors. *Health Psychol.* 1999;18(6):555–560.

6. Koopman C, Butler LD, Classen C, et al. Traumatic stress symptoms among women with recently diagnosed primary breast cancer. *J Trauma Stress.* 2002;15(4):277–287.

7. Janoff-Bulman R, Frieze IH. A theoretical perspective for understanding reactions to victimization. *J Soc Issues.* 1983;39(2):1–17.

8. Taylor SE. Adjustment to threatening events: a theory of cognitive adaptation. *Am Psychol.* 1983;38:1161–1173.

9. Lewis CS. *A Grief Observed.* New York: Barton; 1961.

10. Jim HS, Richardson SA, Golden-Kreutz DM, Andersen BL. Strategies used in coping with a cancer diagnosis predict meaning in life for survivors. *Health Psychol.* 2006;25(6):753–761.

11. Tedeschi RG, Calhoun LG. Posttraumatic growth: conceptual foundations and empirical evidence. *Psychol Inq.* 2004;15(1):1–18.

12. Park CL, Cohen LH, Murch RL. Assessment and prediction of stress-related growth. *J Pers.* 1996;64(1):71–105.

13. Davis CG, Nolen-Hoeksema S, Larson J. Making sense of loss and benefiting from the experience: two construals of meaning. *J Pers Soc Psychol.* 1998;75(2):561–574.

14. Zoellner T, Maercker A. Posttraumatic growth in clinical psychology—a critical review and introduction of a two component model. *Clin Psychol Rev.* 2006;26(5):626–653.

15. Schaefer JA, Moos RH. Life crises and personal growth. In: Carpenter BN, ed. *Personal Coping: Theory, Research, and Application.* Westport, CT: Praeger; 1992:149–170.

16. Andrykowski MA, Brady MJ, Hunt JW. Positive psychosocial adjustment in potential bone marrow transplant recipients: cancer as a psychosocial transition. *Psycho-Oncol.* 1993;2:261–276.

17. Collins RL, Taylor SE, Skokan LA. A better world or a shattered vision? Changes in life perspectives following victimization. *Soc Cognit.* 1990;8:263–285.

18. Thompson SC, Pitts J. Factors relating to a person's ability to find meaning after a diagnosis of cancer. *J Psychosoc Oncol.* 1993;11(3):1–21.

19. Tomich PL, Helgeson VS. Is finding something good in the bad always good? Benefit finding among women with breast cancer. *Health Psychol.* 2004;23(1):16–23.

20. Carpenter JS, Brockopp DY, Andrykowski MA. Self-transformation as a factor in the self-esteem and well-being of breast cancer survivors. *J Adv Nurs.* 1999;29(6):1402–1411.

21. Cordova MJ, Cunningham LL, Carlson CR, Andrykowski MA. Posttraumatic growth following breast cancer: a controlled comparison study. *Health Psychol.* 2001;20(3):176–185.

22. Lechner SC, Carver CS, Antoni MH, Weaver KE, Phillips KM. Curvilinear associations between benefit finding and psychosocial adjustment to breast cancer. *J Consult Clin Psychol.* 2006;74(5):828–840.

23. Penedo FJ, Dahn JR, Molton I, et al. Cognitive-behavioral stress management improves stress-management skills and quality of life in men recovering from treatment of prostate carcinoma. *Cancer.* 2004;100(1): 192–200.

24. Tedeschi RG, Calhoun LG. The Posttraumatic Growth Inventory: measuring the positive legacy of trauma. *J Trauma Stress.* 1996;9(3):455–471.

25. Antoni MH, Lehman JM, Kilbourn KM, et al. Cognitive-behavioral stress management intervention decreases the prevalence of depression and enhances benefit finding among women under treatment for early-stage breast cancer. *Health Psychol.* 2001;20(1):20–32.

26. Behr SK, Murphy DL, Summers JA. *User's Manual: Kansas Inventory of Parental Perceptions.* Lawrence: University of Kansas; 1992.

27. Wortman CB. Posttraumatic growth: progress and problems. *Psychol Inq.* 2004;15:81–90.

28. McFarland C, Alvaro C. The impact of motivation on temporal comparisons: coping with traumatic events by perceiving personal growth. *J Pers Soc Psychol.* 2000;79(3):327–343.

29. Taylor SE, Brown JD. Illusion and well-being: a social psychological perspective on mental health. *Psychol Bull.* 1988;103(2):193–210.

30. Albert S. Temporal comparison theory. *Psychol Rev.* 1977;84:485–503.

31. Widows MR, Jacobsen PB, Booth-Jones M, Fields KK. Predictors of posttraumatic growth following bone marrow transplantation for cancer. *Health Psychol.* 2005;24(3):266–273.

32. Weiss T. Posttraumatic growth in women with breast cancer and their husbands: an intersubjective validation study. *J Psychosoc Oncol.* 2002; 20(2):65–80.

33. Manne S, Ostroff J, Winkel G, Goldstein L, Fox K, Grana G. Posttraumatic growth after breast cancer: patient, partner, and couple perspectives. *Psychosom Med.* 2004;66(3):442–454.

34. Klauer T, Ferring D, Filipp S. "Still stable after all this . . . ?": temporal comparisons in coping with severe and chronic illness. *Int J Behav Dev.* 1998;22:339–355.

35. Schulz U, Mohamed NE. Turning the tide: benefit finding after cancer surgery. *Soc Sci Med.* 2004;59(3):653–662.

36. Cruess DG, Antoni MH, McGregor BA, et al. Cognitive-behavioral stress management reduces serum cortisol by enhancing benefit finding among women being treated for early stage breast cancer. *Psychosom Med.* 2000; 62(3):304–308.

37. Carver CS, Antoni MH. Finding benefit in breast cancer during the year after diagnosis predicts better adjustment 5 to 8 years after diagnosis. *Health Psychol.* 2004;23(6):595–598.

38. Helgeson VS, Reynolds KA, Tomich PL. A meta-analytic review of benefit finding and growth. *J Consult Clin Psychol.* 2006;74(5):797–816.

39. Stanton AL, Danoff-Burg S, Sworowski LA, et al. Randomized, controlled trial of written emotional expression and benefit finding in breast cancer patients. *J Clin Oncol.* 2002;20(20):4160–4168.

chapter

6

Sexuality and Intimacy After Cancer

Leslie R. Schover, PhD

ABSTRACT

Currently in the United States, 50% of our approximately 12 million cancer survivors have had breast, prostate, gynecological, or colorectal malignancies. At least half of these 5 million men and women suffer from long-term, severe sexual dysfunction that is directly related to their cancer treatment. The most common problems for men and women include loss of sexual desire, erectile dysfunction (ED) in men, and vaginal dryness, tightness, and pain with sex in women. Although a number of recent studies have demonstrated good results for short-term psychoeducational interventions, most cancer survivors do not have access to expert, multidisciplinary care for their sexual problems.

PREVALENCE AND TYPES OF CANCER-RELATED SEXUAL PROBLEMS

Sexual problems are observed in at least 50% of survivors of breast cancer and gynecological cancer, as well as up to 90% of men treated for prostate cancer.[1,2] After treatment for colorectal cancer, 30% to 70% of patients have impaired sex lives, depending on the surgical procedure, their gender, and their age.[1] According to the National Cancer Institute's Office of Cancer Survivorship, these cancer sites account for 50% of the approximately 12 million cancer survivors alive today in the United

States.[3] Sexual dysfunction rates for cancer sites not involving the pelvis or breast are less, but typically at least 20% of men and women report new sexual problems after cancer treatment.[1]

For both genders, typical dysfunctions include loss of desire for sex and difficulty feeling arousal and pleasure. Erectile dysfunction is the other frequent complaint for men, and sexual changes related to sudden menopause—reduced vaginal expansion and lubrication, and consequent pain during sexual activity—are common for women.[4] Difficulty achieving orgasm is less common for men than for women and is often secondary to having sex with little erotic desire or arousal.[1]

Table 6.1 presents common sexual problems related to cancer and its treatment and the most typical factors that cause them. Most of these problems are related to damage to the hormonal, neurologic, or circulatory systems underlying sexual function. Unfortunately, they tend to be severe and persistent. Unlike emotional distress after cancer, sexual dysfunction does not decrease with time alone but remains a problem unless appropriate interventions take place.[1] In the table, the most frequent causal factors are listed first, with less common factors further down the list.

ᶜ∿ Case Example 6.1

Bob was a 61-year-old African American factory worker, diagnosed with stage B prostate cancer, Gleason grade 6. He had a radical prostatectomy with bilateral nerve-sparing but was very disappointed to find after recovery that he could not achieve firm erections. He experienced only mild swelling with sexual arousal and was unable to maintain even that degree of erection. His urologist prescribed tadalafil, but Bob found it did not improve his erections enough to allow penetration except perhaps on 1 out of 5 tries.

Bob had a long-term relationship with a woman in his apartment building but also occasionally dated others. Before his cancer diagnosis, he had been proud of his success in attracting younger women, but he was now too embarrassed by his ED (and too worried about gossip in his community) to approach new women to date. His girlfriend was pressuring him to get married, but Bob was not ready to make a commitment to her. He described her as a nice lady, but "a good church-going woman" who provided little sexual caressing and believed that normal sex involved intercourse in the missionary position.

Bob discussed his problem with another survivor in his support group and decided to go back to his urologist. After a longer discussion of treatment alternatives, he opted to have surgery to implant an inflatable penile prosthesis. Both the technical and psychosocial results were excellent. Bob felt like a "real man" again. He was somewhat disappointed that his erections remained at least an inch shorter than before his cancer, but he enjoyed the good rigidity and ability to have intercourse in a variety of positions. He did have one negative incident in which he developed some skin irritation on his glans penis, which he disclosed on interview was caused when he had kept on thrusting for 20 minutes after his own orgasm to please his partner. He agreed to focus on quality rather than quantity in future encounters.

OPTIONS FOR DIAGNOSIS AND TREATMENT

Table 6.2 summarizes current diagnostic and treatment options for patients' cancer-related sexual dysfunction. Some services are relevant only at specific times, such as, counseling—in consultation with the primary treating physician—to help patients consider whether a cancer treatment that preserves sexual function is a viable option for them. Other services are relevant across the timeline of cancer treatment, such as evaluating a concern about loss of desire for sex. Because most problems involve an organic deficit as well as the emotional impact of the sexual dysfunction, optimal programs combine gynecologic or urologic consultation with counseling by a mental health professional trained in both psycho-oncology and sex therapy. Unfortunately, such treatment programs may not be well reimbursed by private insurers, particularly for the time-consuming mental health services. It is difficult for survivors to find knowledgeable practitioners outside of major cancer centers or urban areas, and true, multidisciplinary clinics that treat cancer-related sexual dysfunction are extremely rare.

TABLE 6.1 ∽ Cancer-Related Sexual Problems

Problem	Frequent Causal Factors in Men	Frequent Causal Factors in Women
Generalized loss of desire for sex (includes loss of subjective pleasure during sex)	• Distress about erectile dysfunction • Medications: Anti-depressants, anxiolytics, anti-emetics, opiate pain medications, anti-hypertensives • Fatigue • Depression • Anti-androgen therapy for advanced prostate cancer • Hypogonadal after cancer treatment	• Avoidance of sex due to dyspareunia • Medications: Anti-depressants, anxiolytics, anti-emetics, opiate pain medications • Possible loss of androgens with ovarian failure: Bilateral oophorectomy, pelvic radio-therapy, high-dose or alkylating chemotherapy (more common after age 35) • Distress about attractiveness • Depression • Fatigue

(continues)

TABLE 6.1 ∾ Cancer-Related Sexual Problems (*continued*)

Problem	Frequent Causal Factors in Men	Frequent Causal Factors in Women
Erectile Dysfunction (ED) in men and Vaginal dryness, tightness, and pain with sex in women	• Damage to pelvic nerves from radical surgery (radical prostatectomy, radical cystectomy, pelvic exenteration, abdomino-perineal resection) • Damage to penile circulation from radical surgery or pelvic radiotherapy • Hypogonadism (anti-androgen therapy, high-dose chemotherapy, testicular radiation for childhood leukemia) • Interaction with prior damage to circulation from comorbid disorders (diabetes, hypertension, cardiovascular disease)	• Loss of estrogen due to sudden ovarian failure: Bilateral oophorectomy, pelvic radiotherapy, high-dose or alkylating chemotherapy (more common after age 35) • Cessation of estrogen replacement after post-menopausal cancer diagnosis • Local effects of radiotherapy on vaginal mucosa and walls (loss of elasticity, reduced lubrication, radiation ulcers, agglutination or stenosis in vagina) • Acute vaginal mucositis during chemotherapy • Vaginal graft vs. host disease (present in 20% or more of women with the syndrome)

(continues)

TABLE 6.1 ⌒ Cancer-Related Sexual Problems (*continued*)

Problem	Frequent Causal Factors in Men	Frequent Causal Factors in Women
Difficulty experiencing orgasm (pleasure and sensation)	• Inexperienced or unwilling to try to reach orgasm without erection • Reduced arousal and pleasure on anti-androgen therapy for advanced prostate cancer • Tumor in spinal cord or brain interrupting sexual pathways • Loss of erotic zones after total penectomy	• Distracting cancer-related images and cognitions during sex interfere with arousal • Loss of erotic zones after mastectomy or vulvectomy • Tumor in spinal cord or brain interrupting sexual pathways
Orgasm without ejaculation of semen	• Prostate and seminal vesicles removed as part of pelvic surgery (prostatectomy, cystectomy, pelvic exenteration) • Radiotherapy for prostate cancer damages prostate and seminal vesicles so no seminal fluid is produced • Anti-androgen therapy for advanced prostate cancer decreases semen production	• Not applicable to women

(continues)

TABLE 6.1 Cancer-Related Sexual Problems (*continued*)

Problem	Frequent Causal Factors in Men	Frequent Causal Factors in Women
	• Surgery interrupts sympathetic ganglia in retroperitoneum (retroperitoneal lymphadenectomy for testis cancer or resection of residual tumor post chemotherapy) • Surgery damages sympathetic nerves near sigmoid colon	

TABLE 6.2 Diagnostic and Treatment Options for Cancer-Related Sexual Problems

Option	Place in the Timeline of Cancer Treatment		
	Diagnosis to Treatment Disposition	During Active Cancer Treatment	After Active Cancer Treatment
Counseling on choosing cancer treatment that may conserve sexual function	X		
Assessment of sexual history and current function/concerns	X	X	X

(continues)

TABLE 6.2 ᗧ   Diagnostic and Treatment Options for Cancer-Related Sexual Problems (*continued*)

Option	Place in the Timeline of Cancer Treatment		
	Diagnosis to Treatment Disposition	During Active Cancer Treatment	After Active Cancer Treatment
Individual counseling for sexual concerns	X	X	X
Couple counseling for sexual concerns	X	X	X
Peer counseling for sexual concerns	X	X	X
Group counseling for sexual concerns		X	X
Screening for organic erectile dysfunction (penile Doppler, Rigiscan studies, etc.)	X	X	X
Screening for cause of pain during sexual activity (pelvic examination, imaging as needed)	X	X	X

(continues)

TABLE 6.2 Diagnostic and Treatment Options for Cancer-Related Sexual Problems (*continued*)

Option	Place in the Timeline of Cancer Treatment		
	Diagnosis to Treatment Disposition	During Active Cancer Treatment	After Active Cancer Treatment
Screening for factors contributing to loss of desire for sex (hormone profile, depression, fatigue, medication side effects, body image, relationship conflict, etc.)	X	X	X
Medical treatment of erectile dysfunction (ED) (phosphodiesterase type 5-inhibitors, vacuum devices, penile injection therapy, etc.)			X
Surgical treatment of ED (penile prostheses, correction of penile curvature)			X
Counseling to help couples integrate ED treatments into their sex lives			X

(continues)

TABLE 6.2 ∾   Diagnostic and Treatment Options for Cancer-Related Sexual Problems (*continued*)

Option	Place in the Timeline of Cancer Treatment		
	Diagnosis to Treatment Disposition	During Active Cancer Treatment	After Active Cancer Treatment
Medical treatment of dyspareunia (counseling on vaginal lubricants, moisturizers, options for local hormonal therapy, vaginal dilators, use of alpha-blocking medications for men, etc.)			X
Surgical treatment of dyspareunia (lysis of adhesions, vaginal reconstruction, treatment of urethral strictures, etc.)			X
Evaluation and treatment of vaginal scarring in graft vs. host disease			X

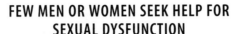

FEW MEN OR WOMEN SEEK HELP FOR SEXUAL DYSFUNCTION

Researchers surveyed over 27,500 adults from 29 countries, unselected for health and aged 40 to 80. The questionnaire asked about the prevalence of sexual problems and whether the respondent sought any medical help for the problem.[5] Rates of sexual problems and of help-seeking did not vary dramatically by geographic region. Overall, 43% of men and 49% of women reported a persistent sexual problem in the past year, but only 18% of men and 19% of women with a sexual problem sought medical help. Even fewer sought psychological help (1% to 12%). Although about half of respondents in English-speaking countries (Canada, United States, Australia, New Zealand, and South Africa) thought doctors should routinely ask patients about their sexual function, only 10% of either gender had been asked about sexuality by a physician in the past year.

Since the advent and popularization of the phosphodiesterase type 5 (PDE5) inhibiting drugs, however, more men have been consulting physicians about ED. A recent survey of 4422 men with ED from 8 industrialized nations found that 58% had seen a physician, with 41% specifically requesting a PDE5-inhibitor.[6] Another multinational survey of 1930 men with ED recruited from physician offices reported that 46% of patients had sought help, including 56% of patients from the United States.[7]

HELP-SEEKING FOR CANCER-RELATED SEXUAL DYSFUNCTION IN MEN

The percentage of men who seek help for ED after cancer treatment appears similar to the rate of help-seeking for ED unrelated to cancer. After localized prostate cancer treatment, of more than 1200 men from a registry at the Cleveland Clinic Foundation, 59% had tried a treatment for ED, with 52% opting for PDE5-inhibitors.[8] The 5-year data from the Prostate Cancer Outcomes Study was quite similar, with a 52% overall rate of help-seeking for ED.[9] Both of these surveys concluded that few prostate cancer survivors were able to use PDE5-inhibitors successfully but that most men remained reluctant to try more invasive therapies. Those who did also had high rates of nonadherence.[8,9] A recent review of this literature concurred with the 2 studies

cited, suggesting that a broader, biopsychosocial model of sexual rehabilitation would be necessary to increase the satisfaction of couples trying treatment for sexual dysfunction after prostate cancer.[10]

INTERVENTIONS FOR MEN

Our own attempt to provide a short-term, comprehensive psychoeducational intervention for sexual dysfunction after prostate cancer has
shown significant increases, at least in the short-term, in sexual satisfaction for both partners and in the percentage of men utilizing a medical
treatment for ED.[11] The intervention included partners and focused on
enhancing sexual communication and expression of affection in the
couple, coping with menopausal symptoms for women, helping partners agree on a medical treatment for ED, and troubleshooting in incorporating new treatments into the couple's sexual routine. We are
currently evaluating an Internet-based version of this program to increase the ease of disseminating it at relatively low cost.

HELP-SEEKING FOR CANCER-RELATED SEXUAL
PROBLEMS IN WOMEN

Barriers to seeking help for sexual problems appear to be even greater
for women. Even in a cohort of well-educated US women who completed an Internet survey, only 40% of those with a sexual problem consulted a healthcare professional.[12] Within that subgroup, less than half
felt the physician was interested in hearing about the problem, and only
14% received some kind of treatment plan. Forty-two percent consulted
gynecologists about the problem, and 24% saw a general practitioner.

Given the added time pressures in a busy oncology clinic, women
cancer survivors are likely to get even poorer care for their sexual problems. A survey of the patient education departments of comprehensive
cancer centers in 2002 revealed that only 14% offered counseling on
sexuality.[13] In a cohort of 166 well-educated women in the Northeast diagnosed with premenopausal breast cancer, only 68% recalled being
informed about premature menopause by one of their physicians, let
alone having a discussion directly about sexual function.[14] In a similar
cohort in Australia, 86% had discussed menopause with an oncologist, but many women were dissatisfied with the amount and timing

of information they received.[15] Interviews of 39 lesbian or bisexual women treated for breast cancer revealed that healthcare providers never inquired about sexual orientation, although 72% of women initiated disclosure with their oncologists.[16] Knowing a woman's sexual orientation is important for her healthcare providers not only for sexual counseling, but because lesbian women are at heightened risk for breast cancer, as well as cardiovascular disease and depression.[17]

The situation in other English-speaking, developed countries is quite similar. In England, a survey of members of multidisciplinary oncology teams showed that the clinical nurse specialist was often the only one to discuss sexual issues.[18] In a study of health care providers for women with ovarian cancer, the same researchers found that only 25% of oncologists and 20% of nurses discussed sexuality with the patients. A major reason for failing to bring up the topic was lack of knowledge or resources for support and referral.[19] A survey of radiation oncology clinics in Australia found that there was not even consistency on prevalence or type of advice given to women on using vaginal dilators after their treatment,[20] despite consensus that dilation may prevent vaginal stenosis.[21] Furthermore, a recent survey of over 200 long-term survivors of vaginal and cervical cancer found that 62% did not recall any discussion of sexuality with their oncology team.[22] These women were more likely to be experiencing severe sexual problems than those who remembered having some counseling, even though the average duration of follow-up was 27 years.

INTERVENTIONS FOR WOMEN

Only a few researchers have tried to intervene to improve sexual function in women after cancer. A Canadian group used support and education to try to increase adherence to vaginal dilation, with some improvement in dilator usage, mainly for younger women.[23] A brief nursing intervention improved sexual function and decreased menopause symptoms in breast cancer survivors.[24] A 3-session peer counseling intervention based on a written workbook had similar results for a cohort of African American breast cancer survivors.[25] A pilot psychoeducational program with handouts and 3 sessions of counseling by a psychologist helped improve sexual function in survivors of early-stage gynecological cancer.[26] Giving women accurate knowledge about sexual anatomy, function, and the impact of cancer treatment is crucial in these programs. Empowering women to ask to have their sexual needs met with a partner is also an important element, as is overcoming fears that having cancer will decrease a woman's sexual attractiveness to her partner.

∽ Case Example 6.2

Jenny was a 59-year-old woman who developed bladder cancer after smoking 2 packs of cigarettes daily for 40 years. She had a radical cystectomy with an ileal conduit urinary diversion. Because her tumor was extensive, her anterior vaginal wall was removed en bloc with her bladder and urethra. Her vagina was reconstructed by sewing the edges together vertically, giving good depth but a narrow caliber.

Jenny and her husband typically had sex once to twice a week and had no difficulties until the cancer diagnosis. When she tried to resume sex after her surgery, she found that she could still enjoy the caressing of her clitoris and was orgasmic, but that penetration for intercourse was dry, tight, and very painful. Because she was postmenopausal, she was prescribed a vaginal ring that released a low dose of estradiol. She also was given a set of 4 vaginal dilators, sized from about the length and diameter of a forefinger up to one about the size of an erect penis. A sexual counselor instructed Jenny on how to recognize the muscles surrounding her vaginal entrance and how to practice tensing and relaxing them. When she felt relaxed, she inserted the smallest vaginal dilator, using a water-based vaginal lubricant to minimize dryness and friction. Over several weeks, she was able to insert larger dilators without pain. She then showed her husband how to put in the lubricated dilators, guiding his hand and trying to stay relaxed. Within 2 months, Jenny was able to enjoy penile-vaginal intercourse again, although she continued to use low-dose vaginal estrogen and felt more in control when the couple used positions that gave her freedom to control the angle and depth of penetration.

CONCLUSION

Despite our improved knowledge about the prevalence and causes of cancer-related sexual problems, and even though many patients demonstrate improved sexual function with short-term counseling, we have a long way to go in making sexual interventions more accessible to cancer survivors.

REFERENCES

1. Schover LR. Reproductive complications and sexual dysfunction in the cancer patient. In: Chang AE, Ganz PA, Hayes DF, et al., eds. *Oncology: An Evidence-Based Approach*. New York: Springer-Verlag; 2005:1580–1600.
2. Schover LR, Fouladi RT, Warneke CL, et al. Defining sexual outcomes after treatment for localized prostate cancer. *Cancer*. 2002;95:1773–1785.
3. Cancer survivorship research. National Cancer Institute Office of Cancer Survivorship Web site. http://www.cancercontrol.cancer.gov/ocs/prevalence/prevalence.html. Accessed November 13, 2008.
4. Ganz PA, Rowland JH, Desmond K, et al. Life after breast cancer: understanding women's health-related quality of life and sexual functioning. *J Clin Oncol*. 1998;16:501–514.
5. Moreira ED, Brock G, Glasser DB, et al. Help-seeking behaviour for sexual problems: the Global Study of Sexual Attitudes and Behaviors. *Int J Clin Pract*. 2005;59:6–16.
6. Rosen RC, Fisher WA, Eardley I, et al. The multinational Men's Attitudes to Life Events and Sexuality (MALES) study: I. prevalence of erectile dysfunction and related health concerns in the general population. *Curr Med Res Opin*. 2004;20:607–617.
7. Shabsigh R, Perelman MA, Laumann EO, Lockhart DC. Drivers and barriers to seeking treatment for erectile dysfunction: a comparison of six countries. *BJU Int*. 2004;94:1055–1065.
8. Schover LR, Fouladi RT, Warneke CL, et al. The use of treatments for erectile dysfunction among survivors of prostate carcinoma. *Cancer*. 2002;95:2397–2407.
9. Stephenson RA, Mori M, Hsieh Y, et al. Treatment of erectile dysfunction following therapy for clinically localized prostate cancer: patient reported use and outcomes from the Surveillance, Epidemiology, and End Results Prostate Cancer Outcomes Study. *J Urol*. 2005;174:646–650.
10. Matthew AG, Goldman A, Trachtenberg J, et al. Sexual dysfunction after radical prostatectomy: prevalence, treatments, restricted use of treatments, and distress. *J Urol*. 2005;174:2105–2110.
11. Canada AL, Neese L, Sui D, Schover LR. A pilot intervention to enhance sexual rehabilitation for couples after treatment for localized prostate cancer. *Cancer*. 2005;104:2689–2700.

12. Berman L, Berman J, Felder S, et al. Seeking help for sexual function complaints: what gynecologists need to know about the female patient's experience. *Fertil Steril.* 2003;79:572–576.
13. Tesauro GM, Rowland JH, Lustig C. Survivorship resources for post-treatment cancer survivors. *Cancer Pract.* 2002;10:277–283.
14. Duffy CM, Allen SM, Clark MA. Discussions regarding reproductive health for young women with breast cancer undergoing chemotherapy. *J Clin Oncol.* 2005; 23:766–773.
15. Thewes B, Meiser B, Taylor A, et al. Fertility- and menopause-related information needs of younger women with a diagnosis of early breast cancer. *J Clin Oncol.* 2005;23:5155–5165.
16. Boemer U, Case P. Physicians don't ask, sometimes patients tell. Disclosure of sexual orientation among women with breast carcinoma. *Cancer.* 2004;101:1882–1889.
17. Case P, Austin SB, Hunter DJ, et al. Sexual orientation, health risk factors, and physical functioning in the Nurses' Health Study II. *J Womens Health (Larchmt).* 2004;13:1033–1047.
18. Catt S, Fallowfield L, Jenkins V, et al. The informational roles and psychological health of members of 10 oncology multidisciplinary teams in the UK. *Br J Cancer.* 2005. http://www.nature.com/bjc/journal/v93/n10/abs/6602816a.html. Published October 18, 2005. Accessed November 13, 2008.
19. Stead ML, Brown JM, Fallowfield L, Selby P. Lack of communication between healthcare professionals and women with ovarian cancer about sexual issues. *Br J Cancer.* 2003;88:666–671.
20. Lancaster L. Preventing vaginal stenosis after brachytherapy for gynaecological cancer: an overview of Australian practices. *Eur J Oncol Nurs.* 2005;8:30–39.
21. Denton AS, Maher EJ. Interventions for the physical aspects of sexual dysfunction in women following pelvic radiotherapy. *The Cochrane Library.* 2003;3:1–26. http://www.cochrane.org/reviews/en/ab003750.html. Published January 20, 2003. Accessed November 13, 2008.
22. Lindau ST, Gavrilova N, Anderson D. Sexual morbidity in very long term survivors of vaginal and cervical cancer: a comparison to national norms. *Gynecol Oncol.* 2007;106:413–418.
23. Jeffries SA, Robinson JW, Craighead PS, Keats MR. An effective group psychoeducational intervention for improving compliance with vaginal dilation: a randomized controlled trial. *Int J Radiat Oncol Biol Phys.* 2006; 65:404–411.
24. Zibecchi L, Greendale GA, Ganz PA. Continuing education: comprehensive menopausal assessment: an approach to managing vasomotor and

urogenital symptoms in breast cancer survivors. *Oncol Nurs Forum.* 2003;30:393–407.

25. Schover LR, Jenkins R, Sui D, et al. A randomized trial of peer counseling on reproductive health in African American breast cancer survivors. *J Clin Oncol.* 2006;24:1620–1626.

26. Brotto LA, Heiman JR, Goff B, et al. A psychoeducational intervention for sexual dysfunction in women with gynecologic cancer. *Arch Sex Behav.* 2008;37(2):317–319.

7

Male Sexuality and Fertility After Cancer

Michael A. Diefenbach, PhD,

Gina A. Turner, PhD,

&

Natan Bar-Chama, MD

ABSTRACT

Human sexuality permeates every facet of our life, and comprises a broad range of behavior and processes. The occurrence of cancer affects sexuality in men in three specific domains or processes: 1) the direct influence of the disease on sexuality; 2) the indirect influence of cancer treatment on sexuality; and 3) psychosocial factors that impact a patient's thoughts and feelings about sexuality. In this chapter, we will discuss three specific areas within the cancer and sexuality literature that have received the most attention and empirical support: the influence of cancer on fertility, erectile dysfunction, and body image. We will introduce approaches and methods commonly used by healthcare providers to address these concerns, and finally, we will discuss the importance of open communication between the patient and their provider.

INTRODUCTION

Human sexuality permeates every facet of our life; it is after all the reason for our existence. Human sexuality comprises a broad range of behavior and processes, including physiological, psychological, social, cultural, and political aspects. Sexuality further extends into philosophical, ethical, moral, theological, legal, and spiritual thinking.

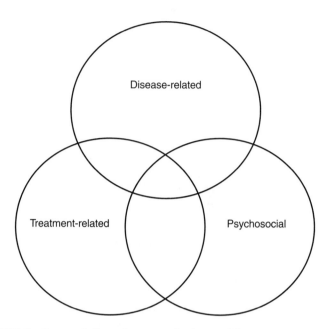

FIGURE 7.1   Factors influencing sexuality in men after cancer.

Men's sexuality after cancer is an important but rather broad area that can be approached from several directions. The Venn diagram in Figure 7.1 provides an outline of our approach for this chapter. In the diagram:

▷ The first circle, labeled "disease-related," represents the fact that cancer might influence sexuality directly. The best example of such a relationship is testicular cancer.

▷ The second circle, labeled "treatment-related," represents the influences of cancer treatment on sexuality; these influences might include the effects of alkylating chemotherapy regimens that have the potential to severely impact a patient's fertility.

▷ The third circle represents psychosocial factors that impact a patient's thoughts and feelings about sexuality. These might include changed body perception, loss of libido, or erectile dysfunction (ED) among men.

The overlap of the three circles (e.g., the intersection of the Venn diagram) represents the area for which considerable research evidence

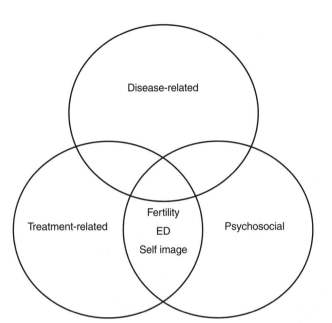

FIGURE 7.2 Inside the Venn diagram—area for which considerable research evidence exists.

exists (Figure 7.2). Other common factors, such as age, that have been found to influence sexuality are subsumed under this organization.

Sexuality and cancer is not only an issue for the elderly, as demonstrated by testicular cancer. This form of cancer on average occurs in men between the ages of 20 and 34 and is highly prevalent. It accounts for 19% of all cancers in this age group. Fortunately, it has a very high cure rate; with radiation and chemotherapy, over 90% of patients will experience remission, with an approximate recurrence rate of only 5% in the contra-lateral testis.

FERTILITY PRESERVATION

Fertility is of particular concern for the young male. Fertility is impacted by the following cancers directly: testicular cancer, lymphoma (e.g., Hodgkin disease and non-Hodgkin lymphoma), and leukemia, and soft-tissue sarcoma. These cancers are associated with varying degrees of potential for azoospermia (zero sperm concentration) or oligospermia (sperm count of less than 20 million sperm per milliliter of semen),[1] as represented in the following list:

▷ 28% among testicular cancer patients
▷ 25% among Hodgkin disease patients
▷ 57% among leukemia patients

An example of fertility preservation can be found in the treatment of testicular cancer patients. Various surveillance protocols have been implemented to avoid or diminish the impact of radiation chemotherapy and additional surgery on future fertility. More recently, in isolated cases a new approach involving testicular-sparing management of testicular masses is considered instead of radical orchiectomy in an attempt to preserve spermatogenesis and hormonal function.[2] But there are additional concerns with this experimental approach, primarily the yet unknown risk of recurrence in the remaining testicular tissue, secondary malignancies, and pulmonary and cardiovascular complications.

For men with testicular cancer who undergo a retroperitoneal lymph node dissection for either prophylactic or diagnostic reasons, as well as for those in whom metastatic disease is documented, injury to the sympathetic nerves feeding the pelvis can occur. While surgical templates have been created and applied when appropriate to minimize this untoward effect, they are not always successful. Injury to the sympathetic system can result in the inability to ejaculate (anejaculation) and, thus, infertility; yet the parasympathetic nerves remain intact, so no alteration in erectile function occurs. Anejaculation and subsequent infertility in this patient population can be successfully treated with either electroejaculation (a procedure, performed under anesthesia, that electrically and directly stimulates the nerves, inducing an ejaculation) or retrieval of sperm directly from the testis. These techniques yield sufficient sperm that can then be utilized with advanced reproductive technologies such as intracytoplasmic sperm injection (ICSI); in ICSI, success is primarily dependent on female age, not sperm source.

THE INFLUENCE OF CANCER TREATMENT ON SEXUALITY

Improvements in therapy have resulted in an increasing number of cancer survivors who are confronted with issues of sexuality and fertility.

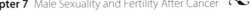

Table 7.1 outlines fertility outcomes associated with various cancers and treatments.[3]

To aid practicing oncologists regarding fertility preservation methods and related issues, the American Society of Clinical Oncology (ASCO) formed a 9-member panel and published a list of guidelines.[4] The panel reviewed 276 articles, consisting of case studies, cohort studies, and small nonrandomized trials; however, there is a paucity of large and/or randomized studies.

First the ASCO panel ascertained whether there is even sufficient interest in fertility preservation among cancer patients and found that fertility preservation is of great importance in this population. Patients want to be able to conceive their own biological children, especially when a patient is disease free after treatment. However, in terms of family planning, there may be concerns about one's own reduced longevity, potential birth defects, or children's risk of cancer. Table 7.2 provides a comparison of different methods that can address the preservation of fertility.[4]

The panel concluded that becoming infertile during cancer treatment is a significant source of distress among cancer survivors. Worry about later infertility can influence the patient's choice of a nonaggressive cancer treatment.

The panel also identified special circumstances for children: Informed consent must be obtained from parents or guardians. Once consent is received, future fertility would be possible for these child patients, by harvesting their semen. This would allow the patients the option of whether or not to conceive children at a later time point.

To preserve fertility, the ASCO panel recommended that cryopreservation (freezing for future possible use) of pretreatment semen should be offered. This is the most successful and empirically validated option. Another option, gonadoprotection through hormonal manipulation (hormonal therapies to protect testicular tissue), is generally ineffective. Other options, such as testicular tissue or spermatogonial cryopreservation and testis xenografting (reimplantation after cancer treatment), are still experimental.

Cryopreserved semen can be used at a later date for intracytoplasmic ICSI. Intracytoplasmic sperm injection involves injecting a single sperm directly into a mature egg. This technique has been successful even with extremely reduced samples.

TABLE 7.1 ∾ Tumor Entity, Treatment, and Post-Treatment Fertility

Tumor Entity	Treatment	Post-treatment Fertility
Testicular cancer	Cisplatin/carboplatin	Prolonged azoospermia in 55%
	Cisplatin 400 mg/m² plus ifosfamide 30 g/m²	Normozooospermia in 64% at 1 yr; 80% at 3–5 yrs
Hodgkin disease	MVPP	Azoospermia in >90%
	MOPP (3 courses)	Recovery significantly higher compared to ≥ 5 courses
	ABVD	Temp azoospermia with normal sperm count at 18 months; 90% normozoospermia after 1 yr
Osteosarcoma	Ifosfamide 46 g/m² plus cisplatin 560 g/m² plus doxorubicin plus methotrexate	Patients who received high-dose ifosfamide showed a higher incidence of azoospermia
Ewing sarcoma or soft tissue sarcoma	CYADIC/CYVADIC	40% of men recovered to normospermic levels by 5 yrs after treatment
Rectal cancer	Pelvic radiotherapy (50 Gy)	High risk of permanent infertility and risk of endocrine failure (hypogonadism)

(continues)

TABLE 7.1 ✎ Tumor Entity, Treatment, and Post-Treatment Fertility (*continued*)

Tumor Entity	Treatment	Post-treatment Fertility
Prostate cancer	Brachytherapy (exposure of 10 mR/h at the symphysis pubis)	No change in semen parameters
	External beam radiotherapy (70 Gy to prostate bed)	Damage on spermatogenesis
Superficial bladder cancer	Intravesical instillation of BCG	Oligozoospermia
Thyroid cancer	Treating with high dose of radioiodine ^{131}I	No evidence of infertility

MVPP (mustine, vinblastine, procarbazine, and prednisolone)

MOPP (mechlorethamine, vincristine, procarbazine, and prednisone)

ABVD (adriamycin, bleomycin, vinblastine, and dacarbazine)

CYADIC (cyclophosphamide, doxorubicin, and dacarbazine)

CYVADIC (cyclophosphamide, vincristine, doxorubicin, and dacarbazine)

BCG (Bacillus Calmette-Guerin)

TABLE 7.2 ✎ Overview of Fertility Intervention Options

Intervention	Definition	Comment	Considerations
Sperm cryopreservation (S) after masturbation	Freezing sperm obtained through masturbation	The most established technique for fertility preservation in men; large cohort studies in men with cancer	Outpatient procedure; approximately $1500 for three samples stored for 3 years; storage fee for additional years*

(continues)

TABLE 7.2 ～ Overview of Fertility Intervention Options (*continued*)

Intervention	Definition	Comment	Considerations
Sperm cryopreservation (S) after alternative methods of sperm collection	Freezing sperm obtained through testicular aspiration or extraction, electroejaculation under sedation, or from a post-masturbation urine sample	Small case series and case reports	Testicular sperm extraction; outpatient surgical procedure
Gonadal shielding during radiation therapy (S)	Use of shielding to reduce the dose of radiation delivered to the testicles	Case series	Possible only with selected radiation fields and anatomy; expertise is required to ensure that shielding does not increase dose delivered to the reproductive organs
Testicular tissue cryopreservation; testis xenografting; spermatogonial isolation (I)	Freezing testicular tissue or germ cells and reimplantation after cancer treatment or maturation in animals	Has not been tested in humans; successful application in animal models	Outpatient surgical procedurea

Abbreviations: S, standard; I, investigational.

*Costs are estimates.

In addition, the ASCO Panel recommended that risks to fertility from cancer treatment should be discussed by providers, that questions about fertility preservation and success of cancer treatment need to be addressed, and finally that providers should be open to referring patients to reproductive specialists and psychological service providers.

ISSUES WITH CRYOPRESERVATION

Cryopreservation is the recommended method for male fertility preservation, yet it is not routinely discussed by healthcare providers. Many lack the specific knowledge and the time to address patients' concerns about cryopreservation; they also often prioritize survival concerns of the patient over fertility concerns during consultations; and finally, they are often ill informed about the cost of long-term storage.[5,6]

Barriers to cryopreservation from the patient's standpoint include perceived logistical and psychological constraints. Patients may not want to delay treatment to address the issue of fertility or may worry that it is not a big enough priority to be concerned about at the time of treatment. Lack of information coupled with financial constraints and inadequate insurance coverage often prevent adoption of cryopreservation.

A descriptive study examining sperm cryopreservation among 129 patients with testicular cancer found that 31 men (24%) banked sperm, 2 men (6%) used their sperm to father a child, and 12 men (9%) were able to father children naturally.[7] The study also found that younger men were significantly more likely to bank their sperm. The median cost was $300, with a range of $0 to $1000, and the annual maintenance median cost was $300, with a range of $0 to $1200. Other studies have reported the use of sperm cryopreservation in this population to be as high as 30%.

Another barrier to cryopreservation is the perceived difficulty of communicating effectively about this issue with a healthcare provider. Chapple and colleagues interviewed 21 young men treated for cancer about fertility.[8] Eighteen of these men talked at length about their disease. They expressed that communication about sperm storage was difficult and embarrassing, and that the decision-making process felt often rushed. They also felt there was a lack of counselors.

To summarize, fertility concerns are high among cancer patients. Cryopreservation is a well-established method for fertility preservation, but currently its adoption by patients is fairly low. The low use of cryopreservation may be attributable to the information gap that exists between patients and providers about availability, cost, and use of cryopreservation.

BODY IMAGE AND SEXUAL FUNCTIONING AMONG TESTICULAR CANCER SURVIVORS

Body image and sexual functioning are important concerns to testicular cancer survivors. The impact of testicular cancer in these areas can be seen in a study in which 157 patients received a questionnaire about their sexuality.[9] Out of the 78% of those who responded, 52% mentioned that their body had changed. Although 90% of participants reported being sexually active, they also reported decreases in sexual interest (21%), pleasure (20%), and problems with erections (17%).

Changes in appearance after cancer can also lead to alterations in body image, and even to social withdrawal.[10] A multiple case study of male adolescents who had one of several types of cancer, such as Hodgkin disease or osteosarcoma, revealed altered perceptions of body image. Patients reported such feelings as "I don't look normal," "I look ugly," and "I look sick." These self-images evoke feelings of vulnerability ("people look at me") and can lead to social avoidance and decreased social interactions.[11]

ERECTILE DYSFUNCTION

Erectile dysfunction is defined as the inability to obtain an erection adequate for satisfactory sexual activity.[12] Erectile dysfunction is one of the likely side effects of prostate cancer treatment, as reported in a large study of a multi-ethnic group of American men (39–79 years of age) treated with radical prostatectomy. Of these 1291 men, 59.9% of the patients had ED at 18 months.[13] In another study, following external beam radiation, approximately one-third of these patients had ED; after adjusting for age (mean age of this group was 68), these ED rates were comparable to those of patients who had undergone radical prostatectomy.[14]

Brachytherapy may have less impact on sexual function than other methods of treatment. Mabjeesh and colleagues followed up with 378 patients who underwent permanent prostate brachytherapy.[15] Of these, 131 patients were potent before implantation, and 80% of this group indicated they were satisfied with their sexual function up to 3 years after treatment. Those satisfied were either able to have successful intercourse as before brachytherapy or were able to have successful intercourse after brachytherapy using sildenafil treatment.

COMMUNICATION ABOUT PATIENT SEXUALITY AND INTIMACY

Severe ED measured in a group of 94 men was associated with a number of negative quality of life outcomes: not having a regular sex partner, low positive affect, loneliness, low sexual self-efficacy, poor psychological adjustment, less marital happiness, anxiety during intercourse, and depression.[16] However, even though it is a major contributor to distress, it is difficult for both clinicians and patients to discuss patient sexuality and intimacy issues. In 1 qualitative study, 50 cancer patients and 32 health care professionals were interviewed regarding this issue.[17] Overwhelmingly, patients reported a lack of success in their search for basic information. Patients voiced such concerns as "Can you have sex after chemo? . . . I was looking for a discussion. Now I will never know." Another area of concern was normalcy. During these interviews, patients expressed questions like "Has something gone wrong with my treatment? My body has changed, my mind has changed. Is it normal to feel so ugly?"

Patients wanted straight information from their providers about this crucial issue: "My relationship is the most important part of my life, not just physically, mentally also. Nobody seems to understand this." Patients also felt that providers prioritized survival above their sexuality. Other patients expressed trust in the expert opinions of their providers, assuming that "if it were that important, they would have told me."

Healthcare professionals expressed different concerns. Some mentioned reluctance bringing up issues that were not matters of life or death: "How can I bring up sex? There are more important things to discuss." Health professionals thought that patients would share their focus on combating the disease. Others actively avoid the topic:

"I understand my limitations. Somebody else will address the issue." Avoiding the issue allows them to protect their own authority and shield their own vulnerability: "I come from a strict background where sex is taboo."

There is also concern about the risk involved in bringing up the topic: "I struggle when patients come from another culture. Am I offending them? I feel so ignorant." This concern may also be exacerbated when health professionals make stereotypical assumptions about their patients, based on factors such as age, sex, diagnosis, and culture. Another risk involved is the threat of litigation. Professionals may hide behind medical language and avoid mentioning certain topics because of fear of embarrassment and potential legal consequences.

RECOMMENDATIONS FOR SUCCESSFUL COMMUNICATION

How might health professionals bring up such a sensitive topic with their patients? Successful communication is patient-centered and negotiated; in the words of one health professional: "The more comfortable I am with who I am . . . my own sexuality . . . the more comfortable I can be with patients." There are also techniques and tools that can assist providers in discussing sexuality. When taking a sexual history, healthcare providers should review each phase of the male sexual cycle: desire, excitement, orgasm, resolution. Physicians should use focused questions for each phase, making sure to use common terminology as needed.

Some examples of targeted questions are:

▷ Desire: "Do you still feel in the mood, feel desire, and have sexual thoughts or fantasies?"
▷ Excitement: "Do you have trouble getting or keeping an erection, getting or staying hard? Or both?" "Is this a problem when you touch yourself or only when you are with a partner?"

Asking questions a number of different ways can also help to clarify the problems a patient is experiencing. For example, additional questioning can help to differentiate between premature, delayed, or retrograde ejaculation (release of semen into the bladder rather than through the urethra). Some men may confuse premature ejaculation with ED.

Questions to ask regarding orgasm include:

▷ "Do you feel you ejaculate too quickly?"
▷ "Do you ever have difficulty reaching orgasm or ejaculating?"
▷ "Do you lose your erection before or after you ejaculate?"

SELF-ASSESSMENT IN PRIMARY CARE

The IIEF-5 Erectile Function Test is an abridged, five-item version of the International Index of Erectile Function (IIEF) diagnostic tool for ED[18] and is easily self-administered, or, in the case of visual or literacy impairment, it can be read by the healthcare provider. The test can be incorporated into routine medical history. See Table 7.3 for the five items.

Heruti and associates introduced the Sexual Health Inventory for Men (SHIM) questionnaire at the examination center for career servicemen of the Israel Defense Force.[19] The SHIM questionnaire was incorporated into a computerized questionnaire used to collect the medical history. The platform of a periodic examination offers maximum privacy and emphasizes the importance of sexual health as a natural and

TABLE 7.3 ∿ International Index of Erectile Function (IIEF-5)

Over the past 6 months*:					
1. How do you rate your confidence that you could get an erection?	1	2	3	4	5
2. When you had erections with sexual stimulation, how often were your erections hard enough for penetration?	1	2	3	4	5
3. During sexual intercourse, how often were you able to maintain your erection after you had penetrated (entered) your partner?	1	2	3	4	5
4. During sexual intercourse, how difficult was it to maintain your erection to completion of intercourse?	1	2	3	4	5
5. When you attempted sexual intercourse, how often was it satisfactory for you?	1	2	3	4	5

*Rate on scale 1–5, 1=very low, 5=very high

fundamental constituent of general health, while positioning sexual dysfunction as an early indicator of underlying disease. The concept of adding an ED questionnaire to a screening program may encourage more men to seek treatment, not only for their ED, but also for the underlying disease.

SUMMARY

The influence of cancer on sexuality can be caused by the disease and its treatment. Sexual dysfunction has been associated with stress and anxiety, altered body image, lowered sexual desire, erectile difficulties, diminished sexual satisfaction, decreased frequency of sexual contact, and diminished sexual self-esteem.

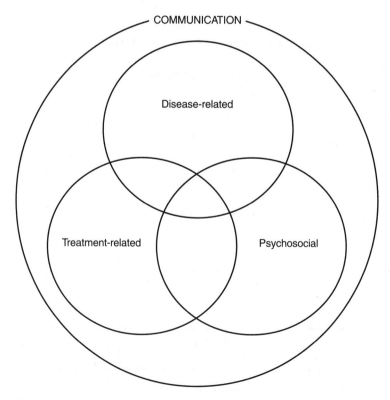

FIGURE 7.3 Communication.

Significant psychological disturbances both in partners and patients can lead to conflict through communication and relationship difficulties. Patients may also feel a lack of support from their health care providers as well as the healthcare system.[20–22]

Open communication between patient and healthcare provider can help to alleviate the impact of cancer on sexuality. Patients cannot rely on physicians to address issues of sexuality, just as physicians cannot expect patients to freely talk about their sexual concerns. Both parties need to proactively bring up this important issue. For their part, healthcare providers can facilitate communication by providing a safe setting and an open atmosphere conducive to discussing concerns about sexuality (Figure 7.3). Patients, on the other hand, might write down their questions and concerns before the meeting. Finally, researchers are challenged to develop and evaluate better ways to enhance communication between patients and healthcare providers.

REFERENCES

1. Chung IJ, Knee G, Efymow B, Blasco L, Patrizio P. Sperm cryopreservation for male patients with cancer. *Eur J Obstet Gynecol Reprod Biol.* 2004;113 (suppl):S7–11.
2. Paduch DA. Testicular cancer and male infertility. *Curr Opin Urol.* 2006; 16:419–427.
3. Trottmann M, Becker AJ, Stadler T, et al. Semen quality in men with malignant diseases before and after therapy and the role of cryopreservation. *Eur Urol.* 2007;52(2):355–367.
4. Lee SJ, Schover LR, Partridge AH, et al. ASCO recommendations on fertility preservation in cancer patients: guideline summary. *J Clin Oncol.* 2006;24(18):2917–2931.
5. Schover LR, Schover KB, Lichtin A, Lipshultz LI, Jeha S. Oncologists' attitudes and practices regarding banking sperm before cancer treatment. *J Clin Oncol.* 2002;20:1890–1897.
6. Reebals JF, Brown R, Buckner EB. Nurse practice issues regarding sperm banking in adolescent male cancer patients. *J Pediatr Oncol Nurs.* 2006; 23(4):182–188.
7. Girasole CR, Cookson MS, Smith JA Jr, Ivey BS, Roth BJ, Chang SS. Sperm banking: use and outcomes in patients treated for testicular cancer. *BJU Int.* 2007;99:33–36.

8. Chapple A, Salinas M, Ziebland S, McPherson A, MacFarlane A. Fertility issues: the perceptions and experiences of young men recently diagnosed and treated for cancer. *J Adolesc Health.* 2007;40(1):69–75.

9. Incrocci L, Hop W, Wijnmaalen A, Slob A. Treatment outcome, body image, and sexual functioning after orchiectomy and radiotherapy for stage I-II testicular seminoma. *Int J Radiat Oncol Biol Phys.* 2002;53:1165–1173.

10. Enskär, K., Carlsson, M., Golsäter, M., Hamrin, E. Symptom distress and life situation in adolescents with cancer. *Cancer Nursing.* 1997;20(1):23–33.

11. Larouche SS, Chin-Peuckert L. Changes in body image experienced by adolescents with cancer. *J Pediatr Oncol Nurs.* 2006;23(4):200–209.

12. Marwick C. Survey says patients expect little physician help on sex. *JAMA.* 1999;281(23):2173–2174.

13. Stanford JL, Feng Z, Hamilton AS, et al. Urinary and sexual function after radical prostatectomy for clinically localized prostate cancer. *JAMA.* 2000;283:354–360.

14. Mantz CA, Song P, Farhangi E, et al. Potency probability following conformal megavoltage radiotherapy using conventional doses for localized prostate cancer. *Int J Radiat Oncol Biol Phys.* 1997;37:551–557.

15. Mabjeesh N, Chen J, Beri A, Stenger A, Matzkin H. Sexual function after permanent 125I-brachytherapy for prostate cancer. *Int J Impotence Res.* 2005;17:96–101.

16. Latini DM, Peson DF, Wallace KL, Lupek DP, Lue TF. Clinical and psychosocial characteristics of men with erectile dysfunction: baseline data from ExCEED. *J Sex Med.* 2006;3:1059–1067.

17. Hordern AJ, Street AF. Communicating about patient sexuality and intimacy after cancer: mismatched expectations and unmet needs. *Med J Aust.* 2007;186:224–227.

18. Rosen RC, Cappelleri JC, Smith MD, Lipsky J, Peña BM. Development and evaluation of an abridged, 5-item version of the International Index of Erectile Function (IIEF-5) as a diagnostic tool for erectile dysfunction. *Int J Impotence Res.* 1999;11:319–326.

19. Heruti RJ, Yossef M, Shochat T. Screening for erectile dysfunction as part of periodic exams—concept and implementation. *Int J Impotence Res.* 2004;16:1–5.

20. Bar-Chama N, Schiff J, Yavorsky R, Diefenbach MA. Erectile dysfunction and infertility. *Curr Sex Health Rep.* 2007;4:20–23.

21. Newton CR, Sherrard W, Glavac I. The fertility problem inventory: measuring perceived infertility-related stress. *Fertil Steril.* 1999;72:54–62.

22. Fassino S, Piero A, Boggio S, Piccioni V, Garzaro L. Anxiety, depression and anger suppression in infertile couples: a controlled study. *Hum Reprod.* 2002;17(11):2986–2994.

8

Fertility and Parenthood in Cancer Survivors

Leslie R. Schover, PhD

ABSTRACT

As cancer survivorship becomes a more salient issue, concerns about interrupted childbearing and infertility for younger men and women have been recognized. New technologies in reproductive medicine are bringing new options for fertility preservation, treating cancer during pregnancy, and utilizing cryopreserved gametes for cancer survivors. The psychosocial impact of interrupted childbearing and using alternative paths to parenthood still requires more attention and research, however.

INTRODUCTION

In the past several years, infertility after cancer treatment has become a high profile issue. In its 2004 report, the President's Cancer Panel recommended that all men, women, and parents of children be informed if a cancer treatment has potential to damage fertility or childbearing potential.[1] As with other aspects of quality of life after cancer, a patient advocacy group, Fertile Hope, deserves a major share of the credit for publicizing the importance of parenthood after cancer. Its Web site, brochures, and conferences offer information and even financial aid to cancer patients and survivors.

The attention to fertility issues has also been fostered by oncology professionals. In 2004, a multidisciplinary conference on parenthood after cancer at the University of Texas M. D. Anderson Cancer Center, organized with a grant from the National Institutes of Health, attracted attendees from 13 countries. The proceedings were published in 2005, with funding from the Lance Armstrong Foundation, as volume 34 of the *Journal of the National Cancer Institute Monographs*. The American Society for Reproductive Medicine now has a special interest group on fertility preservation and has published a consensus report on the ethical implications of established and experimental technologies.[2] The American Society of Clinical Oncology also created an expert panel on cancer and fertility preservation that published practice recommendations for its members.[3]

THE PREVALENCE OF CANCER-RELATED INFERTILITY

According to the National Health Interview Survey of 2001, 2.2% of US adults aged 18 to 44 have been diagnosed with cancer.[4] Extrapolating based on statistics for this age group from the US Census of 2000,[5] approximately 2.5 million adults of childbearing age are cancer survivors. It is more difficult to specify how many have faced infertility, but most probably had treatment with gonadotoxic chemotherapy, and smaller numbers would be at risk of infertility due to surgery or radiation therapy affecting the reproductive system.

Another trend that increases the salience of cancer and fertility is delayed childbearing in American families. Birth rates for women in their thirties have been climbing steadily, reaching a high in 2001 of 95.6 per 1000 women aged 30 to 34 and 41.4 per 1000 women aged 35 to 39.[6] Births to women aged 40 to 44 have more than doubled since 1981 to 8.1 per 1000 women. According to the US Census report for 2000, the percentage of childless women aged 30 to 34 has jumped from 19.8% in 1980 to 28.1% in 2000, and for women aged 35 to 39, it has jumped from 12.1% in 1980 to 20.1% in 2000.[7] Thus more women are pregnant at ages when the incidence of cancer begins to increase. Data on paternal age are not readily available, but in 1995 in the United States, men were on the average 2.7 years older than their brides[8]; thus men would also be more at risk currently to have cancer interfere with their fertility, if only because of their partners' more advanced ages.

FACTORS ASSOCIATED WITH CANCER-RELATED MALE INFERTILITY

Although cancer treatment may cause male infertility, the malignancy itself may be associated with impaired sperm production. Testicular cancer is the most common malignancy in men aged 15 to 40, with about 8000 new cases each year in the United States.[9] It is more common in men who had cryptorchidism (undescended testes), a condition also related to infertility. Even in men whose testes appear normal, many men diagnosed with testicular cancer have tissue abnormalities and reduced sperm production in the contralateral testis.[10] Bilateral testicular cancer occurs in less than 1% of newly diagnosed men, however, and less than 1.9% develop a second, invasive cancer in their remaining testicle in the subsequent 15 years.[11] A Danish registry study found significantly lower fertility in a cohort of 3530 men born between 1945 and 1980 who developed testicular cancer compared to all other Danish men born in the same era.[12] Fertility was particularly reduced in the 2 years leading up to cancer diagnosis and in men with nonseminomatous tumors. In 3847 men in an American infertility clinic who had abnormal semen analyses, the rate of testicular cancer was 20 times higher than expected, reinforcing the need for infertility specialists to be on the lookout for this cancer.[13]

In addition to testicular cancer, other malignancies common in teens and young men include non-Hodgkin lymphoma, Hodgkin disease, leukemia, sarcomas, melanoma, colorectal tumors, and central nervous system tumors.[14] In general, young men diagnosed with cancer are more likely to have reduced sperm counts and motility, perhaps due to recent fevers, anesthesia for diagnostic procedures, or other tumor-related factors.[15] Young teens have semen quality very similar to that of cancer patients in their late teens and 20s.[16]

Tests for DNA damage in sperm measure strand breakage or the condensation of genetic material in the nucleus. The sperm of men recently diagnosed with cancer show more DNA damage than the sperm of healthy men.[17,18] Such abnormalities are associated with poor fertilization rates in natural and assisted conception.[19]

Male Fertility After Cancer Treatment

A number of cancer treatments damage male fertility, either temporarily or permanently. Surgery for pelvic or genital cancers, for example bilateral orchiectomy for testicular cancer or advanced prostate cancer, may remove a critical part of the reproductive organ system. Although we think of men with prostate cancer as beyond reproductive age, their average age of diagnosis has decreased in countries using prostate-specific antigen screening, and some are still interested in having children.[20] Radical surgery for prostate or bladder cancer removes the prostate and seminal vesicles, eliminating semen. When retroperitoneal lymphadenectomy is performed to diagnose the extent of testicular cancer, nerve-sparing techniques can usually prevent retrograde ejaculation, which is an obvious barrier to fertility. However, when similar surgery is performed to remove residual disease after chemotherapy, the nerves are often damaged, resulting in orgasms without semen.[21] Surgery for colorectal cancer may cause similar impairment.[22]

Chemotherapy drugs and radiation therapy aimed close to the testes can impair male fertility.[23,24] Alkylating chemotherapy drugs, including the platinum-based ones,[21] are the most destructive to spermatogenesis. The higher the dose, the greater the chance that all the spermatogonia (stem cells that produce maturing sperm cells) are destroyed, leaving men permanently azoospermic (without sperm cells in the semen). Although some regimens have been designed to spare fertility, such as adriamycin, bleomycin, vinblastine, and dacarbazine for Hodgkin disease, recurrent or advanced disease may necessitate treatment with a more toxic regimen.[25]

The higher the dose of radiation the testes receive, the greater the damage to spermatogenesis. Men who have total body irradiation before bone marrow transplant commonly experience permanent azoospermia.[24] Testicular radiation in prepubertal boys with leukemia is also quite destructive to fertility.[26] Recently, however, good recovery of spermatogenesis has been reported in men treated with brachytherapy for prostate cancer.[27,28]

Cancer survivors as a group tend to have decreased sperm counts and motility after chemotherapy or pelvic radiotherapy.[24,29] The degree of damage to sperm counts and motility before cancer does not accurately predict recovery of fertility after cancer treatment, however. Men with testicular cancer have the lowest sperm concentrations (count per mL of semen) pretreatment, but are most likely to have some sperm cells in their semen after treatment.[29] However, those men with the lowest sperm counts after treatment did have the longest times to recovery. Ultimately, in a recent study of 42 men who were azoospermic at cancer diagnosis and were followed for a median of 9 years, 12 of 17 who wanted to father a child achieved that goal.[30]

Sperm DNA damage also worsens after cancer treatment,[18,19] although DNA repair also occurs. Most defects are found in sperm exposed directly to cancer treatment, with diminishing abnormalities over the next 2 years.[31] Thus, sperm banking is not recommended once a man has been exposed to chemotherapy or pelvic radiotherapy. Most oncologists suggest waiting 6 to 12 months after cancer treatment to try to conceive.[19] When 33 long-term survivors of childhood cancer were compared to 66 healthy controls, no excess DNA abnormalities were found in their sperm.[26] However, 30% of the cancer survivors were azoospermic, and only 33% had normal semen quality.

The Underutilization of Sperm Banking

Sperm banking has been available to men before cancer treatment for many years but became much more practical with the success in the early 1990s of in vitro fertilization with intracytoplasmic sperm injection, because only a few live sperm needed to survive freezing and thawing to be used in assisted reproductive treatments.[32,33] Cancer treatment does not need to be delayed, because adequate semen samples can be collected daily. Even 1 stored ejaculate can often provide a man with the future chance of having biological offspring. Adolescents as young as 12 often have the physical capacity and emotional maturity to provide semen samples and should be informed routinely of this option.[34] Yet, a survey of over 200 male patients seen in major cancer centers revealed that only half recalled being told about sperm banking. The most common reason for not banking sperm (other than having already completed all family building at the time of cancer diagnosis) was not having been informed in time; 25% of men who did not bank sperm gave this reason.[33] A companion survey of oncology faculty and fellows revealed that despite almost universal agreement that sperm banking should be mentioned to all cancer patients whose treatment might impair fertility, 48% either never mentioned it or informed less than 10% of their eligible patients.[35]

The major barriers to referring men for sperm banking, cited by half of physician respondents, included lack of time to discuss the topic in a busy clinic, the belief that most patients could not afford to bank sperm (a problem cited only by 7% of men who did not bank sperm),[33] and not knowing where to find a convenient sperm bank. Hematologist/ oncologists were also less likely to discuss sperm banking with men who needed rapid cancer treatment or had a poor prognosis, which includes most patients with acute leukemia or high-grade lymphoma. As with many other aspects of cancer care, men who had a referral from a physician were significantly more likely to bank sperm than those who found out about it on their own.[33] Clearly, educational materials are needed to facilitate communication between healthcare providers and patients on this important topic.

ᴄᴡ Case Example 8.1

Bill, a 15-year-old high school student, was diagnosed with acute leukemia. He was referred to begin chemotherapy as quickly as possible. Bill and his mother were told by his oncologist that he might have infertility in the future and could bank sperm. Bill's mother thought this was an excellent idea, and because both parents were dentists, the family could afford the out-of-pocket costs. Bill, however, was reluctant to go to the sperm bank. He had never discussed masturbation with either of his parents and was a shy teen who had not yet had a dating relationship. He had been running a high fever, and sex was the last thing on his mind.

The oncologist told Bill he had only 1 day to produce a semen sample, which could mean the difference in the future between the option of having a biological child and having to choose between donor insemination or adoption. Bill's mother drove him to the sperm bank and sat in the waiting room while a grim-faced nurse showed Bill into an exam room. She gave him a sterile cup to collect his semen along with a small pile of dog-eared men's magazines. After 20 minutes of trying, Bill found he was unable to even maintain an erection, much less ejaculate. He left the sperm bank in tears to return to the hospital.

CANCER-RELATED INFERTILITY IN WOMEN

A recent evidence-based review of the link between infertility and cancer risk concluded that borderline ovarian tumors are slightly more common in women diagnosed with infertility.[36] It is less clear whether infertile women are at increased risk for invasive ovarian cancer, but rates may be elevated in those who never achieve a pregnancy or among women with endometriosis. In contrast, infertility does not appear to be a risk factor for breast cancer.[36] Most cohort and case-control studies have not demonstrated a link between using ovarian-stimulating drugs to treat female infertility and subsequent cancer risk for any site.[37]

Female Fertility After Cancer Treatment

Surgical treatment for pelvic cancer may remove a critical part of the reproductive organ system, as seen in bilateral oophorectomy as part of treatment for gynecological malignancies or as prevention for breast or ovarian cancer in women with BRCA mutations.[38] Radiation therapy to the pelvis damages fertility because developing gametes and ovarian follicles, like cancer cells, are more likely to be in the genetically vulnerable, proliferative state.[39] Patients treated for cervical cancer, or those who have total body irradiation as preparation for bone marrow transplant, are the most common groups to experience radiation-associated infertility.

Chemotherapy drugs also interfere with gametogenesis because maturing oocytes are vulnerable to the toxins that damage rapidly growing cancer cells.[40,41] Alkylating drugs (including the platinum-based chemotherapies) are most likely to damage fertility. The likelihood of permanent ovarian failure in women increases with cumulative dose and age, and is manifested as decreased numbers of follicles, atretic follicles, and fibrotic changes in the ovary.[42] Unfortunately, most research has depended on resumption of menses as a rough marker of fertility. We still lack a more precise predictor of ovarian reserve, but promising results are now available with combined ultrasound measurements and the chemical marker anti-müllerian hormone (AMH).[43] A mathematical function predicting ovarian reserve using age at cancer treatment, radiation dose, and fractionating schedule, however, has also shown some utility.[44]

Options to Preserve Female Fertility

Fertility options for women are still quite experimental, except for the option of freezing fertilized embryos before cancer treatment.[23] Women who do not require urgent treatment may undergo a cycle of in vitro fertilization before cancer treatment and cryopreserve embryos, but the chance of a pregnancy with future use is still limited, and patients without a male partner have to use donor sperm to take advantage of this option.[45] Women with breast cancer can utilize new protocols that may limit exposure of cancer cells to high estrogen levels by using aromatase inhibitors or tamoxifen to the ovarian-stimulating drugs.[46] Cryopreservation of mature, unfertilized oocytes is another experimental choice, but only about 200 children have been born worldwide from this technique, and concerns remain about the genetic integrity of the spindle and the optimal freezing technique.[45,47,48] Centers around the world have begun harvesting ovarian tissue for cryopreservation in the hopes that autotransplantation or even xenotransplantation of the tissue will result in the development of healthy, mature oocytes.[45,47,48] For some malignancies, cancer cells could theoretically be harbored in the ovarian tissue. One published birth from autotransplanted, cryopreserved ovarian tissue has been questioned because the patient had signs of recovered activity in her remaining ovary on the other side.[49] Further attempts at autotransplantation are ongoing, however, and cryopreservation of the entire ovary, rather than just of cortical tissue strips, has been suggested recently as an alternative.[48,50]

Another controversial area is whether the ovary can be protected during cancer treatment by using GnRH-agonists to create a temporary menopause.[45,47,48] Some promising results have been published, but methodological limitations of the studies and uncertainty about the mechanism of the protective effect remain. In the future, chemoprotection may utilize small molecule compounds that inhibit ovarian apoptosis.

Women with very early stage or low-grade gynecologic cancer may be able to preserve fertility by having limited surgery, such as conservation of the uterus and contralateral ovary for women with ovarian cancer or radical trachelectomy (preservation of the uterus despite removal of most of the cervix) for cervical cancer.[47,48] Lateral transposition of

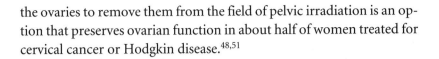

the ovaries to remove them from the field of pelvic irradiation is an option that preserves ovarian function in about half of women treated for cervical cancer or Hodgkin disease.[48,51]

Informing Women About Fertility Preservation

Given this array of experimental options, most of which are not covered in the United States by insurance, it is no surprise women are often poorly informed about fertility preservation. Two recent studies of young women treated for breast cancer found a great deal of distress about infertility and dissatisfaction with communication with hematologist/oncologists on this issue.[52,53] In a survey of affluent, well-educated women belonging to an advocacy organization for premenopausal women with breast cancer, 72% had discussed fertility with their hematologist/oncologist, but often the topic was brought up by the patient. Only 51% felt their concerns had been adequately addressed.[53] In a more diverse sample of 166 young breast cancer patients, only 34% recalled discussing fertility with their oncology team.[52]

NEED FOR PRACTICE GUIDELINES FOR MEN AND WOMEN

Table 8.1 lists the types of services that could be helpful to cancer patients facing impaired fertility. Not only is better communication about fertility preservation strongly needed between patients and hematologist/oncologists, but organizations need to develop practice guidelines on when it is appropriate to bring up infertility, how to discuss new modalities that remain experimental and often involve large out-of-pocket costs to the patient, and what options should be offered by cancer centers. The ethics committee of the American Society for Reproductive Medicine published guidelines on cancer and fertility in 2005.[2] A technical panel of the American Society of Clinical Oncology published practice guidelines on fertility preservation in 2006.[3] The organization Fertile Hope has developed high-quality patient education materials that are easily accessible on its Web site and also offers financial help to patients unable to afford fertility preservation or treatment procedures (www.fertilehope.org).

TABLE 8.1 ⚬ Diagnostic and Treatment Options Relevant to Fertility and Cancer

Option	Place in the Timeline of Cancer Treatment		
	Diagnosis to Treatment Disposition	During Active Cancer Treatment	After Active Cancer Treatment
Counseling on choosing cancer treatment that may conserve fertility	X		
Counseling on deciding whether to cryopreserve gametes or embryos	X		
Individual counseling for infertility-related distress	X	X	X
Couple counseling for infertility-related distress	X	X	X
Peer counseling for infertility-related distress	X	X	X
Group counseling for infertility-related distress		X	X

(continues)

TABLE 8.1   Diagnostic and Treatment Options Relevant to Fertility and Cancer (*continued*)

Option	Place in the Timeline of Cancer Treatment		
	Diagnosis to Treatment Disposition	During Active Cancer Treatment	After Active Cancer Treatment
Evaluation of ovarian reserve (ovarian ultrasound, hormones, AMH menstrual history, etc.)	X		X
Evaluation of male fertility (semen analysis, physical examination, etc.)	X		X
Screening for genetic factors that could affect health of future offspring, and referral for genetic counseling as appropriate	X	X	X
Sperm-banking	X		
Banking of spermatogonia or testicular tissue	X		
Exploration of testes for sperm in azoospermic men	X		X

(continues)

TABLE 8.1 ᖶ   Diagnostic and Treatment Options Relevant to Fertility and Cancer (*continued*)

Option	Place in the Timeline of Cancer Treatment		
	Diagnosis to Treatment Disposition	During Active Cancer Treatment	After Active Cancer Treatment
Referral for pre-treatment in vitro fertilization and embryo or oocyte freezing	X		
Cryopreservation of ovarian tissue	X		
Counseling on experimental protocols of chemoprotection of the gonads during cancer treatment	X		
Referral for screening by high-risk obstetrician prior to attempts to conceive (ultrasound of uterus, cardiac & lung function testing, etc.)			X
Counseling on adoption or third-party reproduction	X		X

COUNSELING ABOUT NONBIOLOGICAL PARENTHOOD AFTER CANCER

Another set of issues relates to options for becoming a parent when fertility persists after cancer treatment. Use of third-party reproductive options (e.g., donated sperm or oocytes, or gestational carrier) and barriers to adoption for cancer survivors are areas very much in need of research, although third-party options and adoption are already in practice clinically.[54] Research on pregnancy complications in cancer survivors and health of offspring is also increasing.[55] Mental health practitioners with expertise in infertility counseling can help individuals or couples explore the emotional and practical complications in adoption and third-party reproduction. This type of counseling is very helpful in ensuring that both partners are in agreement about their choice and are prepared for such issues as when or how much to inform their potential child about his or her history of nontraditional conception, concerns about a gamete donor who has a genetic link to the child, how to deal with questions or disapproval from their extended family, or whether to consider not having children.

Most importantly, reproductive health after cancer is only increasing in importance as the number of cancer survivors multiplies and the length of their survival also improves. Sexual function and fertility can no longer be regarded by hematologist/oncologists as frivolous or irrelevant issues, because our current cancer therapies damage reproductive health in ways that are profound and often permanent. Interventions that prevent or reverse these problems will greatly improve the quality of life of our patients.

REFERENCES

1. Reuben SH. Living beyond cancer: finding a new balance: President's Cancer Panel 2003–2004 Annual Report. National Cancer Institute Web site: http://deainfo.nci.nih.gov/advisory/pcp/pcp03-04rpt/Survivorship.pdf. Published May 2004. Accessed November 14, 2008.
2. The Ethics Committee of the American Society for Reproductive Medicine. Fertility preservation and reproduction in cancer patients. *Fertil Steril.* 2005;83:1622–1628.

3. Lee SJ, Schover LR, Partridge AH, et al. American Society of Clinical Oncology recommendations on fertility preservation in cancer patients. *J Clin Oncol.* 2006;24:2917–2931.

4. Lucas JW, Schiller JS, Benson V. Summary health statistics for United States adults: National Health Interview Survey, 2001. *Vital Health Stat.* 2004;10(218).

5. United States Census Bureau. *US Summary 2000: Census 2000 Profile.* Washington, DC: US Census Bureau; 2002:Government publication C2KPROF00US.

6. MacDorman MF, Minino AM, Strobino DM, et al. Annual summary of vital statistics—2001. *Pediatrics.* 2002;110:1037–1052.

7. Bachu A, O'Connell M. *Fertility of American Women: June 2000.* Washington, DC: US Census Bureau; 2001:Current Population Reports, P20-543RV.

8. World Marriage Patterns 2000 (Wall Chart). United Nations Population Division of the Department of Economic and Social Affairs. United Nations Web Site: http://www.un.org/esa/population/publications/world marriage/worldmarriage.htm. Accessed November 14, 2008.

9. Garner MJ, Turner MC, Ghadirian P, et al. Epidemiology of testicular cancer: an overview. *Int J Cancer.* 2005;116:331–339.

10. Hoei-Hansen CE, Holm M, Rajpert-De Meyts E, et al. Histological evidence of testicular dysgenesis in contralateral biopsies from 218 patients with testicular germ cell cancer. *J Pathol.* 2003;200:370–374.

11. Fossa SD, Chen J, Schonfeld SJ, et al. Risk of contralateral testicular cancer: a population-based study of 29,515 U.S. men. *J Natl Cancer Inst.* 2005; 97:1056–1066.

12. Jacobsen R, Bostofte E, Engholm G, Hansen, et al. Fertility and offspring sex ratio of men who develop testicular cancer: a record linkage study. *Hum Reprod.* 2000;15:1958–1961.

13. Raman JD, Nobert CF, Goldstein M. Increased incidence of testicular cancer in men presenting with infertility and abnormal semen analysis. *J Urol.* 2005;174:1819–1822.

14. Pearce MS, Parker L, Windebank KP, et al. Cancer in adolescents and young adults aged 15–24 years: a report from the North of England young person's malignant disease registry, UK. *Pediatr Blood Cancer.* 2005;45: 687–693.

15. Chung K, Irani J, Knee G, et al. Sperm cryopreservation for male patients with cancer: an epidemiological analysis at the University of Pennsylvania. *Eur J Obstet Gynecol Reprod Biol.* 2004;113(suppl 1):S7–S11.

16. Wallace WHB, Anderson RA, Irvine DS. Fertility preservation for young patients with cancer: who is at risk and what can be offered? *Lancet Oncol.* 2005;6:209–218.

17. Kobayashi H, Larson K, Sharma RK, et al. DNA damage in patients with untreated cancer as measured by the sperm chromatin structure assay. *Fertil Steril.* 2001;75:469–475.

18. O'Donovan M. An evaluation of chromatin condensation and DNA integrity in the spermatozoa of men with cancer before and after therapy. *Andrologia.* 2005;3:83–90.

19. Morris ID. Sperm DNA damage and cancer treatment. *Int J Androl.* 2002;25:255–261.

20. Varenhorst E, Garmo H, Holmberg L, et al. The National Prostate Cancer Register in Sweden 1998–2002: trends in incidence, treatment and survival. *Scand J Urol Nephrol.* 2005;39:117–123.

21. Saxman S. Doctor . . . will I still be able to have children? *J Natl Cancer Instit.* 2005;97:1557–1559.

22. Havenga K, Maas CP, DeRuiter MC, et al. Avoiding long-term disturbance to bladder and sexual function in pelvic surgery, particularly with rectal cancer. *Semin Surg Oncol.* 2000;18:235–243.

23. Agarwal A, Allamaneni SS. Disruption of spermatogenesis by the cancer disease process. *J Natl Cancer Inst Monogr.* 2005;34:9–12.

24. Howell SJ, Shalet SM. Spermatogenesis after cancer treatment: damage and recovery. *J Natl Cancer Inst Monogr.* 2005;34:12–17.

25. Grigg A. The impact of conventional and high-dose therapy for lymphoma on fertility. *Clin Lymphoma.* 2004;5:84–88.

26. Thomson AB, Campbell AJ, Irvine DS, et al. Semen quality and spermatozoal DNA integrity in survivors of childhood cancer: a case-control study. *Lancet.* 2002;360:361–367.

27. Grocela J, Mauceri T, Zietman A. New life after prostate brachytherapy? Considering the fertile female partner of the brachytherapy patient. *BJU Int.* 2005;96:781–782.

28. Mydlo JH, Lebed B. Does brachytherapy of the prostate affect sperm quality and/or fertility in younger men? *Scand J Urol Nephrol.* 2004;38: 221–224.

29. Bahadur G, Ozturk O, Muneer A, et al. Semen quality before and after gonadotoxic treatment. *Hum Reprod.* 2005;20:774–781.

30. Ragni G, Arnoldi M, Somigliana E, et al. Reproductive prognosis in male patients with azoospermia at the time of cancer diagnosis. *Fertil Steril.* 2005;83:1674–1679.

31. Wyrobek AJ, Schmid TE, Marchetti F. Relative susceptibilities of male germ cells to genetic defects induced by cancer chemotherapies. *J Natl Cancer Inst Monogr.* 2005;34:31–35.
32. Ragni G, Somigliana E, Restelli L, et al. Sperm banking and rate of assisted reproduction treatment: insights from a 15-year cryopreservation program for male cancer patients. *Cancer.* 2003;97:1624–1629.
33. Schover LR, Brey K, Lichtin A, et al. Knowledge and experience regarding cancer, infertility, and sperm banking in younger male survivors. *J Clin Oncol.* 2002;20:1880–1889.
34. Bahadur G, Ling KL, Hart R, et al. Semen quality and cryopreservation in adolescent cancer patients. *Hum Reprod.* 2002;17:3157–3161.
35. Schover LR, Brey K, Lichtin A, et al. Oncologists' attitudes and practices regarding banking sperm before cancer treatment. *J Clin Oncol.* 2002;20: 1890–1897.
36. Venn A, Healy D, McLachlan R. Cancer risks associated with the diagnosis of infertility. *Best Pract Res Clin Obstet Gynecol.* 2003;17:343–367.
37. Doyle P, Maconochie N, Beral V, et al. Cancer incidence following treatment for infertility at a clinic in the UK. *Hum Reprod.* 2002;17:2209–2213.
38. Kauff ND, Satagopan JM, Robson ME, et al. Risk-reducing salpingo-oophorectomy in women with a BRCA1 or BRCA2 mutation. *N Engl J Med.* 2002;346:1609–1615.
39. Meirow D, Nugent D. The effects of radiotherapy and chemotherapy on female reproduction. *Hum Reprod Update.* 2001;7:535–543.
40. Tilly JL, Kolesnick RN. Sphingolipids, apoptosis, cancer treatments and the ovary: investigating a crime against female fertility. *Biochim Biophys Acta.* 2002;1585:135–138.
41. Blumenfeld Z. Preservation of fertility and ovarian function and minimalization of chemotherapy associated gonadotoxicity and premature ovarian failure: the role of inhibin-A and -B as markers. *Mol Cell Endocrinol.* 2002;187:93–105.
42. Minton SE, Munster PN. Chemotherapy-induced amenorrhea and fertility in women undergoing adjuvant treatment for breast cancer. *Cancer Control.* 2002;9:466–472.
43. Lutchman Singh K, Muttukrishna S, Stein RC, et al. (2007) Predictors of ovarian reserve in young women with breast cancer *BR J Cancer.* 2007;96:1808–1816.
44. Wallace WHB, Thomson AB, Kelsey TW. The radiosensitivity of the human oocyte. *Hum Reprod.* 2003;18:1171–1121.
45. Roberts JE, Oktay K. Fertility preservation: a comprehensive approach to the young woman with cancer. *J Natl Cancer Inst Monogr.* 2005;34:57–59.

46. Sönmezer M, Oktay, K. Assisted reproduction and fertility preservation techniques in cancer patients. *Curr Opin Endocrinal Diabetes Obes.* 2008;15:514–522.

47. Seli E, Tangir J. Fertility preservation options for female patients with malignancies. *Curr Opin Obstet Gynecol.* 2005;17:299–308.

48. Kim SS. Fertility preservation in female cancer patients: current developments and future directions. *Fertil Steril.* 2006;85:1–11.

49. Oktay K, Tilly J. Live birth after cryopreserved ovarian tissue autotransplantation. *Lancet.* 2004;364(9451):2091–2093.

50. Imhof M, Hofstetter G, Bergmeister H, et al. Cryopreservation of a whole ovary as a strategy for restoring ovarian function. *J Assist Reprod Genet.* 2004;21:459–465.

51. Duffy CM, Allen SM, Clark MA. Discussions regarding reproductive health for young women with breast cancer undergoing chemotherapy. *J Clin Oncol.* 2005;23:766–773.

52. Gershenson D. Fertility-sparing surgery for malignancies in women. *J Natl Cancer Inst Monogr.* 2005;34:43–47.

53. Partridge AH, Gelber S, Peppercorn J, et al. Web-based survey of fertility issues in young women with breast cancer. *J Clin Oncol.* 2004;22:4174–4183.

54. Rosen A. Third-party reproduction and adoption in cancer patients. *J Natl Cancer Inst Monogr.* 2005;34:91–93.

55. Nagarajan R, Robison LL. Pregnancy outcomes in survivors of childhood cancer. *J Natl Cancer Inst Monogr.* 2005;34:72–76.

Treatment Choices and Quality of Life Among Prostate Cancer Patients

Michael A. Diefenbach, PhD

&

Gina A. Turner, PhD

ABSTRACT

Quality of life (QOL) refers to the extent to which one's usual or expected physical, social, and emotional well-being are affected by a medical condition or its treatment. Prostate cancer is a significant health problem that affects 33% of men in the United States. This disease has a major impact on both disease-specific QOL (such as urinary, sexual, and bowel functioning) and general QOL (such as fatigue, physical limitations, social and emotional functioning, and pain). Clinicians and patients may perceive what exactly QOL entails in different ways; how much time a treatment can add to a patient's life, versus how much patients' lives are impacted by the disease and its treatment in those added years. Yet the most common treatments also produce many side effects that have the potential to significantly impact QOL. In this chapter, we will discuss treatment options, their possible side effects and impact on quality of life; and the process of decision making about treatment.

INTRODUCTION

Quality of life (QOL) refers to the extent to which one's usual or expected physical, social, and emotional well-being are affected by a medical condition or its treatment.[1] The quality of one's life may be considered in a number of domains, such as physical ability or disability, social and family connections, and emotional state of mind. Quality of life has particular meaning when discussing the impact of a disease such as prostate cancer on specific health areas such as urinary, sexual, or bowel functioning.

Quality of life is an important construct both for clinicians and for patients; however, clinicians and patients may perceive what exactly QOL entails in different ways. For clinicians, the major concern may be how much time a treatment can add to a patient's life, without much consideration of the quality of the time spent. On the other hand, the most important factor for patients may be how much their life is impacted by the disease and its treatment in those added years. Research has shown that QOL is of great concern to patients and that it influences their treatment selections.[2]

Prostate cancer is a significant health problem that affects 33% of men in the United States.[3] This disease has a major impact on both disease-specific QOL (such as urinary, sexual, and bowel functioning) and general QOL (such as fatigue, physical limitations, social and emotional functioning, and pain).[4] For example, urinary and sexual problems were more prevalent in men treated for prostate cancer than in men the same age without the disease.

Men who have been diagnosed with localized prostate cancer will generally live many years following treatment. Yet the most common treatments also produce many side effects that have the potential to significantly impact QOL.[2] Thus QOL is a significant issue for most prostate cancer patients when deciding on treatment. It is important for patients (and their doctors) to understand how the different treatment options may impact their QOL, during, immediately after, and long after treatment. Before we discuss the results from various studies examining QOL further, we will introduce the most common treatment options.

TREATMENT MODALITIES

There are several treatment options available for prostate cancer patients. Patients may be directed toward a particular treatment option by their physician, or may be inclined toward a particular option for personal reasons (see Table 9.1). Four treatment modalities are discussed below.

Radical Prostatectomy

Radical prostatectomy is considered the gold standard in prostate cancer treatment, and it is one of the most common procedures. A radical prostatectomy is a complex and demanding procedure usually requiring general anesthesia. This surgery takes 2 to 4 hours, during which time the prostate and surrounding tissues are removed. If possible, the doctor will perform a "nerve-sparing technique" to avoid cutting or

TABLE 9.1 In Their Own Words: Treatment Choices

Surgery: "My doctor recommended surgery. Although, at first, I didn't like the idea of needing an operation, my wife and I thought it would be better to get the cancer out of my body."
External Beam Radiation: "I talked to my urologist and a radiation oncologist. My urologist thought I was a good candidate for surgery, but I was concerned about the higher rates of side effects some men have. My radiation oncologist told me that I had the same chances for a cure with radiation without those side effects."
Brachytherapy: "I chose the seeds because it was the most convenient option for my situation. I spent only 1 night in the hospital and was able to return to work within 2 days."
Watch and Wait: "My doctor told me that my prostate cancer is slow growing and that I can live many years without the cancer becoming a problem. I have to get checked every 6 months, but that's still better to me than having to deal with side effects from some of the treatments."

stretching the two bundles of nerves and blood vessels that are close to the prostate. This procedure can be done if the cancer is not too close to or has not spread to the nerves, which are needed for an erection.

Many patients choose prostatectomy because the surgeon physically removes the cancer from the body. For many patients, this can be a reassuring thought. Surgery also does not require a long-term commitment to a treatment schedule like radiation therapy does and thus is considered by some patients to be more convenient.

Laparoscopic and robotic surgeries are the newest type of surgical tools and procedures used in prostatectomies. In a laparoscopic prostatectomy, all or part of the prostate is removed with the aid of a laparoscope, which is a thin, tubelike instrument with a light and a lens that allows the surgeon to see a highly magnified image of the prostate. The surgeon makes a small incision near the navel through which the laparoscope is inserted, and several other small incisions are made in the abdomen through which the surgeon can insert additional surgical instruments to remove the prostate. If a robotic system is used to control the instruments, the surgery is called robotic radical prostatectomy. These surgeries would be performed under the guidance of a highly trained surgeon.

External Beam Radiation Therapy

External beam radiation therapy can go by several alternative names: radiation therapy, radiotherapy, x-ray therapy, or irradiation. This therapy is a localized treatment that uses high-energy rays to kill cancer cells and generally involves treatments 5 days a week over the course of 6 to 7 weeks. As opposed to surgery, external radiation therapy is painless, and patients do not hear, see, or smell the radiation. Radiation therapy takes about 30 minutes per appointment, depending on the treatment, but only 1 to 5 minutes are devoted to administering the radiation. Shields are used during the procedure to help protect normal tissues and organs.

External beam radiation therapy has a survival rate similar to that of radical prostatectomy. There are several benefits to this choice when compared to surgery. The chances of impotence and incontinence are lower for radiation than for surgery. Radiation treatment is an outpatient procedure and does not require overnight stays in the hospital; nor does it require anesthesia or blood transfusions, and it avoids the risk of surgical complications. For some patients, there may be some treatment-related fatigue, but most are able to work and remain active during the weeks of treatment.

Brachytherapy

Brachytherapy, or seed implantation, is a form of radiation in which small radioactive pellets made of palladium or iodine ("seeds") are placed directly into the prostate to kill the malignant tumor from the inside out. The implantation is generally performed as an outpatient procedure, and the use of local, rather than general anesthesia leads to a quicker recovery.

Some doctors choose to implant more powerful, temporary radioactive seeds. These seeds are placed into the prostate for a period of several days and are then removed. Such temporary implants require a short stay in the hospital. Otherwise, if permanent seeds are used, the patient usually goes home the same day.

Seeding has a survival rate comparable to other treatment methods, such as other forms of radiation therapy or surgery. There are several benefits to this treatment method. Permanent seeding simply requires a single outpatient treatment procedure. Patients can usually return to normal activities within 2 to 3 days following implantation or release from the hospital, and there is minimal pain or discomfort during and after the procedure.

Watchful Waiting

Doctors may suggest watchful waiting for early stage prostate cancer, older patients, and those who have other serious health problems. Men in their 70s and 80s also may not be as willing to undergo surgery or radiation therapy as younger men. Those who choose watchful waiting will still have regular exams, including regular prostate-specific antigen (PSA) tests and DREs (digital rectal exams). Further decision making may be based on the symptoms getting worse, increases in PSA level, or the potential of new treatments with fewer side effects.

TREATMENT MODALITIES AND QUALITY OF LIFE ISSUES

Patients often wonder "are there different side effects (or patterns of side effects) associated with different treatment modalities?" Studies that examine side effects among prostate cancer patients show that there are.[4]

Radical Prostatectomy

Urinary and sexual problems are worse in men treated with prostatectomy, compared to those who opted for radiation treatment (external beam radiation or brachytherapy).[5–7] Significant urinary symptoms may last up to 34 months after treatment among prostatectomy patients,[8] and in some men, these symptoms may persist after prostatectomy for as long as 5 years. In a study involving 1,288 men with localized prostate cancer, 14% still experienced frequent urinary leakage or no urinary control, and only 28% could achieve erections sufficient for intercourse.[9] When the "nerve-sparing technique" is performed, the likelihood of erectile dysfunction is decreased; however, erectile dysfunction may still occur, which can be temporary or permanent. Many older men may become permanently impotent.

Compared with other types of prostatectomy, the laparoscopic and robotic surgeries may result in fewer side effects. A patient can expect shorter hospital stays, a faster recovery period, and less blood loss and pain. He can also expect a greater possibility of preserving sexual and urinary function. There should be less impact on these functions because the surgeon has a larger, more detailed view of the surgical area; in addition, robotic tools allow for more control. This additional surgical precision can provide an increased likelihood that nerves will be spared. One thing for a patient to keep in mind, however, is that because these methods of surgery are newer, researchers have not had the chance to follow their effectiveness for as long as they have for standard surgery.

Some other, more general QOL issues experienced by men who choose the prostatectomy include the need for a catheter, which drains urine for 10 days to 3 weeks after surgery. It is also common for the patient to feel tired or weak for a few weeks after the operation. In addition, with surgery, there is the small risk for patients to experience complications, such as bleeding (requiring a blood transfusion), blood clots, heart attack, or infection. Lastly, men do not produce semen after a radical prostatectomy; therefore, they have dry orgasms, which may influence their sexual enjoyment.

External Beam Radiation Therapy

Bowel problems are more prevalent in men treated with external beam radiation than in men treated with prostatectomy.[10] Also, a large group of men (n = 709) were contacted approximately 6 years following external beam radiation therapy; those with treatment reported higher rates of incontinence and more issues with sexual QOL than participants in a control group.[11]

For those who choose this treatment modality, many factors can influence their chances of experiencing erectile dysfunction. One important factor is the size and location of the tumor. The larger the tumor, or the closer it is located to the nerves that control erections, the greater the chances of dysfunction after treatment. The greater a person's ability to have and sustain an erection before treatment, the more likely he is to retain this ability. However, because radiation can damage nerves that control erections and arteries that carry blood to the penis, about 40% to 60% of men treated will develop some degree of erectile dysfunction. These effects may develop over 1 to 2 years after treatment has been completed; side effects are often not immediate.

There are other QOL issues with external beam radiation therapy. Patients are often tired during treatment. Also, the skin in the treated area may become irritated, and temporary or permanent hair loss in the treated area may occur, depending on the dosage of radiation. Cystitis, an inflammation of the bladder, is occasionally diagnosed, as is proctitis, an inflammation of the rectum.

Brachytherapy

Side effects of brachytherapy may include fatigue as well as bowel and bladder problems, such as urgency (e.g., a sudden need to go to the bathroom), more frequent urination during the day and nights, and burning sensations while urinating. Patients also may notice blood in their urine for about 1 week after the implantation. These side effects usually lessen with time, and do not occur frequently.

Erectile dysfunction is less likely to occur with radiation seeding than with external beam radiation. After brachytherapy, erectile dysfunction occurs in a small percentage of men under age 70 and is slightly more common in men over age 70. One study measured erectile function and continence at three points.[12] Of 98 patients receiving brachytherapy, 73% were capable of erections, and 93% were continent at baseline. At 6 months following treatment, 56% were capable of erections, and 86% were continent. Finally, at 1 year after treatment, 59% were capable of erections, and 99% were continent. If a man has satisfactory erections prior to the procedure, chances are high he will not experience difficulties after the procedure. However, erectile problems before the procedure are predictive of problems after the procedure.

One additional issue with brachytherapy is that implant patients emit low-energy radiation and therefore need to avoid close and prolonged contact with children less than 2 years of age and pregnant women for 2 to 4 weeks following treatment.

Watchful Waiting

Some of the benefits of watchful waiting are that there are no side effects such as bladder and bowel control or impotence with this treatment. It is not likely to affect a patient's sex life, and a patient can decide to begin treatment at any time. Many men who choose watchful waiting live for years with no signs of disease. A number of studies have found that for 5, 10, or even 15 years, the life expectancy of men treated with watchful waiting (mostly older men with early stage prostate cancer) is not that different from the life expectancy of men treated with surgery or radiation.[13]

On the other hand, during the watchful waiting period, the cancer may grow faster than expected and could grow outside of the prostate. If the cancer spreads outside the prostate, the patient will no longer be able to have surgery to take out the cancer. Also, it may get harder for the patient to cope with surgery and radiation therapy as he gets older. He will need more tests and procedures. A PSA blood test and DRE are usually required every 6 months along with a yearly biopsy of the prostate.

Some specific QOL decreases can occur during watchful waiting. In a study, 310 men with localized prostate cancer reported significant decreases in seven out of eight general QOL domains (and four out of six domains controlling for age), and the declines in sexual domains were steeper than would be expected with aging.[14]

Taken together, studies looking at different treatment modalities for prostate cancer have indicated that prostate cancer and its treatment significantly affect patients' urinary, sexual, and bowel functions, and the risk for urinary and sexual problems is significant regardless of modality. However, despite these effects on disease-specific domains, cross-sectional studies showed few significant effects of prostate cancer and its treatment on patients' general QOL.[4,15]

DECISION-MAKING PROCESSES FOR PATIENTS DIAGNOSED WITH EARLY STAGE PROSTATE CANCER

A cancer diagnosis, treatment, and accompanying symptoms are highly distressing and have the potential to disrupt a patient's life. Studies show that the increased experience of physical and psychological symptoms among patients suffering from prostate, colon, breast, and ovarian cancer was related to diminished QOL and elevated distress.[16] Sexual dysfunction in particular is associated with significant levels of distress in prostate cancer patients.[17]

Elevated levels of distress are important when making a decision and in adherence to treatment regimens in general. Both low and high levels of anxiety can interfere with the processing of threatening information. Low levels of anxiety can lead a person to ignore the threat,[18] while high levels of anxiety can lead to denial and avoidance.[19] We also know that knowledge is one of the most significant factors affecting men's postoperative adjustment.[20]

Patients diagnosed with early stage prostate cancer are not only coping with the emotional trauma of a cancer diagnosis, but they are also expected to digest complicated and often threatening information about treatment procedures. The most common treatment options (prostatectomy and radiation therapy) both carry the risk of significant side effects. In addition, physicians often do not agree with one another in treatment recommendations, suggesting treatments they are the most familiar with. Thus, a person's decision making will be increasingly influenced by his own beliefs and attitudes about disease and treatment.

Patient perceptions of prostate cancer treatment (e.g., perceived convenience of the treatment or perceived problems with urinary and sexual functioning) are important contributors in the decision-making process, especially because the pros and cons of each treatment modality have so much overlap and there is no one clear path to take. In situations like this, a "preference-sensitive decision" (as compared to an "effectiveness-based decision") is required, and the role of personal goals and values takes on increasing importance.[21] Preference-sensitive decisions largely depend on an individual's values, whereas effectiveness-based decisions depend on clear, evidence-based information that supports a particular course of action, such as the use of aspirin for patients at risk for a myocardial infarct.

DECISION MAKING AND REGRET

The elements that contribute to the difficulty of arriving at a decision can also contribute to the likelihood of regret about the decision. Regret has been defined in several ways:

▷ "Painful cognitive and emotional state of feeling sorry for losses, shortcomings, or mistakes"[22]
▷ "A psychological reaction to making the wrong decision"[23]
▷ Interplay of ruminative thoughts and negative feelings, distinct from negative affect, which involves comparison of the actual event with another one that "might have taken place"[24]

Negative thoughts and emotions, triggered by thinking about a past decision regarding a treatment choice, can be common among prostate cancer patients. Among 349 patients surveyed 12 to 48 months after treatment for localized prostate cancer, 16% reported regret of therapeutic choice.[25] In another study, these findings were replicated, and 16% of 96 patients previously treated for early stage prostate cancer expressed regret.[26]

It is important to note that regretful men were more likely to have worse general and disease-specific health-related QOL compared to men without regret. Similarly, levels of regret among prostate cancer patients with metastatic disease were even higher; 23% of these patients expressed regret, and higher levels of regret were significantly associated with surgical versus chemical castration, the occurrence of nausea, and lower level of QOL.[27]

Another study has indicated that higher levels of regret are related to increased difficulty making the initial treatment decision and with decreases in both satisfaction with treatment decisions and overall QOL.[28] Similarly, in another study,[29] we found that feelings of decisional regret increased significantly in the 6 to 12 months following diagnosis and treatment, especially in those treated with prostatectomy.

How Can We Improve Quality of Life and Reduce the Probability of Regret?

First-rate clinical care aims to help patients improve their decision-making process by fostering realistic expectations and beliefs. Doctors should work with patients to ensure that they are recommending treatments in line with patients' values and goals. This may require doctors to explore patients' illness beliefs and models. Also, it is important that doctors work to prepare patients for the emotional and social ramifications of treatment and its consequences; hopefully this preparation will help lead to lower levels of regret. Davison and colleagues determined that providing individualized information to 74 couples in which the men had been newly diagnosed with prostate cancer lowered the men's levels of psychological distress and helped them, and their partners, to become more active participants in their treatment decision making.[30]

Doctors should bear in mind that considering the way information is delivered (such as the timing and method of providing information, the complexity of medical information, and certainly patients' anxiety level) can help patients retain this information.[31-33] Moreover, doctors should remind patients of their responsibility for gathering as much information as possible, including asking for second and even third opinions, so that they feel comfortable with their own levels of knowledge.

In addition, patients should talk to family members, soliciting help both in the decision-making process and for emotional support during this difficult process. But talking alone will not guarantee that patients will not experience regret; therefore, patients may consider listing the pros and cons of various treatment options based on the information they have gathered. This technique may allow patients to more clearly compare and contrast the relevant issues. See Figure 9.1 for an example

My concerns about treatment	How I rate this treatment in terms of each concern: 1 = Not so good; 2 = About average; 3 = Good			
	Surgery	EBRT	Brachytherapy	Watchful Waiting
1.				
2.				
3.				
4.				
5.				
6.				
7.				
8.				

FIGURE 9.1   Decision Aid

of a grid patients could use to aid their decision making. In this decision aid grid, patients would list specific concerns, such as the likelihood of postoperative erectile dysfunction, and then rate treatment methods based on the chances of this concern happening. For example, in the case of possible erectile dysfunction following treatment, surgery would be rated the lowest and watchful waiting would be the highest. It is important to note that patients list their own concerns and expectations, and rate them according to their impression of how the different treatment options may address these concerns. Once completed, patients can take the grid to their physician for further discussion. An approach such as the one suggested here is currently being evaluated with a prostate cancer patient population.

Finally, clinicians should reassure their patients that they indeed have time to make their decisions. It goes without saying that consultations should be conducted in an open, trusting atmosphere and that clinicians should talk in plain language, avoiding excessive medical jargon. Given the important role of patients' knowledge, beliefs, and expectations in treatment selection, it is crucial that clinicians explore these beliefs and expectations up front. This exploration will not only help physicians to better understand their patients' subsequent decisions and behavior, but it will also enable them to address misconceptions and unrealistic beliefs. It is important that clinicians be sensitive when probing beliefs and expectations; some individuals may feel uncomfortable sharing their thoughts because they may fear that the physician will belittle or discount their beliefs. And perhaps most importantly, clinicians need to be aware of different emphases that they and their patients may have regarding QOL.

CONCLUSION

Patients newly diagnosed with prostate cancer face many difficult decisions that can have serious implications for their QOL. Clinicians can guide patients through this process by presenting necessary treatment-related information and by exploring patients' beliefs and values regarding their treatment and future QOL as prostate cancer survivors.

REFERENCES

1. Cella, D.F. 1995. Measuring quality of life in palliative care. *Seminars in Oncology*, *22*(2 Suppl 3), 73-81.
2. Diefenbach, MA, Dorsey J, Uzzo, RG, et al. Decision making strategies for patients with localized prostate cancer. *Semin Urol Oncol.* 2002;20(1): 55–62.
3. Cancer Facts & Figures 2007. American Cancer Society Web site. http://www.cancer.org/downloads/STT/CAFF2007PWSecured.pdf. Accessed November 15, 2008.
4. Eton DT, Lepore SJ. Prostate cancer and quality of life: a review of the literature. *Psycho-Oncol.* 2002;11:307–326.
5. Brandeis JM, Litwin MS, Burnison CM, Reiter RE. Quality of life outcomes after brachytherapy for early stage prostate cancer. *J Urol.* 2000;163:851–857.

6. Eton DT, Lepore SJ, Helgeson VS. Early quality of life in patients with localized prostate carcinoma. *Cancer.* 2001;92:1451–1459.

7. Yarbro CH, Ferrans CE. Quality of life of patients with prostate cancer treated with surgery or radiation therapy. *Oncol Nurs Forum.* 1998;25: 685–693.

8. Hollenbeck BK, Dunn RL, Wei JT, McLaughlin PW, Han M, Sanda MG. Neoadjuvant hormonal therapy and older age are associated with adverse sexual health-related quality-of-life outcome after prostate brachytherapy. *Urology.* 2002;59:480–484.

9. Penson DF, Feng Z, Kuniyuki A, et al. General quality of life 2 years following treatment for prostate cancer: what influences outcomes? Results from The Prostate Cancer Outcomes Study. *J Clin Oncol.* 2003;21: 1147–1154.

10. Shrader-Bogen CL, Kjellberg JL, McPherson CP, Murray CL. Quality of life and treatment outcomes: prostate carcinoma patients' perspectives after prostatectomy or radiation therapy. *Cancer.* 1997;79:1977–1986.

11. Miller DC, Sanda MG, Dunn RL, et al. Long-term outcomes among localized prostate cancer survivors: health-related quality-of-life changes after radical prostatectomy, external radiation, and brachytherapy. *J Clin Oncol.* 2005;23(14):2772–2780.

12. Feigenberg S, Lee W, Desilvio M, et al. Health-related quality of life in men receiving prostate brachytherapy on RTOG 98-05. *Int J Radiat Oncol Biol Phys.* 2005;62(4):956–964.

13. Holmberg L, Bill-Axelson A, Helgesen F, et al. A randomized trial comparing radical prostatectomy with watchful waiting in early prostate cancer. *N Engl J Med.* 2002;347:781–789.

14. Arredondo S, Downs T, Lubeck D, et al. Watchful waiting and health related quality of life for patients with localized prostate cancer: data from CaPSURE. *J Urol.* 2004;172(5):1830–1834.

15. Tefilli MV, Gheiler EL, Tiguert R, et al. Quality of life in patients undergoing salvage procedures for locally recurrent prostate cancer. *J Surg Oncol.* 1998;69:156–161.

16. Portenoy RK, Thaler HT, Kornblith AB, et al. Symptom prevalence, characteristics and distress in a cancer population. *Qual Life Res.* 1994;3(3): 183–189.

17. Helgason AR, Adolfsson J, Dickman P, Fredrikson M, Arver S, Steineck G. Waning sexual function—the most important disease-specific distress for patients with prostate cancer. *Br J Cancer.* 1996;73:1417–1421.

18. Leventhal H. Findings and theory in the study of fear communications. In: Berkowitz L, ed. *Advances in Experimental Social Psychology.* Vol 5. New York: Academic Press; 1970:120–186.

19. Miller SM, Roussi P, Altman D, Helm W, Steinberg A. Effects of coping style on psychological reactions of low-income, minority women to colposcopy. *J Reprod Med.* 1994;39:711–718.

20. Burt J, Caelli K, Moore K, Anderson M. Radical prostatectomy: men's experiences and postoperative needs. *J Clin Nurs.* 2005;14(7):883–890.

21. O'Connor AM, Legare F, Stacey D. Risk communication in practice: the contribution of decision aids. *Br Med J.* 2003;327(7417):736–740.

22. Landman J. *Regret: The Persistence of the Possible.* New York: Oxford University Press; 1993.

23. Bell DE. Disappointment in decision making under uncertainty. *Operat Res.* 1985;33:1–27.

24. Connolly T, Reb J. Regret in cancer-related decisions. *Health Psychol.* 2005;24:29–34.

25. Clark JA, Inui TS, Silliman RA, et al. Patients' perceptions of quality of life after treatment for early prostate cancer. *J Clin Oncol.* 2003;21:3777–3784.

26. Hu J, Kwan L, Saigal CS, Litwin MS. Regret in men treated for localized prostate cancer. *J Urol.* 2003;169:2279–2283.

27. Clark JA, Wray NP, Ashton CM. Living with treatment decisions: regrets and quality of life among men treated for metastatic prostate cancer. *J Clin Oncol.* 2001;19:72–80.

28. Brehaut JC, O'Connor AM, Wood TJ, et al. Validation of a decision regret scale. *Med Decis Making.* 2003;23(4):281–292.

29. Diefenbach MA, Mohamed NE. Regret of treatment decision and its association with disease-specific quality of life following prostate cancer treatment. *Cancer Invest.* 2007;25:449–457.

30. Davison BJ, Goldenberg SL, Gleave ME, Degner LF. Provision of individualized information to men and their partners to facilitate treatment decision making in prostate cancer. *Oncol Nurs Forum.* 2003;30(1):107–114.

31. Moore KN, Estey A. The early post-operative concerns of men after radical prostatectomy. *J Adv Nurs.* 1999;29:1121–1129.

32. Valanis BG, Rumpler CH. Helping women choose breast cancer treatment alternatives. *Cancer Nurs.* 1985;8:167–175.

33. Egiker SA, Kirscht JP, Becker MH. Understanding and improving patient compliance. *Ann Intern Med.* 1994;100:258–268.

10

Genetic Counseling and Testing for Cancer Survivors

Ellen T. Matloff, MS

ABSTRACT

Genetic counseling and testing for cancer are now recognized as critical tools in guiding surgical decision making, chemoprevention, and surveillance for patients at high risk for a hereditary cancer syndrome. However, most cancer survivors were not offered this relatively new technology at the time of their diagnosis. This information could be important for their future management and the management of their family members. All cancer survivors should be reassessed at their follow-up visits for factors that place them at risk for hereditary cancer; those deemed high risk should be educated about their options for genetic counseling and testing.

INTRODUCTION

As the field of oncology evolves, more and more technology is available to help manage cancer patients. Many of these advancements, such as chemotherapy, radiation, and new surgical techniques, are most important at the time of diagnosis and treatment of the initial cancer. Genetic counseling and testing are important when constructing an initial treatment plan; however, in high-risk patients, these services are also crucial in the long-term management of the cancer patient and his or her entire family. If patients were not offered genetic counseling and testing at diagnosis or early in treatment, they can still be offered these options months, years, or even decades later to help them reduce their risk for future cancers and, importantly, to help their family members identify cancer risk. Unlike some medical options, genetic counseling and testing remain relevant in elderly and terminally ill patients. For this reason, follow-up care of the cancer survivor should include risk assessment for hereditary cancer. Patients at increased risk should be referred for genetic counseling, no matter how far out they are from their cancer diagnosis.

ELICITING A GENETIC PEDIGREE

Only 5% to 10% of most cancers are due to mutations within inherited cancer susceptibility genes.[1] A detailed family history can help the clinician decipher which patients are at greatest risk for hereditary cancer. Optimally, a family history should include at least three to four generations; however, patients do not always have accurate information about their relatives, and this family history may require some research. For each individual affected with cancer, it is important to document the primary site and age of diagnosis. Treatment and environmental exposures (e.g., radiation, occupational exposures, cigarettes, other agents) can also be important.[2] Past surgical history, such as a total hysterectomy at a young age, should also be documented because such surgeries can artificially alter the chance that a person will later develop certain cancers, such as ovarian, uterine, and breast cancer. All cancer diagnoses should be confirmed with pathology reports whenever possible because a high rate of misreporting has been documented.[3] It is common for patients to report a uterine cancer as an ovarian cancer, or a colon polyp as an invasive colorectal cancer. These differences, although seemingly subtle to the patient, can make a tremendous difference in risk assessment.

The most common misconception in family history taking is that somehow a maternal family history of breast, ovarian, or uterine cancer is more significant than a paternal history.[4] Conversely, many still believe that a paternal history of prostate cancer is more significant than a maternal history. These beliefs are completely inaccurate. Maternal and paternal histories are equally significant, and both must be explored thoroughly.

A detailed family history should also include consanguinity (inbred relationships), genetic diseases, birth defects, mental retardation, multiple miscarriages, and infant deaths. A history of certain recessive genetic diseases (e.g., ataxia telangiectasia or Fanconi anemia) can indicate that healthy family members who carry just 1 copy of the genetic mutation may be at increased risk to develop cancer.[5,6] Other genetic disorders (such as hereditary hemorrhagic telangiectasia (HHT)), can be associated with a hereditary cancer syndrome (as HHT is with juvenile polyposis) caused by a mutation in the same gene.[7]

A complete pedigree includes the spouse's personal and family history of cancer. This component has bearing on the cancer status of common children but may also determine if children are at increased risk for a serious genetic disease such as Fanconi anemia.[6] Children who inherit 2 copies of a BRCA2 mutation are now known to have this serious disorder characterized by defective DNA repair and high rates of birth defects, aplastic anemia, leukemia, and solid tumors.[6] Patients should be encouraged to report changes in their family history over time (e.g., upon new cancer diagnoses or genetic testing results in relatives), because this may change their risk assessment and counseling.[4]

ᗐ Case Example 10.1

John is a 65-year-old colon cancer survivor who is 30 years out from his colon cancer diagnosis. He was seen for his regular follow-up appointment with his gastroenterologist who mentioned that if John were diagnosed with colon cancer at age 35 today, he would be referred for genetic counseling. John decided he would like to go for genetic counseling to learn if his children are at increased risk for colon cancer.

At his first visit, John immediately reported to his genetic counselor that he has absolutely no family history of colon cancer. The genetic counselor elicited a full pedigree and learned that John's mother was an only child, and he therefore had no maternal aunts, uncles, or cousins. John's mother died at age 55 of ovarian cancer, and his only sibling, a brother, died at age 25 in a car accident. John's maternal grandmother was diagnosed with uterine cancer at age 65 but died many years later of heart disease.

(continues)

Case Example 10.1 (*continued*)

John was not aware that both ovarian and uterine cancers can be part of the hereditary colorectal cancer spectrum. He had genetic testing for mutations within *MSH2* and *MLH1* and learned that he carries a mutation in *MLH1*. John's four adult children were then tested, and one son was found to carry the familial *MLH1* mutation and will be followed carefully by a gastroenterologist. John's three daughters do not carry the familial mutation and are now at population risk for colorectal, uterine, and ovarian cancers.

RISK ASSESSMENT FOR THE CANCER SURVIVOR

There are 7 critical risk factors that help the clinician decipher who is at greatest risk for hereditary cancer, [4] as presented in the following list:

1. **Early age of cancer onset.** This risk factor, *even in the absence of a family history*, is associated with an increased frequency of germline mutations in many types of cancers.[8] For example, this risk factor could be overlooked in a 40-year-old cancer survivor who is now 20 years out of a breast cancer diagnosis. However, her risk to carry a mutation is the same as a woman diagnosed with the same cancer today at that age; therefore, this cancer survivor should be offered the same options in terms of genetic counseling and testing.

2. **Presence of the same cancer in multiple affected relatives on the same side of the pedigree and within the same bloodline.** These cancers do not need to be the same histological type in order to be caused by a single mutation. Many clinicians obtain a family history at the time of the first clinical visit. In cancer survivors, this history should be updated *on an annual basis*, as the family history changes. Patients may not recognize that evolving family history is critical to their own follow-up, and therefore the clinician must initiate this discussion.

3. **Clustering of cancers known to be caused by a single gene mutation in one family** (e.g., breast/ovarian/pancreatic cancer, colon/ovarian/uterine cancer, breast/thyroid/rare skin tumors). It is important for the clinician to recognize these patterns and to specifically ask the patient about these other cancers in the family. The patient may not know, for instance, that his mother's history of

uterine cancer is in any way connected to his own diagnosis of early-onset colon cancer.

4. **Multiple primary cancers in an individual.** This risk factor applies to an individual with multiple primary breast or colon cancers as well as to an individual with separate cancers known to be caused by a single gene mutation (e.g., breast and ovarian cancer, or colon and uterine cancer, in a single individual).

5. **Ethnicity.** Individuals of Jewish ancestry are at increased risk to carry 3 specific mutations in the *BRCA1* and *BRCA2* genes[9] and the APCI1307K allele.[10] It is clear that each breast, ovarian, and pancreatic cancer patient should be asked *specifically* if he or she is of Jewish ancestry. This information should not be assumed based on patients' last names or the religion they have listed as part of their medical intake form.

6. **Cancer with an unusual presentation** (e.g., male breast cancer or multiple colon polyposis). This risk is important even when isolated. Retinoblastoma, medullary thyroid cancer, and adrenocortical carcinomas are rare cancers that are often hereditary, and all require a genetics work-up.[11]

7. **Pathological findings.** Pathology is a new and evolving way of assessing cancer risk. It appears that certain types of cancer are overrepresented in hereditary cancer families. For example, medullary breast cancer appears to be overrepresented in BRCA1 families,[12] and early data suggest that the triple negative breast cancer phenotype (ER-, PR-, her-2–) may also be overrepresented in BRCA1 families[13]; however, breast cancer patients without these pathological findings are *not* necessarily at lower risk to carry a mutation. In contrast, patients with a borderline or mucinous ovarian carcinoma appear to be at lower risk to carry a BRCA1 or BRCA2 mutation.[14] It is already well established that medullary thyroid carcinoma, sebaceous adenoma or carcinoma, and adrenocortical carcinoma before the age of 25, or multiple adenomatous, hamartomatous, or juvenile colon polyps are indicative of other rare hereditary cancer syndromes.[11,15]

These risk factors should be viewed in the context of the entire family history and must be weighed in proportion to the number of individuals who have not developed cancer. Risk assessment is often limited in families that are small or have few female relatives; in such families, a single risk factor may carry more weight.[16]

A less common, but extremely important, finding is the presence of unusual physical findings or birth defects associated with rare hereditary cancer syndromes. Examples include benign skin findings and thyroid disorders in Cowden syndrome, ontogenic keratocysts in Gorlin syndrome,[17] and desmoid tumors or dental abnormalities in familial adenomatous polyposis (FAP).[2] Again, it is critical that the clinician is aware of these associations and specifically asks the cancer survivor about these findings when taking the family history, because they can change the genetic testing that should be ordered.[4]

CANCER GENETIC COUNSELING

Cancer genetic counseling provides clients with an assessment of the chance that the cancers in their family are hereditary—and, if so, which gene is most likely mutated. Aggressive advertising by genetic testing companies paints the testing process as a simple one that can be carried out by clinicians with no formal education in the field. However, there are many genes (other than *BRCA1* and *BRCA2*) involved in cancer, and the interpretation of test results is often complicated. For example, a patient with early-onset breast cancer whose family history is positive for thyroid cancer, thyroid disease, and rare skin findings may actually be at greater risk to carry a *PTEN* mutation than a *BRCA1* or *BRCA2* mutation.[18]

Several studies have now demonstrated that misinterpretation of genetic test results is a common occurence.[19,20] The ramifications of result misinterpretation for the patient and the patient's entire family, and the associated liability for the healthcare providers, are great. Therefore, it is important to utilize a cancer genetics provider who has graduate training in this area (as opposed to a few hours of training by the testing company selling testing kits) whenever possible (Table 10.1).

Informed consent for each patient *before* testing should include the risks, benefits, and limitations of testing. If the patient is interested in pursuing testing, the counselor will identify a lab that offers appropriate genetic testing, will obtain insurance pre-authorization (important for a test that often costs more than $3000), and will facilitate

TABLE 10.1 Cancer Genetic Counseling Resources

CancerNet
(800) 4-CANCER
http://www.cancer.gov/search/geneticsservices/
A free service designed to locate providers of cancer risk counseling and testing services.
National Society of Genetic Counselors
(312) 321-6834
http://www.nsgc.org
For a listing of genetic counselors in your area who specialize in cancer.

sample collection, shipping, and result interpretation. The result session will include detailed counseling about medical management options for early detection and risk reduction, and may include referrals to prevention trials, surveillance programs, and medical specialists.

The cancer risks given are not absolute but change over time as the family and personal history changes and the patient ages. The risk reduction options available are often radical (e.g., chemoprevention or prophylactic surgery) and are not appropriate for every patient at every age. The surveillance and management plan must be tailored to the patient's age, childbearing status, menopausal status, risk category, ease of screening, and personal preferences. The ultimate goal of cancer genetic counseling is to help the patient and his or her physicians construct a management plan best suited to the patient's personal situation, needs, and circumstances; this management plan often needs to be evaluated and modified over time.[4]

INFORMATIVE GENETIC TESTING

In order to pinpoint the mutation in a family, an *affected* individual most likely to carry the mutation should be tested first, whenever possible. This person is most often the family member affected with the cancer in question at the earliest age. Test subjects should be selected with care, because it is possible for a person to develop sporadic cancer in a hereditary cancer family. For example, in an early-onset breast cancer family, it would not be ideal to first test a woman diagnosed with breast cancer at age 68, because she may represent a sporadic case.

Unfortunately, the opportunity to test the key person in the family is often missed if that person is critically ill, elderly, or in the midst of treatment. Clinicians and family members are often, and appropriately, focused on the care of the person with cancer. However, if that person dies before testing is ordered, the opportunity to perform informative testing on other family members may be lost forever. When approached, these key family members are often grateful for the opportunity to help their family members. A family member who has already been diagnosed with cancer is also more likely to have insurance coverage for full genetic testing than is an unaffected relative.

If a mutation is detected in an affected relative, other family members can be tested for the same mutation with a great degree of accuracy, and this testing is much less expensive than the full testing initially performed to search for the familial mutation (e.g., $430 vs $3200). Family members who do not carry the mutation in their family are deemed "true negative," and their cancer risks usually drop to the general population risk. Family members who test positive for the mutation in their family will be provided with more definitive information about their cancer risks, as well as options for surveillance and risk reduction.[4]

If a mutation is not identified in the affected relative, it usually means that either the cancers in the family (a) are not hereditary, or (b) are caused by an undetectable mutation or a mutation in a different gene. A careful review of the family history and the risk factors will help to decipher which interpretation is more likely. Additional genetic testing may need to be ordered at that point. In cases in which the cancers appear hereditary and no mutation is found, DNA banking should be offered to the individuals being studied for a time in the future when improved testing may become available (Table 10.2). A letter indicating exactly who in the family has access to the DNA should accompany the banked sample.

TABLE 10.2 DNA Banking Resources

GeneTests™: Genetic Testing Resource

(206) 616-4033

http://www.genetests.org

Offers current information on laboratories and testing, including DNA banking facilities.

Selected DNA Banks

Oregon Health Sciences University

(503) 494-5400

Prevention Genetics

www.preventiongenetics.com

(715) 387-0484

University of Medicine and Dentistry of New Jersey

(973) 972-3170

 Case Example 10.2

Joy is a 45-year-old unaffected woman whose mother, Linda, was recently diagnosed with stage III ovarian cancer at age 77, had a total abdominal hysterectomy, and is now undergoing aggressive chemotherapy. After her mother's diagnosis, Joy requested a prophylactic bilateral salpingo-oophorectomy (BSO) from her obstetrician/gynecologist (OB/GYN) to re-duce her own risk of developing ovarian cancer. The OB/GYN took a family history and learned that Joy's maternal aunt died of breast cancer at age 48, and her maternal grandfather died of pancreatic cancer at age 70. Based on this history, the physician referred Joy for genetic counseling. After reviewing the case, the genetic counselor suggested that testing begin with Linda because she is the most likely person in the family to carry a mutation. Joy was reluctant to involve her mother because she was going through treatment, feeling sick and depressed, and Joy was afraid that her mother would feel guilty that the cancers in the family could be hereditary. The counselor explained that in order to pinpoint the mutation in the family, it is most accurate to begin testing with Linda and that this information would benefit Joy, her 2 siblings and 6 maternal cousins, as well as the grandchildren in the family.

(continues)

> ### Case Example 10.2 (*continued*)
>
> Joy agreed to approach her mother about testing and explained to her that this process could help all of the other family members reduce their chances of developing cancer. Linda initially felt overwhelmed but decided she wanted to do what she could to help her family. Her insurance agreed to cover BRCA1 and BRCA2 testing, and Linda had her blood drawn and sent for testing. She learned that she carried a mutation in the *BRCA2* gene and that she had done nothing to cause her ovarian cancer diagnosis. Joy's insurance company then agreed to pay for testing because she had a first-degree relative who was a mutation carrier, and she subsequently learned that she did not carry the mutation. She was deemed a "true negative," and her cancer risks dropped to general population level. Several female relatives tested positive for the familial mutation and chose high-risk breast surveillance and prophylactic BSO. One male relative tested positive and will have breast and prostate surveillance; he also learned that his 25-year-old daughter should have testing.

LIFETIME CANCER RISKS

Each hereditary cancer syndrome is associated with its own risks and options for surveillance and risk reduction. An outline of these syndromes has been published in the *Journal of Clinical Oncology*.[21] The following outlines two of the most common hereditary cancer syndromes: breast and ovarian cancer syndrome (the majority of which is caused by mutations in the *BRCA1* and *BRCA2* genes) and hereditary nonpolyposis colorectal cancer (HNPCC) syndrome.

Female carriers of BRCA1 and BRCA2 mutations have a 50% to 85% lifetime risk to develop breast cancer and a 15% to 60% lifetime risk to develop ovarian cancer.[9,22,23] The risks of both breast and ovarian cancer increase with the age of the patient, although the average age of diagnosis is lower than the average in the general population.[21,24] Cancer of the fallopian tubes and primary peritoneal carcinoma also fall within this syndrome, although the risks of each are relatively small.[25,26] BRCA2 carriers also have an increased lifetime risk of male breast cancer and pancreatic cancer.[27,28] Carriers of an HNPCC (also known as Lynch syndrome) mutation have a 65% to 85% lifetime risk to develop colon cancer, and female carriers have at least a 40% to 60% lifetime risk of uterine cancer and as great as a 10% to 12% risk of ovarian cancer.[29,30]

OPTIONS FOR SURVEILLANCE AND RISK REDUCTION

Patients who carry a mutation for a hereditary cancer syndrome have options for earlier and more aggressive surveillance, chemoprevention, and prophylactic surgery.

Surveillance recommendations are evolving constantly with newer techniques and additional long-term data. It is recommended that female carriers of BRCA mutations have annual mammograms beginning between ages 25 and 35, undergo annual or semi-annual clinical breast examinations, and perform monthly breast self-examinations.[31] It appears that breast magnetic resonance imaging (MRI) may also play an important role in surveillance of this population.[32]

BRCA carriers may take tamoxifen in hopes of reducing their risks of developing breast cancer. Tamoxifen has proven effective in women at risk due to a positive family history of breast cancer.[33,34] There are limited data on the effectiveness of prophylactic tamoxifen in BRCA carriers[35–37]; however, there are some data to suggest that BRCA carriers taking tamoxifen as treatment for a breast cancer reduce their risk of a contralateral breast cancer.[38] Additionally, the majority of BRCA2 carriers who develop breast cancer develop an estrogen-positive form of the disease,[39] and it is hoped that this population will respond especially well to chemoprevention. Further studies in this area are necessary before drawing conclusions about the efficacy of tamoxifen in this population.

Prophylactic bilateral mastectomy appears to reduce the risk of breast cancer by more than 90% in women at high risk for the disease.[40] Before genetic testing was available, it was not uncommon for entire generations of cancer families to have at-risk tissues removed without knowing if they were *personally* at increased risk for their familial cancer. Fifty percent of individuals in hereditary cancer families will *not* carry the inherited predisposition gene and can be spared prophylactic surgery or invasive high-risk surveillance regimens. Therefore, it clearly is not appropriate to offer prophylactic surgery until a patient is referred for genetic counseling and, if possible, testing.[4,41]

Women who carry BRCA1/2 mutations are also at increased risk to develop second contralateral and ipsilateral primaries of the breast.[42] These data bring into question the option of breast-conserving surgery in women at high risk to develop a second primary within the same breast. For this reason, BRCA1/2 carrier status can have a profound impact on surgical decision making,[41] and many patients have genetic counseling and testing immediately after diagnosis and before surgery or radiation therapy. Those patients who test positive and opt for prophylactic mastectomy can often be spared radiation and the resulting skin side effects that can complicate reconstruction.

Women who carry BRCA1/2 mutations are also at increased risk to develop ovarian, fallopian tube, and primary peritoneal cancer, even if no one in their family has developed these cancers. Surveillance for ovarian cancer is complex, with the recommended interventions being annual transvaginal ultrasounds and testing of CA-125 levels beginning between the ages of 25 and 35.[31] The effectiveness of such surveillance in detecting ovarian cancers at early, more treatable stages has not been proven in any population. Some data have indicated that oral contraceptives reduce the risk of ovarian cancer in women carrying BRCA mutations.[43] Recent data indicate that the impact of this intervention on increasing breast cancer risk, if any, is low.[37,44] Given the difficulties in screening and treatment of ovarian cancer, risk/benefit analysis likely favors the use of oral contraceptives in young carriers of BRCA1/2 mutations[45] who are not yet ready to have their ovaries removed.

Prophylactic BSO is currently the most effective means to reduce the risk of ovarian cancer and is recommended to BRCA1/2 carriers by the age of 35 or when childbearing is complete.[46] This prophylactic surgery is highly effective in reducing the subsequent risk of ovarian cancer in BRCA1/2 carriers[47]; however, even women who have had this procedure have a small residual risk of developing a primary peritoneal carcinoma.[4,25,48] The risk of ovarian cancer *increases* with age and, contrary to common belief, does not decrease or disappear when a woman goes through menopause.

A secondary, but important, reason for female BRCA carriers to consider prophylactic oophorectomy is that it also significantly reduces the risk of a subsequent breast cancer, particularly if they have this surgery before menopause.[49,50] The reduction in breast cancer risk remains even if a healthy premenopausal carrier elects to take low-dose hormone replacement therapy after this surgery.[51] Early data suggest that tamoxifen in addition to premenopausal oophorectomy in BRCA carriers may have little additional benefit in terms of breast cancer risk reduction.[52] Research is needed in balancing quality of life issues secondary to estrogen deprivation with cancer risk reduction in these young female BRCA1/2 carriers.

The standard surveillance method in carriers of HNPCC mutations is full colonoscopy to the cecum every 1 to 3 years beginning between the ages of 20 and 25.[31] While several studies are investigating chemopreventive options for colorectal cancer, no agents are currently approved for clinical use. Prophylactic subtotal colectomy with ileorectal anastomosis is an option for HNPCC carriers, and a decision analysis revealed that this procedure may offer slightly greater gains in life expectancy for young HNPCC carriers than surveillance alone.[53] Quality of life issues must be weighed against the rate of detecting cancer at an early, treatable stage with surveillance alone.

Options for endometrial cancer surveillance include endometrial aspirate and transvaginal ultrasound beginning between the ages of 25 and 35. The efficacy of such surveillance in HNPCC carriers is unknown. Oral contraceptives are known to reduce the risk of both ovarian and endometrial cancer in the general population,[54] but the impact of this intervention in HNPCC carriers, or on colon cancer risk, is currently unknown. Prophylactic total hysterectomy is also an option. Recent data suggest that this surgery is effective in significantly reducing the risk of both ovarian and uterine cancer in women with HNPCC syndrome and should be considered after the age of 35 or once childbearing is completed.[4,30]

Genetic counseling and testing are also available for many rare cancer syndromes, including von Hippel-Lindau, multiple endocrine neoplasias, and FAP. Surveillance and risk reduction for patients who are known mutation carriers for such conditions may decrease the associated morbidity and mortality of these syndromes.[4]

INSURANCE DISCRIMINATION

When cancer genetic testing was first introduced into routine clinical practice, one of the most common concerns cited by both patients and providers was that of insurance discrimination.[55,56] Fortunately, it appears that the risks of health insurance discrimination were overstated and that almost no such discrimination has been reported.[57] Cancer survivors are likely at the lowest risk for insurance discrimination due to genetic testing because their own personal histories of cancer are already well documented in their medical records.

Most patients now submit their genetic counseling and testing charges to their health insurance companies. In the past few years, more insurance companies have agreed to pay for counseling and testing,[58] perhaps in light of decision analyses that show these services and subsequent prophylactic surgeries to be cost-effective.[59] The risk of life insurance discrimination, however, is possible for patients who have never been diagnosed with cancer. Patients should be counseled about such risks before they pursue genetic testing.

PSYCHOSOCIAL ISSUES FOR THE CANCER SURVIVOR

The process of cancer genetic counseling and testing is accompanied by a multitude of psychosocial issues for most patients, because they realize that the cancers in their family may in fact be hereditary. The simple process of drawing a pedigree can, in fact, be overwhelming for some patients who see the pattern of cancers in their family in a graphic form for the first time.

Genetic testing in the cancer survivor, however, can be associated with some unique psychosocial issues. The emotional process can be particularly complicated in patients who are 5 or more years out from their cancer diagnosis and feel that their treatment, management, and cancer risks are behind them. The following list summarizes some key concerns that patients may have and suggests discussion points for the clinician to address.

> ▷ *Patient:* Why would I want genetic testing now? I'm a cancer survivor. This problem is in my outbox. Why would I want to open Pandora's box?
>
> *Clinician:* It must be surprising and upsetting to hear that your cancer may be hereditary, especially a few years out from your diagnosis; however, you deserve to know about new options as they become available, particularly if those options can reduce your risk of developing a new cancer and can help your family members.
>
> ▷ *Patient:* What do you mean I might be at risk for other cancers?
>
> *Clinician:* This is understandably an upsetting thought for any cancer survivor. However, you are not at high risk for every cancer,

and this information can help us reduce the risk that you will ever develop cancer again. If we know this information ahead of time, we can change the odds.

▷ *Patient:* I've already been through surgery, chemotherapy, and radiation. I don't want to have prophylactic surgery.

Clinician: You have been through a lot, and it is understandable that you don't even want to think about having another surgery. However, prophylactic surgery is only *one* of the options available. Having genetic testing does not mean that you have to have prophylactic surgery, although we should review those options in detail if we learn you carry a mutation. Close surveillance, even closer than you receive now, and medications used to reduce cancer risk are also options for many patients.

▷ *Patient:* I can't believe that my children, grandchildren, siblings, and other relatives might also carry this mutation. I feel so guilty that I may have passed this mutation on to them.

Clinician: We all pass on both positive characteristics and genetic mutations to our children. We just happen to know about this information in your case! This information is power. It is a gift that you are giving to the next generation. With this information, your relatives can reduce the chance that they will ever get cancer. You are changing the legacy of cancer in your family for the better.

CONCLUSION

Genetic counseling and testing have become parts of routine clinical practice for patients newly diagnosed with cancer. These services can be of great benefit for the cancer survivor in terms of reducing the risk of a new cancer and for helping the entire family. The clinician should elicit and update a full family pedigree from all cancer survivors to determine if they are at high risk for a hereditary cancer syndrome; if so, they should be offered genetic counseling and testing and/or DNA banking.

Acknowledgments

Special thanks to Danielle Campfield, MS, and Martha Steadman Matloff, MD, for their insightful reviews of this chapter.

REFERENCES

1. Claus E, Schildkraut J, Thompson W, Risch N. The genetic attributable risks of breast and ovarian cancer. *Cancer.* 1996;77:2318–2324.
2. Schneider K. *Counseling About Cancer: Strategies for Genetic Counseling.* 2nd ed. New York: John Wiley & Sons, Inc; 2002.
3. Love R, Evan A, Josten D. The accuracy of patient reports of a family history. *J Chronic Dis.* 1985;38:289.
4. Matloff E. Genetic counseling. In: DeVita VT, Lawrence T, Rosenberg S, eds. *Cancer: Principles & Practice of Oncology.* 8th ed. Philadelphia: Lippincott Williams & Wilkins Publishers; 2008.
5. Thompson D, Duedal S, Kirner J, McGuffog L, et al. Cancer risks and mortality in heterozygous ATM mutation carriers. *J Natl Cancer Inst.* 2005;97:813–822.
6. Alter B, Rosenberg P, Brody L. Clinical and molecular features associated with biallelic mutations in FANCD1/BRCA2. *J Med Genet.* 2007;44:1–9.
7. Korzenik J, Chung D, Digumarthy S, Badizadegan K. Case 33-2005: a 43-year-old man with lower gastrointestinal bleeding. *N Engl J Med.* 2005; 353:1836–1844.
8. Loman N, Johannsson O, Kristoffersson U. Family history of breast and ovarian cancers and BRCA1 and BRCA2 mutations in a population-based series of early-onset breast cancer. *J Natl Cancer Inst.* 2001;93:1215.
9. Struewing J, Hartge P, Wacholder S. The risk of cancer associated with specific mutations of BRCA1 and BRCA2 among Ashkenazi Jews. *N Engl J Med.* 1997;336:1401–1408.
10. Gryfe R, Nicola N, Lal G, Gallinger S, Redston M. Inherited colorectal polyposis and cancer risk of the APCI1307K polymorphism. *Am J Hum Genet.* 1999;64:378–384.
11. Plon S, Nathanson K. Inherited susceptibility for pediatric cancer. *Cancer.* 2005;11:255–267.
12. Eisinger F, Jacquemier J, Charpin C, et al. Mutations at BRCA1: the medullary breast carcinoma revisited. *Cancer Res.* 1998;58:1588–1592.
13. Kandel M, Stadler Z, Masciari S, et al. Prevalence of BRCA1 mutations in triple negative breast cancer (BC). In: *2006 42nd Annual ASCO Meeting.* Atlanta, GA; 2006:508.
14. Risch H, McLaughlin J, Cole D, et al. Population BRCA1 and BRCA2 mutation frequencies and cancer penetrances: a kin-cohort study in Ontario, Canada. *J Natl Cancer Inst.* 2006;98:1694–1706.
15. Matloff E, Brierley K, Chimera C. A clinician's guide to hereditary colon cancer. *Cancer J.* 2004;10:280–287.

16. Weitzel J, Lagos V, Cullinane C, et al. Limited family structure and BRCA gene mutation status in single cases of breast cancer. *JAMA*. 2007;297: 2587–2595.
17. Gorlin R. Nevoid basal-cell carcinoma syndrome. *Medicine*. 1987;66: 98–113.
18. Eng C. Cowden syndrome. *J Genet Counsel*. 1997;6:181–192.
19. Giardiello F, Brensinger J, Petersen G. The use and interpretation of commercial APC gene testing for familial adenomatous polyposis. *N Engl J Med*. 1997;336:823–827.
20. Brierley K, Kim K, Matloff E. Obstetricians' and gynecologists' knowledge, interests, and current practices with regard to providing breast and ovarian cancer genetic counseling. *J Genet Counsel*. 2001;10:438.
21. Garber J, Offit K. Hereditary cancer predisposition syndromes. *J Clin Oncol*. 2005;23:276–292.
22. Ford D, Easton D, Bishop D. Risks of cancer in BRCA1 mutation carriers. *Lancet*. 1994;343:692–695.
23. Antoniou A, Pharoah P, Narod S. Average risks of breast and ovarian cancer associated with BRCA1 or BRCA2 mutations detected in case series unselected for family history: a combined analyses of 22 studies. *Am J Hum Genet*. 2003;72:1117.
24. Robson M, Offit K. Clinical practice. Management of an inherited predisposition to breast cancer. *N Engl J Med*. 2007;357:154–162.
25. Piver M, Jishi M, Tsukada Y. Primary peritoneal carcinoma after prophylactic oophorectomy in women with a family history of ovarian cancer. *Cancer*. 1993;71:2751–2755.
26. Aziz S, Kuperstein G, Rosen B. A genetic epidemiological study of carcinoma of the fallopian tube. *Gynecol Oncol*. 2001;80:341.
27. van Asperen C, Brohet R, Meijers-Heijboer, et al. Cancer risks in BRCA2 families: estimates for sites other than breast and ovary. *J Med Genet*. 2005;42:711–719.
28. Breast Cancer Linkage Consortium. Cancer risks in BRCA2 mutation carriers. *J Natl Cancer Inst*. 1999;91:1310–1316.
29. Aarnio M, Mecklin JP, Aaltonen L. Lifetime risk of different cancers in hereditary non-polyposis colorectal cancer (HNPCC) syndrome. *Int J Cancer*. 1995;64:430–433.
30. Schmeler K, Lynch H, Chen L, et al. Prophylactic surgery to reduce the risk of gynecologic cancers in the Lynch syndrome. *N Engl J Med*. 2006; 354:261–269.
31. Burke W, Daly M, Garber J, Botkin, et al. Recommendations for follow-up care of individuals with an inherited predisposition to cancer. II.

BRCA1 and BRCA2. Cancer Genetics Studies Consortium. *JAMA*. 1997; 277:997–1003.

32. Warner E, Plewes D, Hill K, Causer, et al. Surveillance of BRCA1 and BRCA2 mutation carriers with magnetic resonance imaging, ultrasound, mammography, and clinical breast examination. *JAMA*. 2004;202: 1317–1325.

33. Powles T, Ashley S, Tidy A, Smith I, Dowsett M. Twenty-year follow-up of the Royal Marsden randomized, double-blinded tamoxifen breast cancer prevention trial. *J Natl Cancer Inst*. 2007;99:283–290.

34. Cuzick J, Forbes J, Sestak I, et al. Long-term results of tamoxifen prophylaxis for breast cancer: 96 month follow-up of the randomized IBIS-I trial. *J Natl Cancer Inst*. 2007;99:272–282.

35. Fisher B, Constantino J, Wickerman D. Tamoxifen for the prevention of breast cancer: report of the National Surgical Adjuvant Breast and Bowel Project P-1 Study. *J Natl Cancer Inst*. 1998;90:1371–1388.

36. King M, Wieand S, Hale K. Tamoxifen and breast cancer incidence among women with inherited mutations in BRCA1 and BRCA2. *JAMA*. 2001;286:2251.

37. Narod S, Brunet J, Ghadirian P. Tamoxifen and risk of contralateral breast cancer in BRCA1 and BRCA2 mutation carriers: a case-control study. *Lancet*. 2000;356:1876.

38. Metcalfe K, Lynch H, Ghadirian P, et al. Contralateral breast cancer in BRCA1 and BRCA2 mutation carriers. *J Clin Oncol*. 2004;22: 2328–2335.

39. Lakhani S, van de Vijver M, Jacquemier J, et al. The pathology of familial breast cancer: predictive value of immunohistochemical markers estrogen receptor, progesterone receptor, HER-2, and p53 in patients with mutations in BRCA1 and BRCA2. *J Clin Oncol*. 2002;20:2310–2318.

40. Hartmann L, Schaid D, Woods J. Efficacy of bilateral prophylactic mastectomy in women with a family history of breast cancer. *N Engl J Med*. 1999;340:77–84.

41. Matloff E. The breast surgeon's role in BRCA1 and BRCA2 testing. *Am J Surg*. 2000;180:294.

42. Turner B, Harold E, Matloff E. BRCA1/BRCA2 germline mutations in locally recurrent breast cancer patients after lumpectomy and radiation therapy: implications for breast-conserving management in patients with BRCA1/BRCA2 mutations. *J Clin Oncol*. 1999;17(10):3017–3024.

43. McLaughlin J, Risch H, Lubinski J, et al. Reproductive risk factors for ovarian cancer in carriers of BRCA1 or BRCA2 mutations: a case-control study. *Lancet*. 2007;8:26–34.

44. Milne R, Knight J, John E, et al. Oral contraceptive use and risk of early-onset breast cancer in carriers and noncarriers of BRCA1 and BRCA2 mutations. *Cancer Epidemiol Biomarkers Prev.* 2005;14:350–356.
45. Olopade O, Weber B. Breast cancer genetics: toward molecular characterization of individuals at increased risk for breast cancer. Part II. *PPO Updates.* 1998;12:1–8.
46. Domchek S, Friebel T, Neuhausen S, et al. Mortality reduction after risk-reducing bilateral salpingo-oophorectomy in a prospective cohort of BRCA1 and BRCA2 mutation carriers. *Lancet Oncol.* 2006;7:223–229.
47. Finch A, Beiner M, Lubinski J, et al. Salpingo-oophorectomy and the risk of ovarian, fallopian tube, and peritoneal cancers in women with a BRCA1 or BRCA2 mutation. *JAMA.* 2006;296:185–192.
48. American College of Obstetrics and Gynecology. Breast-ovarian cancer screening. *Am J Obstet Gynecol.* 1996;176:1–2.
49. Rebbeck T, Lynch H, Neuhausen S. Prophylactic oophorectomy in carriers of BRCA1 or BRCA2 mutations. *N Engl J Med.* 2002;346:1616.
50. Kauff N, Satagopan J, Robson M. Risk-reducing salpingo-oophorectomy in women with a BRCA1 or BRCA2 mutation. *N Engl J Med.* 2002;346:1609.
51. Rebbeck T, Friebel T, Wagner T, et al. Effect of short-term hormone replacement therapy on breast cancer risk reduction after bilateral prophylactic oophorectomy in BRCA1 and BRCA2 mutation carriers: the PROSE study group. *J Clin Oncol.* 2005;23:7804–7810.
52. Gronwald J, Tung N, Foulkes W, et al. Tamoxifen and contralateral breast cancer in BRCA1 and BRCA2 carriers: an update. *Int J Cancer.* 2006;118(9):2281–2284.
53. Syngal S, Weeks J, Schrag D. Benefits of colonoscopic surveillance and prophylactic colectomy in patients with hereditary nonpolyposis colorectal cancer mutations. *Ann Intern Med.* 1998;129:787–796.
54. Silverberg S, Makowski E. Endometrial carcinoma in young women taking oral contraceptive agents. *Obstet Gynecol.* 1975;46:503–506.
55. Bluman L, Rimer B, Berry D. Attitudes, knowledge, and risk perceptions of women with breast and/or ovarian cancer considering testing for BRCA1 and BRCA2. *J Natl Cancer Inst.* 1999;17:1040–1046.
56. Matloff E, Shappell H, Brierley K, Bernhardt B, McKinnon W, Peshkin B. What would you do? Specialists' perspectives on cancer genetic testing, prophylactic surgery and insurance discrimination. *J Clin Oncol.* 2000; 18:2484–2492.
57. Hall, M. Genetic discrimination. In: *North Carolina Genomics & Bioinformatics Consortium.* North Carolina; 2003.

58. Manley S, Pennell R, Frank T. Insurance coverage of BRCA1 and BRCA2 sequence analysis. *J Genet Counsel.* 1998;7:A462.
59. Grann V, Whang W, Jabcobson J, Heitjan D, Antman K, Neugut A. Benefits and costs of screening Ashkenazi Jewish women for BRCA1 and BRCA2. *J Clin Oncol.* 1999;17:494–500.

chapter

11

The Challenges of Parenting During Survivorship

Vaughn L. Mankey, MD

&

Paula K. Rauch, MD

ABSTRACT

A substantial number of cancer survivors are parents of children who depend on them. A child's well-being and development are of paramount importance for parents, and many survivors wonder how their illness will affect their children. This chapter elucidates some of the common parenting concerns and questions that arise throughout the various phases of cancer survivorship. An individual child's temperament and developmental stage are also considered in providing recommendations to address these concerns. Emphasis is placed on the need for clinicians to acknowledge the central role parenting plays in the survivorship experience. Practical tips are provided for clinicians to help them guide parents through the challenging circumstances of cancer survivorship.

INTRODUCTION

In 1992, the National Cancer Institute estimated that approximately 24% of people with cancer have a child at home who is 18 years old or younger.[1] Since that time, there have been innumerable improvements

143

and innovations in the treatment of many types of cancer, and the number of cancer survivors is fortunately on the rise. It is safe to assume, therefore, that the absolute number of parents living with cancer who have dependent children at home is also increasing. Clinical experience teaches that one of the first thoughts parents have after receiving a cancer diagnosis involves a worry about their children. Indeed, many parents soon wonder, "What am I going to tell my children?" or "Will my having cancer ruin my child's life?" Despite the growing number and relative universality of parenting concerns surrounding a cancer diagnosis, there is relatively little attention, research, or services targeted specifically at this topic.

It has been well documented that cancer is associated with significant psychosocial stress for patients and their families. Parents with cancer not only have to contend with illness-related symptoms and difficult treatment protocols, but they also have the added task of caring for dependent children. Among patients, parents often suffer from more distress than do non-parents.[2] There is a wealth of data that shows varying types of psychosocial distress can impede a parent's ability to parent optimally. This distress can have negative and lasting effects on children. For example, a parent's depression has been shown to have a number of deleterious effects on children in social, psychological, and cognitive domains.[3,4] While depression may be on the more severe end of the psychosocial distress spectrum, most children are perceptive of even subtle nuances in their parents' behaviors and attitudes. It is clear that having dependent children can add to the psychosocial stress of having cancer and that parental distress can negatively impact children.

Every person and family's experience with cancer is unique, and the course of survivorship is equally distinct. A broad definition of survivorship, beginning from the time of a cancer diagnosis and continuing as long as the patient is alive, allows for the inclusion of all varieties of experiences families may have with cancer. Some parents may never achieve remission and may face ongoing active treatment to maintain the most optimal length and quality of life possible. Such a course may present the consistent challenges of treatment and recurrent uncertainty about one's prognosis. Other parents may achieve remission but continue to worry about a possible recurrence. They may find themselves in a cyclical pattern of anticipatory apprehension followed by relief or joy after an encouraging follow-up scan or visit. If recurrence happens, some parents might go on to face future cycles of treatment and all the associated struggles and doubts. For other parents, remission may be maintained for many years, but a lingering worry about their health or the health of their children may persist. These are just some of the countless possible permutations of a survivor's course.

There are often common challenges that parents and families face at different phases of the cancer illness, such as during diagnosis, active treatment, remission, recurrence, or end of life. There are also some shared interventions that parents, families, and the clinicians who care for them can integrate into the survivorship experience. One should keep in mind that both challenges and interventions can vary according to a family's structure, as well as the age and developmental composition of the children. The temperamental predisposition of each child is also an important consideration when parents and clinicians examine children's responses to a parent's illness and develop a plan to safeguard their resiliency.

The clinician's role in addressing these challenges may vary depending on the primary identified treatment relationship. Yet all clinicians will be better prepared to care for patients if they acknowledge and address the important role that children play in the lives of parents who are cancer survivors. Knowing, anticipating, and addressing some of their common concerns and questions will undoubtedly be helpful to parents living with cancer and to their dependent children. To this end, the following goals have been established for this chapter:

1. To discuss some of the common concerns and questions parents have as they face cancer and the complex road of survivorship beginning at the time of diagnosis.
2. To reinforce the central role that children play in the cancer survivor's life, thereby explicating the need for clinicians to inquire about children and family in the very first meeting.
3. To emphasize the importance of each child's developmental stage and temperament as one guides parents to foster communication and support.
4. To provide practical tips to clinicians for working with parents who have children at home during the challenges of survivorship.

COMMON CONCERNS AND QUESTIONS

There is a dearth of empirical standardized data elucidating the specific effects of a parent's cancer on his or her children and family during the various phases of cancer survivorship. However, this chapter attempts to combine some of the available data with the collective clinical experience of the Marjorie E. Korff Parenting At a Challenging Time (PACT) Program at the Massachusetts General Hospital in Boston. This parent guidance program is unique, with 11 years of experience helping to address the common challenges and needs of parents with cancer throughout the survivorship course.*

New Diagnosis

Receiving the news that one has cancer can be overwhelming and can initiate a domino effect of concerns for parents who may worry about how their illness will affect their children. They may have concerns about what to say to their children regarding the diagnosis, when to say it, or whether or not they should inform their children at all. Many well-intending parents have the protective impulse to shield their children from the news and effects of cancer. However, not sharing the cancer diagnosis often leads to the opposite of the desired outcome and can be harmful to children instead of helpful. For example, children can feel excluded, worried, or confused when they are not informed of a parent's diagnosis. Rosenheim and Reicher described how children who were not told of a parent's cancer diagnosis were more anxious than children who knew.[5]

Some parents may wonder if valiant efforts on their parts can hide the illness, therein rendering it unnecessary to tell their children. However, as keen observers and astute listeners, children are usually aware of even small changes in a parent or the home dynamic, and often overhear adult conversations. When they are not given information to explain these changes, children are left to imagine and worry about their cause alone, without adult guidance. They can make an endless number of faulty assumptions about the cause, meaning, and prognosis of an illness, often varying with their age and temperament. For example, a gre-

---

* For more information about the Marjorie E. Korff PACT Program, visit www.mghpact.org.

garious 5-year-old boy might worry that he made his mother sick with the frog he had defiantly brought into the house. An inhibited 9-year-old girl might think the mystery illness is contagious and start avoiding family members, as to not contract it.

Overhearing important news about a parent from others can be upsetting and alienating for a child. Some children assume that the illness must be severe if their parents are not sharing information about it with them. Others ascribe personal meaning to being left out of the information and communication channels, and a child may think parents do not feel like he or she is important enough to tell or smart enough to understand. This process can set up a dynamic of mistrust, secrecy, and a host of unspoken feelings between children and their parents. Everyone in the family deserves to know important information that can ultimately have a significant impact on family life.

Parents who share the specific diagnosis, including the word "cancer" and even subtypes of cancer, with children set the stage for open, honest communication. Using the real names of the illness also helps to avoid confusion because euphemisms like "boo boo," "lumps and bumps," or even "feeling sick" are common ways children express their own experiences when they are not feeling well. It is important to make clear that the parent's cancer is distinct from the types of ailments that are routine for children, and using distinct, specific names helps to do this.

Some parents will wonder about the timing of giving this news. For example, children may be facing big exams or major life events around the time of the parent's diagnosis, and the family may wish to postpone the discussion. While briefly postponing the discussion about a new diagnosis is sometimes reasonable for a given family's circumstances, the guiding principle is that news should be shared in a timely, honest, and age-appropriate manner with the children. Parents may want to wait to share the news until a diagnosis is made and an initial treatment plan is established, which can provide some specific information and reassurance to children. However, if a parent's appearance or functional status has changed, or if the household is experiencing a different schedule, children will begin to wonder why. Even if all the information regarding the specific diagnosis and treatment plan is not available, children's observations and questions can be validated. Children can be informed about what is currently known and about the plan to find more answers. In some cases, parents might explain that a full investigation of the cancer is necessary prior to deciding on the best plan of action and that this may take some time. Reassuring children that the parents and doctors plan to do all they can to treat the cancer is helpful. Once the conversation has begun in an honest fashion, ongoing communication regarding the parent's illness can be maintained throughout the rest of the illness course and beyond.

Active Treatment

Clinicians and patients alike know that cancer treatment courses can be taxing in many ways. The physical burden of toxic medications, stress of multiple hospital visits, altered schedules and roles at home and work, and psychological distress are just a few of the challenges associated with treatment. Parents report feeling that their illness and treatment could be a burden on their children as well. They may wonder who will care for their children when they are too sick to do so either from illness-related symptoms or side effects of medications or radiation. Parents with significant symptoms often worry about how best to support their children in their usual activities and how to provide for their typical physical and emotional needs. These concerns are heightened for single parents who have less consistent help available through a present co-parent. However, it is important to recall that caregivers of cancer patients also experience significant distress and morbidity,[6,7] and caregiving duties often fall to the co-parent in dyadic couples. Therefore, even in families with two parents, the level of distress for each parent can be significant and can affect the children at home.

During a serious illness, a parent and family's support network is extremely important. It is not uncommon that there is an initial outpouring of help offerings, which may or may not persist throughout the entire course of survivorship. When assistance can be accepted and is effective, it can buoy a family during these challenging times. The particular type of assistance the family needs may not be apparent to well-wishers. For some parents, just trying to organize volunteers and field phone calls can feel like a full-time job and an added burden. Families should be encouraged to have a small support management team with a few key members who can help with these tasks. A "Captain of Kindness" and "Minister of Information" can be established using a close friend or relative outside the nuclear family.[8] These point people can offload some of the tasks of organizing volunteers, meals, carpools, and so on, and can provide information to concerned community members with an update approved by the parent. This approach not only decreases the amount of energy and effort needed to manage and communicate with supports, but also helps to increase protected family time, which parents and children need and appreciate.

Parents should also be encouraged to maintain the normal household schedule and routines as much as possible, minimizing the alterations in the daily lives of their children. Structure and predictability usually help provide a sense of calm and security among children of all ages. The specifics of doing this, however, vary greatly depending on the age of the children. For example, infants need their basic needs to be met and to have consistent caregivers with whom they can form and maintain healthy attachments. Therefore, having only a small number of additional caregivers who can be called upon regularly and who can become accustomed to the infants' routines (e.g., feeding, napping, soothing) is optimal. However, a teenager might be most concerned with not missing athletic practice or games, and having a friend on the team who can help with transportation may be key.

Parents also often have concerns about how their children will react to physical changes. Parents in active treatment may experience such side effects as hair loss, drastic fluctuations in weight, and skin changes. They may also have other somatic symptoms like nausea, vomiting, and fatigue. Once again, children starting as young as toddlerhood will likely notice many of these changes, and their reactions can vary based on age and temperament. One 4-year-old might be frightened to see a parent without hair, while another might love the way the parent's bald head feels and want to keep touching it. One of the best approaches for these sorts of changes is advanced preparation. Clinicians often talk about possible side effects and risks with patients, and some of these (especially those that are most likely to occur and are noticeable) can be explained to children by the parents in an age-appropriate way.

For example, if a father and his 10-year-old boy have a routine of shooting basketball hoops together, but the father lies on the couch watching TV for 2 days following chemotherapy without explanation, the son can begin to worry. He might think his father is angry with him or that he just does not want to play with him anymore; or he might think the cancer is getting worse and his father might die soon. On the other hand, the father could explain in advance that he will be tired for the 2 days following chemotherapy because the medicine is so strong, and he will not have energy to do the usual activities that he loves doing with his son. This could result in greater understanding and less distress for the son. In addition, the father can remind the son that he values their time together, that he cannot wait to resume their usual routines once he feels better again, and that one of the main reasons he is taking such strong medicine is to fight the cancer so that he can hopefully feel well more regularly. Similar advanced preparation is helpful for other changes in the parent's appearance and behavior.

Continuing honest, open, age-appropriate communication throughout active treatment is important and can readily flow once the children know the diagnosis and initial plan. Advanced preparation is part of this communication, but additional important components include providing children with health and treatment updates, asking what changes the children have noticed and how they feel about them, and asking the children if they have worries, concerns, or questions about what is happening. Parents are encouraged to welcome all questions warmly and positively. Children may give surprising responses and may have questions a parent has never thought about or cannot answer. To such questions, parents can say, "That's a great question, and I'm so glad you asked. I'm not sure of the answer right now. Let me think about it (or talk to the doctor, nurse, social worker, etc.) and get back to you."

Some parents also have concerns regarding their children's behavior during active treatment or other phases of survivorship. Some changes within a typical range might be expected when a parent is ill. A child who seems occasionally sadder or more nervous during a parent's illness, while remaining highly functional overall, is likely to be experiencing the normal range of emotions associated with a parent's illness. However, some significant changes in a child's mood or behavior may be a sign that the child is struggling to cope with the parent's illness. When changes are pronounced and prolonged, they may serve as warning signs for parents that the child needs additional support.

Development and temperament play a role in understanding behavior changes as well. A sensitive 8-year-old boy might become a bit clingy toward his mother while she is sick, which is not necessarily problematic. However, if he has trouble separating from her, stops wanting to go to school, or will not go over to friends' houses like he used to, he likely needs more help in coping during these times. An outgoing and social 16-year-old girl who seems to be spending more time with friends since her father became ill may be fine. However, if she begins breaking curfews, becomes increasingly isolated from family, or starts getting in trouble at school, she may be having difficulties dealing with her father's illness.

For children who are typically more stoic and less inclined to discuss their feelings, relative silence regarding the illness and their feelings about it can be common. In such cases, the child's behavior and functioning are often the main clues by which parents can gauge how well their child is coping. It is important that clinicians working with ill parents are familiar with local resources that can provide support for children when needed. Some sources for additional support may include schools, pediatricians, or community centers. If a child seems to be suffering from depression or anxiety, or has had a significant alteration in functional status, the child should be referred to a mental health professional. Risk-taking behavior or any safety concerns should also lead to an immediate mental health evaluation (Table 11.1).

During Remission

While achieving remission can be a great relief, it does not typically lead to an immediate dissolution of all worry or concern about cancer. Parents might continue to be vigilant about their physical health and monitor their bodies closely for any signs or symptoms of recurrent illness. Many will have ongoing concern about whether or not the cancer will return and will feel uncertain about the future.[9] Some parents might also wonder if their children are more likely to develop cancer because of their own history, and they might become increasingly sensitive to any symptoms the child has. The question of whether or not a child should have genetic testing also becomes relevant in certain cancers, and parents may have concerns or questions about this also. A referral to a genetic counselor may be helpful in thinking about the medical risks, but parents and clinicians should be mindful of the potential emotional and developmental impact on children that test results can have. Often, testing children is most helpful when results will have an impact on screening tests and treatment for them.[8] The pros, cons, and motivations for testing children should be carefully considered prior to testing.

TABLE 11.1   ∾   Referring a Child for Additional Help

When:

- The child's attitudes or mood seems different for a few weeks.
- The child's behavior, daily habits, or functioning at school, at home, or with friends has changed.
- The child is consistently having severe conflict with a parent.
- The child demonstrates signs of worsening or recurring difficulties from a pre-existing condition.
- The child requests additional support.
- The child has engaged in risky behaviors or there are other safety concerns, such as suicidal thoughts. If safety is a concern, an immediate evaluation is necessary.

By:

- Asking the child's pediatrician to recommend an appropriate mental health clinician.
- Calling the insurance plan to learn about clinicians available in the area.
- Requesting support from the child's school.
- Accessing local community support services. It is helpful for clinicians to know local resources that provide children with support.
- Having the child evaluated immediately (e.g., in an emergency room) when safety is a concern.

While still in the shadow of stress from a cancer diagnosis and its treatment, parents may feel an additional strain from the cycle of intermittent testing, waiting for results, and adjusting to the outcome during remission. The anticipatory anxiety and emotional ups and downs can be significant. Some parents worry that children perceive these fluctuations and may even have their own correlating emotional cycles. Keeping the children's schedules and household rules the same, despite approaching follow-up visits, can help to preserve a sense of routine and security for them.

Another potential stressor during the time of remission can occur if a parent decides to make a significant life change that affects the whole family. For example, a parent in remission may decide to take a job that is more meaningful but translates to a lower income. This parent may worry about the impact the decision will have on the children. However, children often inherently admire their parents and look to them for guidance. When parents anticipate and explain significant household changes to their children, they can often understand. Some children may prefer things the way they were prior to the changes, and it can be helpful for parents to learn what specific things each child misses and what compromises from the past and present may be established.

Some parents are also concerned when children have a hard time believing or accepting that they are feeling better. Children might continue to worry about the parent, citing the need for follow-up visits as justification for their apprehension. Parents in remission can tell children that the cancer is gone, but the doctors want to keep checking to make sure it stays away. Parents can let children know that they will continue to provide updates on their status and that the children will be informed of any changes. While reassuring children that there is no current worrisome news, it can be helpful to preemptively ask them how, when, where, and from whom they would like to hear any negative news if it were to occur.

After a Recurrence or a Secondary Cancer

Learning that cancer has returned or that a new cancer has occurred is news no patient wants to receive. Parents may have many of the same concerns and questions about what will happen to them and their children in this scenario as they did with the initial diagnosis. Some parents may experience even more stress related to a recurrence, because they may fear it means their ultimate prognosis is worse. Feelings of guilt or failure are also common.[10] Other parents, however, report that they are less anxious during recurrence,[11] and they may feel comforted by knowing what to expect. It is important for clinicians to keep in mind that the level of parental concern may or may not be directly related to the actual medical status or prognosis associated with the recurrence. Asking parents again about their concerns regarding themselves and their families is necessary at this phase, just as in previous phases, because concerns change over time and with shifting circumstances.

Ideally, parents will ask their children how they would like to hear potential bad news at a time when there is none, such as during remission or a phase of treatment when the parent is feeling well. This earlier discussion prepares the parents to deliver the news of a recurrence, or other bad news, in a manner that is most comfortable for each child individually. It is useful to know if a child away at college would like to wait a few weeks to hear difficult news if big exams are approaching, or if a junior high student would prefer to be told on a weekend evening when the family is all together. Some children will want to know immediately regardless of the circumstances, while others may want to hear only at certain times, in certain ways, from certain people. Respecting children's preferences allows them to receive bad news in a manner that may minimize secondary strain. However, if a parent's condition is worsening precipitously, it may not be possible to wait for the nearest opportune time, and children should be informed right away.

Parents and children alike may also wonder in what ways the recurrence or secondary cancer is the same as or different from the initial cancer. For example, sometimes the location of the tumor is different, which may result in a whole different set of symptoms for the parent. Parents and children may have worries about another round of treatment or the meaning of the recurrent or secondary cancer with regard to prognosis. Just as clinicians provide information to parents to help clarify these questions, parents should again be encouraged to communicate the facts surrounding recurrent or secondary illness to their children in an open, honest, and age-appropriate manner. Both an understanding of the cancer and a plan for next steps will be helpful for children.

End of Life

Cancer survivors who remain in remission may not have to face end-of-life issues prematurely. Other survivors, whose course with cancer and its treatment may be either swift or protracted, may face this difficult last phase of survivorship earlier than they and their families had hoped. Many parents wonder how to discuss death with their children and how to answer the question "Are you going to die?" This question can be difficult for so many reasons. The emotional distress parents may experience regarding thoughts of dying and leaving their children can seem overwhelming. Existential questions and issues of faith may also present greater challenges in this phase. There is the additional dilemma of explaining death and what comes thereafter to children of different ages in ways they can each understand. Because these concepts require abstract thinking, a child's understanding of death is significantly affected by his or her developmental stage. Preschoolers often think death is reversible and think a parent might return. Elementary school-aged children might understand death is permanent but might not comprehend the various layers of meaning and losses that will follow. Adolescents have the capacity to understand death in the complex way that adults do.[12]

When children ask about death, one of the first steps in answering the question is to try to clarify exactly what and why they are asking. A parent should attempt to learn what the question behind the question is. Asking, "What got you thinking about that?" can be a good way to begin clarification. A 4-year-old boy may really want to know who is going to read to him at night if his mother, who usually does this, is no longer there. A 15-year-old girl may wonder if the family will have to move if her dad dies and they can no longer afford the mortgage. Sometimes understanding the real question can allow parents to answer the underlying concern directly, without providing more details and complexities than the child actually wanted to know or can understand.

During the end-of-life stage of survivorship, parents often struggle again with a desire to protect their children, as well as a wish and need to prepare them. Even parents who are rated as good communicators by their children are not likely to disclose the probability of death.[13] It is important to point out to parents that, within uncertainty, being hopeful and optimistic can still coincide with being realistic and honest. Parents can start by establishing a safety zone of time in which the clinical team feels that death is unlikely. This safety zone can be shared with the child, which often helps to allay anxieties for that amount of time, even if cancer will be the most likely cause of the parent's death in the future. In such a case, a parent might say, "The treatments haven't worked as well as we hoped they would, and the doctors think I will eventually die from this cancer. But they don't think that will happen in the next month." Parents can also provide information about the most likely changes in their appearance and functioning that the children will observe in the coming days in order to prepare them.

Other practical worries that some parents have during this stage of survivorship are legal and financial. A single parent will need to ensure that formal custody plans are established and that each child has parental

figures in place. Financial documents should also be organized and reviewed by parents to ensure that they are accurate, up-to-date, and en-
trusted to another adult who can carry out the dying parent's wishes.
Children might also be wondering about these issues privately, and wel-
coming their questions about these topics is strongly encouraged. Even
if they have no specific questions, children can be reassured knowing
their physical and emotional needs will be met by specific adults. Some
children may even be mature enough and want to participate in making
some of these plans, such as which family member a 16-year-old son of
a single mother might live with when she dies.

There is also the issue of treatment decisions at this late stage of
survivorship, which can become complicated and increasingly difficult
to make. If additional treatment can possibly provide a cure, then parents can share that they are still trying to do everything they can to get
better and that they are following the clinicians' advice carefully. If the
treatment is palliative, parents can explain that additional treatment will
likely not cure them, but it can help to give their family more time together. Palliative treatment may also treat the parents' symptoms so
they can be more functional.

Each family has its own constellation of factors that affect the decision to end active treatment. It is important to note that being a parent
with children at home seems to be a factor that influences treatment decisions, and many parents are willing to trade quality of life to gain a
survival advantage.[14] Discussing the factors affecting a parent's treatment
at this stage can be helpful in elucidating his or her true worries and concerns. Sometimes clinicians recommend avoiding additional treatment
when it will provide neither additional quality of life nor extended survival and may only lead to detrimental side effects. Explaining when and
why treatment has ended to children is helpful, because many children
value knowing that their parent tried all reasonable treatments and actively sought healing.

Parents often struggle with decisions about hospice care and how
their choice might affect their children. Some parents worry that if they
choose to die at home, the children will be traumatized by the experience. Others worry that if they choose to die in an inpatient facility, they
will not be able to spend their last days in the comfort of home with their
family, and their children will not know what happened to them. There
is no easy answer to this question, and the right course depends on the

family and circumstances. Open communication and preparation, as well as consideration of the developmental stage and temperament of the children, are again helpful principles in making this decision. For a fearful, anxious 7-year-old girl, knowing that her father is dying in the bedroom next to her may be over-stimulating and scary despite communication and preparation. On the other hand, a cuddly 3-year-old boy might like to go into the bedroom to give his mother a hug even though she cannot hug back. He might accept the explanation that the brain cancer makes his mother sleepy all the time. When home hospice is chosen, it is best for the dying parent to be made comfortable in a bedroom or a room with a door that closes instead of a main living area so that the children can choose when they would like to visit.

Parents who are dying often express worries that their children will not know or remember them as they grow up. Long after a parent's death, however, many children can continue to benefit from appropriate and loving legacy gifts from the deceased parent, which serve as lasting memories. Letters, albums, videos, and similar personal items can be treasures when they express who the parent is, how much the child is loved, what the parent likes about parenting the child, and what specific traits and strengths the parent admires in the child. Designating family and friends who can retell the deceased parent's life story is a sort of living legacy to which children can return throughout their lives. As they continue to develop, children may have specific questions about a parent at different stages of life. Loved ones can often help to paint a detailed picture of the deceased parent's life story through shared experiences.

PRACTICAL TIPS FOR CLINICIANS

Clinicians who care for parents with cancer may find it challenging to address their parenting concerns for a variety of reasons. Some clinicians worry that asking parents about their children is too personal or irrelevant. Others may have concerns about not knowing what to ask, or how to respond to questions parents may have about their children. Others feel constrained by time, and worry that a conversation about a patient's children may open a "Pandora's Box" of feelings. While any host of challenges may exist for a given clinician, it is clear that most parents with cancer have concerns about how their illness might affect their children. These concerns may influence the psychosocial health of parents, and cancer's wide-reaching effects can touch the entire family—at times making additional support necessary. Therefore, clinicians who can overcome the challenges of addressing parenting concerns will be able to provide better, more complete care. The following practical tips are meant to assist clinicans in this process and to provide them with basic guidelines for approaching this discussion with parents.

1. Ask if a patient has children. This question should be considered part of routine screening. As with many screening questions, a "yes" should prompt the clinician to ask additional follow-up questions. The clinician can start with trying to learn a little about each child from the parent's perspective. Asking about age, temperament, coping style, hobbies, school, activities, social scene, and so forth can be helpful information to the clinician in assessing a child's overall functional status. Parents often hesitate to initiate conversations about family with their clinicians even though a vast majority would like to talk about this.[15] A clinician's efforts to discuss a patient's family can help to build a deeper alliance with each parent. Being a parent may also drive treatment decisions, such as an increased willingness to trade quality of life for a survival advantage,[14] which is important information for clinicians.

2. Encourage parents to communicate with their children throughout the course of survivorship. As members of the family, children will have a vested interest in how a parent's illness is progressing. Children deserve to know age-appropriate, honest information about the illness, and open communication from parents is the best way for them to hear it. This communication enhances trust, security, and cohesion within the family, which are all essential during these difficult circumstances. Children should be encouraged to ask their parents any and all questions. Trying to determine what children are really asking can help parents understand their children's needs. If a specific answer is unknown, parents can validate the question, let the child know they will seek the answer, and then return to the child with more information.

3. Consider each child's developmental stage and individual temperament. This practice is extremely important when providing guid-

ance for parents because these key concepts will inform how a child understands and processes information about the parent's illness and what types of support are likely to be most helpful. These concepts also help clinicians to differentiate between typical, expected responses from children and those that may require additional evaluation.

4. Recommend that parents maintain the routine structure and schedule for their children. Children generally feel more secure and relaxed when they know what to expect. Sometimes, families may need to call in reinforcements for this to happen, such as additional help with carpooling for the adolescent soccer player, or a close friend or relative who can act as a babysitter on a regular basis for the energetic toddler.

5. Help parents optimize the family's support system. Parents who are well supported are better able to adhere to treatment and are better able to support their children. There are many available resources through which parents can obtain support. Clinicians can facilitate referrals to social workers, support groups, online blogs, reading materials, clergy, therapists, and psychiatrists. Clinicians can also encourage parents and families to ask others for help, letting them know that support is available and appropriate to use during such challenging times.

6. Encourage the family to establish an organized system for friends and loved ones to contribute in a way that is not overwhelming or intrusive. Having uninterrupted family time is essential and can be difficult when well-intending supporters are often calling or coming by.

7. Ask parents directly whether they have any concerns about how a child is doing. This question can be useful in determining if a child may need additional support. If a child's typical functioning has declined, such as school performance, athletic participation, social interest, behavior, attitude, mood, appetite, or sleep, then additional support may be needed. Problems in these areas can be signs that the child's usual coping mechanisms are overwhelmed. Clinicians can seek additional assistance for children from a variety of sources, such as child mental health specialists, pediatricians, and schools (Table 11.2).

TABLE 11.2   ∽   Practical Tips for Clinicians

- Screen for children who depend on the patient.
- Encourage honest, age-appropriate communication with all children in the family.
- Consider development and temperament.
- Recommend maintaining the usual routine and structure as much as possible.
- Optimize and organize the family's support system.
- Screen for at-risk children, and refer as appropriate.

CONCLUSION

The number of patients with cancer who are also parents of children living at home is significant and growing. Having children at home can add stress to the extremely challenging circumstances of having cancer throughout the course of survivorship. Many parents who have cancer have a primary concern about how their children will be affected by their illness. Having children may affect a parent's distress level and treatment decisions. Therefore, learning whether or not a patient has children is an essential piece of a complete psychosocial assessment. The Institute of Medicine recommends initial psychosocial assessment and care, as well as follow-up reevaluation and adjustment in services as needed throughout a cancer survivor's course.[16] It follows that asking about a parent's children should be done routinely. Such a practice not only benefits parents who are the primary patients but also could identify and triage children having difficulties to appropriate sources of additional support.

Many of the common concerns and questions parents have during the course of cancer survivorship have been addressed, as have some of the best practices and guidelines for how to manage them. While the challenges are substantial, families facing these circumstances can be extremely resilient. Clinicians can play a key role in bolstering the inherent resiliency of parents and children by fostering communication, preparedness, and continued cohesion within the family and encouraging the seeking and organization of outside supports. Many families share the sense that the lessons learned while standing together through cancer survivorship provide valuable guiding principles for facing additional challenges throughout their lives.

Acknowledgments

Cynthia W. Moore, PhD, Anna C. Muriel, MD, MPH, Susan S. Swick, MD, MPH, and Stephen Durant, EdD

REFERENCES

1. National Cancer Institute. *National Health Interview Survey. Division of Cancer Control and Population Sciences.* Washington, DC: Office of Cancer Survivorship; 1992.
2. Bloom JR, Kessler L. Risk and timing of counseling and support interventions for younger women with breast cancer. *J Natl Cancer Inst Monogr.* 1994;16:199–206.
3. Beardslee WR, Versage EM, Gladstone TRG. Children of affectively ill parents: a review of the past 10 years. *J Am Acad Child Adolesc Psychiatry.* 1998;37(11):1134–1141.
4. Burke L. The impact of maternal depression on familial relationships. *Int Rev Psychiatry.* 2003;15:243–255.
5. Rosenheim E, Reicher R. Informing children about a parent's terminal illness. *J Child Psychol Psychiatry.* 1985;26:995–998.
6. Braun M, Mikulincer M, Rydall A, Walsh A, Rodin G. Hidden morbidity in cancer: spouse caregivers. *J Clin Oncol.* 2007;25(30):4829–4834.
7. Northouse LL, Mood DW, Montie JE, et al. Living with prostate cancer: patients' and spouses' psychosocial status and quality of life. *J Clin Oncol.* 2007;25(27):4171–4177.
8. Rauch PK, Muriel AC. *Raising an Emotionally Healthy Child When a Parent Is Sick.* New York, NY: McGraw-Hill; 2006.
9. Lee-Jones C, Humphris G, Dixon R, Hatcher MB. Fear of cancer recurrence—a literature review and cognitive formulation to explain exacerbation of recurrence fears. *Psycho-Oncol.* 1997;6(2):95–105.
10. Mahon SM, Cella DF, Donovan MI. Psychosocial adjustment to recurrent cancer. *Oncol Nurs Forum.* 1990;17(suppl 3):47–52.
11. Yang HC, Thornton LM, Shapiro CL, Andersen BL. Surviving recurrence: psychological and quality-of-life recovery. *Cancer.* 2008;112(5): 1178–1187.
12. Muriel AC, Rauch PK. Talking with families and children about the death of a parent. In: Hanks G, Cherny N, Kaasa S, Portenoy R, Christakis N, Fallon M, eds. *Oxford Textbook of Palliative Medicine.* 4th ed., Section 7. UK: Oxford University Press. In press.

13. Siegel K, Raveis V, Karus D. Patterns of communication with children when a parent has cancer. In: Baider L, Cooper C, Kaplan DeNour A, eds. *Cancer in the Family.* Chichester, England: John Wiley & Sons, Ltd; 1996:109–128.

14. Yellen SB, Cella DF. Someone to live for: social well-being, parenthood status, and decision-making in oncology. *J Clin Oncol.* 1995;13:1255–1264.

15. Detmar SB, Aaronson NK, Wever LDV, Muller M, Schornagel JH. How are you feeling? Who wants to know? Patients' and oncologists' preferences for discussing health-related quality-of-life issues. *J Clin Oncol.* 2000;18:3295–3301.

16. Institute of Medicine of The National Academies. *Cancer Care for the Whole Patient: Meeting Psychosocial Health Needs.* Washington, DC: National Academies Press; October 2007.

12

Family and Caregivers of Cancer Survivors: Being a Strengthened Ally— A Community Perspective

Mitch Golant, PhD

&

Natalie V. Haskins, MAT

ABSTRACT

Patient care has changed significantly over the past 10 years. In a recent survey of over 500 people with cancer, 61% continued working while in treatment.[1] Moreover, hospital stays are shorter due to an increased demand on cancer resources, specifically doctors and nurses. Today, nearly 85% of cancer patients are being treated in community-based medical facilities. However nationally, most research and survivorship centers are located at large, comprehensive cancer centers designated by the National Cancer Institute.[2] There is tremendous need for supportive care services to be delivered where patients are actually receiving treatment. The good news is survivorship rates are increasing, and cancer patients are living longer, fuller lives.

INTRODUCTION

The trend toward community-based medical facilities, shorter hospital stays, and growing survivorship rates is creating a burden on family caregivers—spouses, children, friends, partners, parents, siblings—the people who are on the frontlines battling cancer alongside their diagnosed loved one. This chapter focuses on the *primary* caregiver (the person who is directly involved with providing care) to a loved one affected by cancer.

To understand the context in which this information will be presented, it is important to understand what The Wellness Community (TWC) is. Founded in 1982, TWC is a free program of psychosocial support for cancer patients and their families that now exists in 24 locations as well as abroad and on the Internet through The Wellness Community Online. All programs at TWC are provided free of charge and are facilitated by an array of healthcare professionals that includes social workers, psychotherapists, nurses, and psychologists.

The Wellness Community addresses the needs of caregivers along with those of their loved ones with cancer. We include caregiver information in patient education materials and programs, as well as through weekly support groups specifically for caregivers. Interestingly, on average our brick-and-mortar facilities provide four patient support groups for every one caregiver group. On the other hand, online at TWC Online there is a 2 to 1 ratio of patient to caregiver groups.

Why is there such a significant difference in the ratio of caregiver support groups online versus face-to-face? This question is a profoundly important one for us to consider and will be answered by this chapter and by the results of our two surveys that explore cancer in the workplace and cancer caregiving. But, perhaps this is due, in part, to the profound changes in health care over the last 10 years. As caregiver burden increases, access to care through these emerging technologies is one way to address patients' needs.

CAREGIVING IS STRESSFUL

Cancer survivorship rates are increasing and leading more medical professionals to approach it as a chronic disease. Depending on the stage of the disease and treatment, this approach requires more long-term treatment and presents numerous physical and psychological demands on patients and their caregivers. Diminishment in the patient's functional ability, organ function, appearance, career, family and social role, and self-image directly impacts the caregiver. Advances in screening create earlier diagnosis, improvements in treatment, and increased survival rates and the trend toward outpatient treatment. As a result, informal caregivers are likely to provide more complex care for a longer period of time.[3]

Most research analyzes caregiving along a continuum of physical, emotional, social, and/or economic demands based upon the specific needs of the patient. The demands are not sequential and may burden the caregiver all at once or selectively, depending on the most pressing needs of the patient.[4,5]

According to many researchers, a caregiver's burden is also linked to one of three specific phases in the cancer experience.[6] During the initial or acute phase, the family—caregiver(s) and patient—are under siege. They are active as a unit to adjust to the diagnosis. The chronic phase follows, wherein primary treatment has been administered and the patient is dismissed from the hospital. Caregivers are left to take on additional responsibilities in this phase; some are complex, such as supporting outpatient treatment protocol, and others may be simple but tedious, such as more housework, errands, and new transportation routines. The final phase is resolution, when the family must begin the survivorship or bereavement process.[3]

For many cancer patients, the most significant psychosocial stressors are unwanted aloneness, loss of control, and loss of hope. **Unwanted aloneness** occurs at the time of diagnosis—just imagine what it feels like when a patient hears the words from the doctor, "You have cancer." In effect, not only do patients feel different from others in their social network, but this experience also may create shifts in intimacy between them and the family caregiver. **Loss of control** is often reflected in feelings of helplessness, especially when patients realize that cancer is in their bodies and are unsure of the right course of treatment when faced with conflicting treatment options. **Loss of hope** is associated with the ups and downs of treatment and the side effects from treatment (fatigue, pain, and nausea) and is especially likely when one receives bad news.

Caregivers face parallel challenges. However, too often caregivers do not find outlets to express these anxieties, and instead emotions are suppressed and can create a divide or resentment toward the loved one with cancer. As one participant in an online caregiver group put it, "[Sometimes I feel] as though [my] whole life revolves around his illness and I don't matter except to take care of him." Over the 26 years that TWC has been providing support services to cancer patients and their caregivers, we have learned that sharing these concerns with others in a safe, supportive group setting helps to normalize feelings and concerns.

In a longitudinal study involving cancer patients and their spouses (who are often the primary caregivers), Oberst and James showed that while patient distress did diminish over time, that of the caregiver did not.[7] Janice Kiecolt-Glaser and Ronald Glaser of Ohio State University presented a study to The National Academy of Sciences that found a critical chemical pathway through which the human immune system is weakened by chronic stress.[8] This study reinforced earlier research that showed long-term caregivers suffer from impaired immunity for as long as 3 years after their caregiving role ended, suggesting that people who care for those with chronic illnesses such as cancer are at an increased risk for developing their own serious health problems.[8]

OUR RESEARCH FINDINGS

In May 2007, TWC, in conjunction with KRC Research, conducted a national online survey of 202 cancer patients, survivors, and caregivers (137 interviews with cancer patients/survivors; 65 interviews with caregivers) to gain insight into the specific stressors and concerns caregivers face when caring for a loved one. Sixty-eight percent of cancer patients stated their spouse or partner was their primary caregiver. Nearly three-quarters (73%) reported receiving assistance from a caregiver on a daily basis. Twenty percent of caregivers reported being a caregiver for more than 4 years, and 61% were caring for cancer patients with advanced or metastatic cancer.[9]

Eight in ten cancer patients/survivors and caregivers agree that patients were able to focus on their treatment because their caregiver took on additional responsibilities. In addition, respondents agreed that caregivers provide support in a variety of ways that are invaluable to the well-being of the cancer patient (Table 12.1).

However, these additional responsibilities are taxing on the caregiver's own well-being. Survivors/patients and caregivers differed in

TABLE 12.1 The Roles of a Caregiver

	Cancer Patients/ Survivors	Caregivers
		% Complete/Significant/Some Involvement
Providing emotional support	93% (58% complete involvement)	100% (69% complete involvement)
Providing transportation	92% (33% complete involvement)	84% (39% complete involvement)
Preparing meals	88% (26% complete involvement)	90% (36% complete involvement)
Performing household chores	86% (28% complete involvement)	95% (37% complete involvement)
Providing financial assistance	68% (39% complete involvement)	59% (23% complete involvement)
Managing or overseeing finances	57% (32% complete involvement)	70% (33% complete involvement)

their assessment of caregivers' level of difficulty in balancing their personal lives (Table 12.2). Cancer patients/survivors were divided as to whether their caregivers regularly experienced personal distress. Nearly half believed their caretakers felt regular distress during their cancer experience (49%), while 45% did not believe their caregivers suffered any regular distress. In stark contrast, 80% of caregivers said they personally experienced regular distress throughout the cancer experience.

While the gap may be startling, it does explain why caregivers are just as likely to report being treated for depression and anxiety as cancer patients and survivors. More than three in ten cancer patients and sur-

TABLE 12.2 ∽ Impact of Caregiving on Caregivers' Personal Lives

	Cancer Patients/ Survivors	Caregivers
	% Extremely/Very/Somewhat difficult for caregivers	
Personal routines	47% (53% not too or not at all difficult)	**84%** (16% not too or not at all difficult)
Friendships	31% (69% not too or not at all difficult)	**73%** (27% not too or not at all difficult)
Physical health	28% (72% not too or not at all difficult)	**80%** (20% not too or not at all difficult)
Career	27% (73% not too or not at all difficult)	**73%** (27% not too or not at all difficult)
Family relationships	28% (72% not too or not at all difficult)	**50%** (50% not too or not at all difficult)
Financial status	23% (77% not too or not at all difficult)	**40%** (46% not too or not at all difficult)
Emotional stability	N/A	**87%** (13% not too or not at all difficult)

vivors report being treated for depression (34%) and anxiety (37%) during their cancer experience, which is nearly equal to the number of caregivers seeking treatment (29% for depression; 31% for anxiety). Perhaps as an explanation of these numbers, caregivers report feeling many of the same anxieties cancer patients do upon diagnosis and treatment (Table 12.3).

Caregiver and cancer patient similarities are reflected in the workplace as well. A 2006 survey conducted by Fleishman-Hillard Research and developed in close collaboration with the National Coalition for

TABLE 12.3 Rankings for the Most Stressful Aspects for Caregivers According to Caregivers and as Observed by Cancer Patients and Survivors

	Cancer Patients/ Survivors	Caregivers
	% Ranked 1 of top 3 most stressful aspects for the caregiver	
Anxiety and nervousness	49%	48%
Maintaining a strong front	*41%*	*56%*
Financial burden	31%	7%
Depression	31%	29%
Sleep deprivation	19%	20%
Lack of personal time	18%	18%
Feeling alone	*7%*	*51%*
Did not observe/ have any caregiver stress	*48%*	*31%*

Cancer Survivorship and TWC investigated the effects of cancer on the careers of cancer patients/survivors and caregivers.[1] The online survey was administered to more than 1,000 people affected by cancer (504 working patients and 500 working caregivers). The study is especially relevant to today's cancer patients, who with shortened hospital stays and the rising cost of health care tend to work throughout their cancer experience. Sixty-eight percent of patients reported that they kept working to keep their healthcare coverage. The study found that cancer patients and caregivers face nearly identical career challenges and make similar career sacrifices. More than 80% of patients and caregivers indicated that they missed some work as a result of fighting cancer, and both groups reported working fewer hours per week on average (Figure 12.1).

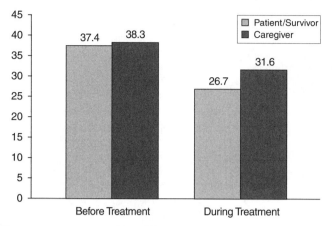

FIGURE 12.1 Average number of hours worked per week before treatment and during treatment.

Nearly half (48%) of caregivers admitted additional responsibilities had some impact on their ability to do their job, and one-fourth (28%) said their caregiver duties had a major impact on their ability to do their job. Caregivers are just as likely—and in some cases more likely—than patients to take days off without pay or to leave early from work (Figure 12.2).

It may come as no surprise that the challenges and sacrifices reflected in our research and supported by the survey data not only affect caregivers' own well-being but also can undermine their best efforts to

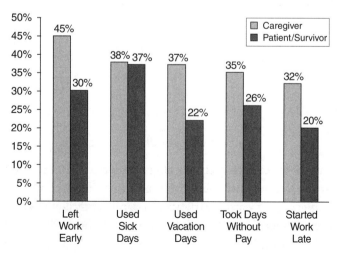

FIGURE 12.2 Actions taken during treatment.

help their loved ones through the cancer journey. It is important to note here that TWC was founded upon the Patient Active Concept, which states, "Patients who participate in their fight for recovery along with their healthcare team, rather than acting as hopeless, helpless, passive victims of the illness, will improve the quality of their lives and may enhance the possibility of recovery." The Wellness Community's Patient Active Concept applies to both patients/survivors and their families, specifically their caregivers. Just as we encourage patients to be proactive in managing their illness, in our caregiver support groups we teach participants to actively cope with their stress.

MANAGING BURNOUT

When counseling caregivers to cope with the demands of their role, we focus on navigating them away from burnout, which is a common occurrence for caregivers. According to burnout expert Dr. Herbert J. Freudenberger, common physical symptoms include headaches, insomnia, backaches, lethargy, lingering colds, gastrointestinal upsets, or cardiovascular problems. Burnout is signaled by emotional components as well, including frustration, anger, insecurity, resentment, and depression.[10] It is critical that caregivers understand that while managing their own stress may seem secondary to the immediate needs of their loved ones with cancer, at some point they must make their own well-being a priority. Before caregivers can be helpful to their loved ones, they need to know how to cope with their own stress.

At TWC we empower caregivers to become strengthened allies (Table 12.4). As strengthened allies, caregivers can provide support through self-care and knowledge, a notion that is reflected in the Patient Active Concept.[11]

CAREGIVER SUPPORT ONLINE

A recent study of the effects of training caregivers in coping skills, not unlike the strategies in Table 12.4, found that family members of a hospice patient with cancer experienced significantly higher quality of life when they employed an active intervention. Despite high levels of interest in support services, it can be extremely difficult for caregivers and family members to attend face-to-face services.[12] In 2003, TWC

TABLE 12.4   ∾   Becoming a Strengthened Ally

- *Get Support.* Join a support group. Research shows that talking to people who share your problems reduces stress and alleviates isolation.

- *Educate Yourself.* Information is power. Understanding the course of cancer, the possibility of relapse, the recommended treatments, and the side effects of medications can help you plan for the future.

- *Keep a Journal.* That's where you can dialogue with yourself to vent frustrations and problem-solve without causing conflict.

- *Maintain Friendships.* Continue contacts with friends and family despite a loved one's illness.

- *Preserve Routines.* Retain as much control over the routines of life as is reasonable.

- *Continue with Hobbies.* Don't abandon favorite pastimes that always give you pleasure.

- *Make Plans for the Future.* Then there is a future in your future.

- *Remember That Life Goes On.* You are a separate person and are entitled to enjoy your own life. Attend classes, start a hobby, go to a movie, make new friends.

- *Learn to "Let Go."* Allow yourself to feel replenished by others' gestures—a card or a kind word left on your answering machine. Music, religious services, or a video can also help you recharge your batteries.

- *Seek Respite.* Realize that you can't do it all. Allow others to do some caring in your stead. Reach out to them.

- *Attend to Your Physical Health.* Eat well and get enough sleep. Tend to any physical ailments that arise.

- *Trigger the Relaxation Response.* Biofeedback, meditation, yoga, listening to music, even washing your car can relieve stress. By focusing on breathing, you trigger the mind–body connection.

- *Deal with Frustration.* A short fuse can be a sign of burnout. You may need more emotional support such as a support group or private therapist.

- *Self-Care and Setting Limits.* Identify when you're feeling overwhelmed and be firm in delineating what you can and can't do.

launched The Wellness Community Online (TWC Online) and began offering online support groups for caregivers who were either too burdened by their mounting caregiver responsibilities or too far from brick-and-mortar facilities to attend face-to-face support groups.

Joining an online support group is a simple, but thorough process. First, caregivers must fill out an online registration form with TWC Online that includes a diagnosis confirmation. Upon proper registration, caregivers participate in a 15- to 30-minute telephone interview with a trained member of our staff. During this brief interview, expectations and goals for participation are discussed. Interviewees are also screened for any psychological problems that may hinder the success of the group as a whole. They then receive literature on the nature of the groups, the TWC philosophy, and a disclaimer explaining that the groups are supportive and educational and are not a substitute for psychotherapy (there is no doctor–patient relationship). Once they have been approved, their final application is sent to the group facilitator, who prepares to integrate new participants into their first meeting.

The online support groups are password secured and are offered weekly for 90 minutes. The caregivers are in a modified chat room setting. The facilitators chosen to lead the groups are all professionals in psychosocial oncology, with an average of 10 years' experience leading face-to-face groups in our brick-and-mortar facilities. In a recent update to the site, participants can now indicate their level of distress on a distress thermometer at the beginning of each session and again at the end. This feature helps facilitators decide to whom they need to be attentive during a session and with whom they may need to follow up after a session. Participants can also use emoticons to express their fluctuating emotions throughout the session.

Because these online support groups are text-based, transcripts are key in measuring their value. From these thousands of transcripts, we have learned, similar to other research findings, that caregivers do not have the time, geographical proximity, or resources to attend a face-to-face support group elsewhere. For example, a young mother warned her fellow participants that some of her text may turn into gibberish when the infant on her lap occasionally reached out to pound on the keyboard. Another woman commented that she could be in group for no more than 30 minutes while a hospice nurse watched over her dying husband. Other participants noted that they might be pulled away from the session when their loved one is feeling particularly ill.[13]

Above all, the transcripts confirmed that the benefits of face-to-face support groups extended to online groups. This result can best be appreciated by reviewing a sample group transcript. The transcript below (Table 12.5) puts into context the feelings of the caregiver mentioned earlier (who admitted she sometimes felt like everything revolved around her husband's illness and that she only mattered in her role as a caregiver). In it you will notice the level of trust members have built with one another.

TABLE 12.5 ∽ Online Caregiver Group Transcript (from TVWC)

Participant 1 (Maggie): Jane [the Facilitator], if I might segue to a new subject—I find myself intensely angry at my husband. He is doing really well, but because my life has been turned upside down, I am finding myself so resentful. Is anyone else feeling this way?

Participant 2 (Rita): While things are good at the moment, I have felt that way . . . as though our whole life revolves around his illness and I don't matter except to take care of him. Fortunately, it doesn't last long for me.

Participant 3 (Ken): I feel that way too.

Participant 4 (Marcia): I was pretty resentful last week when I wasn't able to be here.

Facilitator (Jane): That's a strong thing that Rita said—"as though our whole life revolves around his illness and I don't matter except to take care of him." Sounds like you all feel that way sometimes.

Participant 1: My husband decided to retire when he found out about his illness. I had a part-time career and just let it go. The first few months have been so chaotic, but things have returned to normal, but I am not sure of my husband's expectations.

Participant 4: His expectations with regard to what?????

Participant 5: What do you mean?

Participant 3: You should ask him.

Participant 1: I also feel my whole life revolves around his illness. I have asked him but it is hard to get a clear answer. I am a very independent person and traveled both with him and with friends. I am having to figure out how to redefine my life while he is feeling well.

Facilitator: Is it important for all of you to also know what your expectations are—not just your loved one's?

Participant 1: That's it Jane! What are my expectations? I am trying to figure that out.

Participant 4: When we found out that the experimental drug had shrunk my husband's tumors, everyone was ecstatic but me, it seemed. I thought, well this is just great—I've been trying to figure out how we are going to get through this and now it looks like things are better. I've prepared myself for the worst and now what am I supposed to do?

Participant 3: This also goes back to our other conversation where we talked about taking care of ourselves too. If you give up what is important to you, your feelings of resentment and anger will only get worse.

Facilitator: Do you all feel it is okay for you to have expectations?

Participant 2: Personally, I feel that my life is in a holding pattern, since we can't make long-term plans or dream too far ahead.

Participant 4: Yes, everything is on hold . . . waiting to see what happens. My nephew is getting married in October, and I don't know if we will be able to go.

Facilitator: Like, it's a longer haul than you expected?

Participant 4: I don't think my husband will be able to go, but my daughter wants to. I don't think I'll be able to leave him.

Facilitator: In the deepest part of your heart, are there moments for any of you when you just want it to all be over?

Participant 4: And you're wondering how long you are going to have to deal with the most horrible thing in the world.

Participant 2: Yes, although I never admit it to anyone. Now that my husband is doing well, I don't think that way as much.

Participant 3: I want my mom to get well so it's all over but not if I have to lose her.

(continues)

TABLE 12.5 ∾ Online Caregiver Group Transcript (from TVWC) (*continued*)

> **Participant 4:** Rita, I don't think you are feeling or thinking anything that we all haven't felt at one time or another.
>
> **Facilitator:** What trust, Rita, to share that with us—a tribute to this group.
>
> **Participant 2:** When this started again for the 3rd time and his time looked short and so dismal, I felt so guilty for just wanting it to be over fast. Some of the thinking was that I didn't want him to suffer, but some of it was also that I just didn't know how much longer I could deal with it. Thankfully, those feelings have passed, he's feeling good, and for now, his treatments are working to buy him more time.
>
> **Participant 1:** Not being sure how much time my husband has and despite the fact he is feeling well, I feel compelled to put his needs first and then I am angry.
>
> **Facilitator:** I suspect that all of you have practical solutions to these kinds of situations but get stuck in wondering if it is okay to think about yourselves and have needs—yes?
>
> **Participant 4:** Yes.

This transcript also supports our research and survey findings that caregivers often put their well-being second to that of their loved ones who have cancer. Outside of this very sacred space in their support groups, most caregivers would cringe if you referred to their caregiving role as a burden or even a responsibility. Their love for their ill family member fuels support, energy, and hope for recovery.

CONCLUSION

While this chapter highlights the challenges of caregiving, it is important to remember the opportunity cancer can bring to some families. As one caregiver explained to us:

My father's terminal brain cancer diagnosis was an opportunity for tremendous growth for my family. Throughout my life, my dad traveled weekly and usually only came home 2 weekends a month. He was proactive in his battle and relished the opportunity to coach Little League, pick us up from school, and spend the summer traveling with us to distant friends and family. Partnering with our doctor, Ruth Fredericks, he defied expectations and lived 2½ years beyond his initial diagnosis. As caregivers, we were grateful for the opportunity to fight along with him and grow closer as a family.

In 2007, TWC created a space where cancer patients can show their support and appreciation for their inspiring caregivers. The Star Campaign (www.starcampaign.org) is a Web-driven initiative that gives cancer patients and survivors the opportunity to honor and recognize caregivers—the "stars" in their lives who have supported them during their cancer experience, be it family member, doctor, social worker, friend, nurse, or neighbor.

The following is an excerpt from a tribute of one of our participants, a cancer survivor attending support groups in a brick-and-mortar facility, who honored her husband (Table 12.6). This tribute demonstrates how families can become stronger in the face of cancer.

TABLE 12.6 Excerpt from Star Campaign Walk of Fame

I have been diagnosed with cancer three times in the past 23½ years, stage III ovarian cancer in November of 1983, a reoccurrence in October of 1993 and breast cancer in September of 2005. I am very blessed to have my husband Mike as my STAR through all these years.

I believe one of the hardest things caretakers have to do is sit in waiting rooms while their loved one is in surgery. Over the years, I have had 5 major and several minor surgeries in connection with cancer. My STAR has spent too many apprehensive hours waiting for information from surgeons. The surgeon did not have an optimistic prognosis after my first surgery in 1983. Back then, it was almost unheard of to survive ovarian cancer unless caught early and my diagnosis was stage III. Mike remembers thinking I had only 6 months to live. I can only imagine how devastating it must have been for him, but he never let me see his heartache.

I have had 18 chemo treatments in 22 years and my STAR was there giving me comfort through all of them. Mike had to work during the day, but he would come to the hospital every evening with a smile on his face and cheer me up. They did not have effective drugs for nausea in those early years of chemo so eating was difficult. Whenever I felt I could eat something, even if it were midnight, he would go out and get me a milkshake. Sometimes milkshakes were the only thing that tasted good and stayed down . . .

(continues)

TABLE 12.6 ∽   Excerpt from Star Campaign Walk of Fame (*continued*)

> There have been many other STARS in my life. I am very fortunate to have many other family members and friends who are STARS and contributed to my recovery. I will be forever grateful to all of them . . .
>
> *Source:* Star Campaign Walk of Fame (www.starcampaignorg/star)

REFERENCES

1. Fleishman-Hillard Research, National Coalition for Cancer Survivorship, and The Wellness Community. Breakaway from Cancer Survey. Breakaway from Cancer Web site. http://www.breakawayfromcancer.com. Published October 2006. Accessed July 8, 2007.
2. NCI Office of Cancer Survivorship. Cancer Survivorship Research. National Cancer Institute Web site. http://cancercontrol.cancer.gov/ocs/index.html. Updated May 23, 2008. Accessed November 20, 2008.
3. Nijboer C, Tempelaar R, Sanderman R, et al. Patterns of caregiver experiences among partners of cancer patients. *Gerontologist.* 2000;40(6):738–746.
4. Given CW, Given B, Stommel M, Collins C, King S, Franklin S. The Caregiver Reaction Assessment (CRA) for caregivers to persons with chronic physical and mental impairments. *Res Nurs Health.* 1992;15:271–283.
5. Siegel K, Raveis VH, Houts P, Mor V. Caregiver burden and unmet patient needs. *Cancer.* 1991;68:1131–1140.
6. Northouse L, Stetz KM. A longitudinal study of the adjustment of patients and husbands to breast cancer. *Oncol Nurs Forum.* 1989;16:511–516.
7. Oberst MT, James RH. Going home: patient and spouse adjustment following cancer surgery. *Top Clin Nurs.* 1985;7:46–57.
8. Kiecolt-Glaser J, Glaser R. Mechanism Found That Weakens Caregivers' Immune Status. The Ohio State University Research News Web site. http://researchnews.osu.edu/archive/glaserpnas.htm. Updated June 26, 2003. Accessed November 20, 2008.
9. KRC Research and The Wellness Community (May 2007). The Star Campaign Caregiver Survey. Star Campaign Web site. http://www.starcampaign.org/News/resources.php. Accessed November 20, 2008.
10. Golant M, Golant S. *What to Do When Someone You Love Is Depressed?* 2nd ed. New York: Henry Holt and Company; 2007.
11. Golant M. Your role as strengthened ally. In: *Coping with Cancer.* March/April 2002:34.

12. Ostroff J, Ross S, Steinglass P, Ronis-Tobin V, Singh B. Interest in and barriers to participation in multiple family groups among head and neck cancer survivors and their primary family caregivers. *Fam Process*. 2004;43: 195–208.

13. Golant M, Lieberman M, Gessert A, Owen J. Online support groups for caregivers of patients with cancer and Parkinson's disease. In: Talley R, ed. *Building Community Caregiving Capacity*. UK: Oxford University Press; 2007. In press.

PART

3

Epidemiologic Issues

chapter

13

Physical Activity and Breast Cancer Prevention and Prognosis

Melinda L. Irwin, PhD, MPH

ABSTRACT

Observational studies demonstrate that women who exercise have a lower risk of getting breast cancer and dying from breast cancer compared to sedentary women. This chapter discusses the observational and mechanistic studies of physical activity and breast cancer risk/ prognosis and strategies for improving physical activity after a cancer diagnosis.

INTRODUCTION

Breast cancer is the most frequently diagnosed cancer among American women (217,000 new cases in 2005), and incidence rates continue to rise.[1] Approximately 39,000 women in the United States die of breast cancer each year, and an estimated 2.3 million breast cancer survivors in the United States alone are living with the long-term and late effects of the disease.[1] Although advances in therapy have led to improvements in survival in recent years, new therapies are costly, are associated with significant side effects, and may benefit only subsets of those with breast cancer. Alternative approaches are needed to help diminish the morbidity and mortality of breast cancer, as well as its cost to society.

Multiple observational studies over the past 20 years, coming from North America, Europe, Asia, and Australia, have demonstrated that women who exercise regularly have a decreased risk of developing breast cancer compared to sedentary women.[2] This association has been observed in various racial/ethnic minorities as well as in non-Hispanic white women.[2] The evidence for the association between higher levels of physical activity and lower risk of breast cancer has been classified as "convincing," with the degree of protection estimated at about 30% to 40% with 3 to 4 hours per week of moderate- to vigorous-intensity physical activity, such as brisk walking.[2] Furthermore, recent findings from two large prospective cohort studies (also observational) show that women who are physically active after a breast cancer diagnosis are at an approximate 50% lower risk of a recurrence and death due to breast cancer.[3,4] Numerous observational studies also have demonstrated that obesity and weight gain adversely affect primary and secondary breast cancer risk, adding further validity to the hypothesis that physical activity, one of the critical components of energy balance, influences breast cancer risk and prognosis.[3–5]

Given that women who are more physically active after diagnosis may have been similarly active before diagnosis, these studies cannot exclude the possibility that physically active individuals who develop breast cancer acquire tumors that are biologically less aggressive. Therefore, being physically active prior to diagnosis may have been associated with a later diagnosis of breast cancer or earlier disease stage. However, one study examined change in physical activity from before to after breast cancer diagnosis, with an observed improved prognosis associated with increasing physical activity[4]. This finding emphasizes the importance of also participating in physical activity after a diagnosis of breast cancer to gain the maximum benefits of physical activity on survival.

While observational studies have provided an important base of evidence for inferring that physical activity has a protective benefit against breast cancer development, these studies cannot, by definition, show a protective "effect" of physical activity against breast cancer development. At this point, clinical trials are needed to determine whether the independent effect of physical activity prevents the primary and secondary occurrence of breast cancer[1]; clinical trials would also help elucidate the biological mechanisms by which physical activity protects healthy women from developing breast cancer and prevents breast cancer survivors from experiencing recurrence and breast cancer-related mortality.[5] To date, no human intervention studies have examined the effect of physical activity on primary and secondary breast cancer prevention. Conducting such a trial presents many challenges, including the need for a very large sample size, long study duration, and participation from multiple research institutes. Nevertheless, The Women's Health Initiative Trial provides a model for such a study and suggests that such an undertaking is feasible.[6] In addition, two large National Institutes of Health-funded multi-center clinical trials, the Women's Healthy Eating and Living Study and the Women's Intervention Nutrition Study, further demonstrate the feasibility of lifestyle intervention trials in this population.[7,8] Both of these studies tested the effect of a change in dietary composition on recurrence and survival in breast cancer survivors.

BIOLOGICAL MECHANISMS AND INTERMEDIATE ENDPOINTS

Based on the epidemiologic data and current understandings of how physical activity affects several specific biological processes involved in the primary and secondary occurrence of breast cancer, there is good reason to hypothesize that physical activity has a direct causal role in breast cancer incidence, recurrence, and death. A number of potential physiological responses to physical activity have been postulated to be intermediate markers or endpoints in the development and progression of breast cancer.[5] The evidence for each of these effects is summarized in Table 13.1 and Figure 13.1. Exercise may reduce the risk of breast cancer occurrence or recurrence through a reduction in fat mass, leading to a more beneficial metabolic and sex hormone profile in terms of breast cancer risk, as depicted in Figure 13.1. Other mechanisms for a protective effect of exercise on breast cancer risk could exist. For example, exercise may improve immune status, which could in turn decrease risk for breast cancer.

Obesity and Weight Control

Of the possible biological mechanisms mediating an association between physical activity and breast cancer, body fat or weight control may be most important.[5,9,10] Maintenance of normal body weight throughout

TABLE 13.1 ∾ Potential Biological Mechanisms Involved in the Association Between Physical Activity and Breast Cancer

Possible Mechanism Involved	Effect of Mechanism on Breast Cancer	Effect of Physical Activity on Mechanism
Decreased sex hormones	Increases cell proliferation Decreases apoptosis	Delays menarche Reduces number of ovulatory cycles Reduces ovarian estrogen production Reduces fat-produced estrogens Increases SHBG, resulting in less biologically available estrogen and testosterone
Decreased body fat	Fat storage of carcinogens Increases sex hormones Increases insulin levels	Decreases visceral and subcutaneous body fat Prevents weight gain/promotes weight maintenance
Decreased insulin and IGFs	Increases sex hormones Increases cell proliferation	Increases post-receptor insulin signaling Increases glucose transporter protein and mRNA Increases clearance of free fatty acids Increases muscle glucose delivery Changes muscle composition favoring increased glucose disposal

Increase in immune function	Recognizes and eliminates abnormal cells	Increases # and activity of macrophages Increases lymphokine activated killer cells Increases lymphocyte proliferation
Decreased adipocytokines	Promotes angiogenesis Stimulates estrogen biosynthesis	Decreases TNF-α, leptin, CRP, IL-6, and increases adiponectin via decreases in body fat and insulin
Decreased mammographic density	Increases cell proliferation	Decreases sex hormones, insulin, and IGFs, which in turn, may decrease mammographic density
Improved antioxidant defense systems	Free radicals produce DNA damage	Improves free radical defenses and DNA repair by upregulating free radical scavenger enzymes and levels of antioxidants

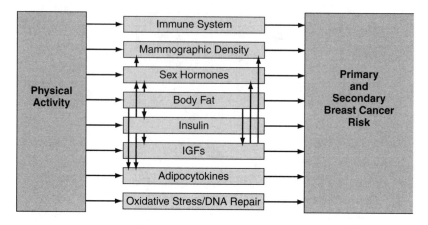

FIGURE 13.1 Hypothesized relationship between physical activity and primary and secondary breast cancer risk.

a woman's adult years is one of the few known modifiable risk factors for breast cancer, and many studies have shown positive associations between obesity and breast cancer risk.[5] Epidemiologic studies have also shown that pre- and postmenopausal women who are overweight or obese when they are diagnosed with breast cancer are more likely to experience a recurrence or die from breast cancer than women who are of a normal weight.[5] Furthermore, some, but not all, studies suggest that women who gain weight after breast cancer diagnosis, regardless of menopausal status, are at increased risk for breast cancer recurrence and death as compared to women who maintain their weight after diagnosis.[5] This finding is especially worrisome given that the majority of women treated for breast cancer gain a significant amount of weight in the year following breast cancer diagnosis, and return to pre-diagnosis weight rarely occurs.[9]

Insulin and Insulin-like Growth Factors

Both physical activity and obesity also influence circulating concentrations of insulin,[5,11] which, in turn, may affect breast cancer risk and prognosis.[5,11] In a study of women with early stage breast cancer, higher insulin levels were associated with a two and three times higher risk of recurrence or breast cancer death, respectively,[11] and in preclinical studies, insulin has a mitogenic effect in normal breast tissue and can stimulate growth of breast cancer cell lines. High insulin levels produce an increase in circulating insulin-like growth factor-I (IGF-I) and a decrease in IGF-binding proteins (increasing the availability of IGF present). IGF-I is thought to have a major role in promoting breast cancer.[5] However, the few trials that have assessed the effect of exercise on IGFs have had variable results.[5] Recently, Ligibel and colleagues observed a 28% reduction in insulin levels in breast cancer survivors randomized to four months of twice-weekly resistance training and 90 min/wk of home-based aerobic exercise compared to a 3% decrease in insulin levels in breast cancer survivors randomized to control.[12] Irwin and colleagues also demonstrated that moderate-intensity aerobic exercise, such as brisk walking, performed on average for 120 min/wk over six months was associated with a borderline statistically significant 21% between-group difference (e.g., comparing women randomized to exercise vs. usual care) in fasting insulin levels ($P = .089$) and statistically significant reductions in IGF-1 ($P < .05$)[13]. Both the Ligibel and Irwin studies observed reductions in insulin without concomitant decreases in body weight or fat.

Sex Hormones

Obesity, a high insulin level, and altered IGF levels are also associated with a less favorable sex hormone profile.[5] Sex steroid hormones have powerful mitogenic and proliferative influences and are strongly associated with the development of breast cancer.[5,14] A recent pooled analysis of nine cohort studies showed that the risk for breast cancer in postmenopausal women increased significantly with increasing concentrations of estradiol, free estradiol, and estrone.[14] Women who were in the highest quintile for these sex hormones were twice as likely to develop breast cancer as women in the lowest quintile. Other findings from epidemiologic studies further support the etiologic role of estrogen in breast cancer, showing that breast cancer risk is associated with early menarche, late menopause, low parity, and use of exogenous estrogens, all of which are linked to prolonged or extensive exposure of breast tissue to estrogen stimulation.[5,14] Finally, a number of clinical trials show that estrogen ablation increases survival following a diagnosis of breast cancer. Changes in sex hormones are perhaps the most consistently cited potential mechanism for the association between physical activity and breast cancer.

Girls who participate in athletics tend to have a later age of menarche and a delay in establishing normal ovarian cyclicity. Later age of menarche and slowed establishment of cycling would decrease the total steroid hormone exposure to the breast.[5] In adult premenopausal women, exercise has been associated with decreased levels of circulating estrogen and progesterone, shortened luteal phase, increased frequency of anovulation, and an increased incidence of oligomenorrhea and amenorrhea.[5] In postmenopausal women, physical activity has been associated with decreased serum estrogens and androgens.[5,15] Increased physical activity also has been associated with increased sex hormone binding globulin, resulting in lower amounts of free, active sex hormones in circulation.[5,15] The primary mechanism of physical activity influencing sex hormones in postmenopausal women is decreased body fat, a substrate for estrogen and testosterone production, which results in less tissue capable of aromatization of the adrenal androgens to estrogens.

Only one randomized controlled exercise trial has been published examining the effect of exercise on sex hormone concentrations.[15] While an overall effect of exercise was significantly associated with decreased sex hormone concentrations in healthy postmenopausal women, a stronger effect was observed among women who lost body fat with exercise compared to women who did not lose body fat with exercise. Because of the paucity of randomized controlled trial data, it is not yet established that change in physical activity can affect sex hormone concentrations independently of an effect of physical activity on adiposity. More randomized trials are required to determine the associations among physical activity, body fat, sex hormones, and breast cancer risk and prognosis.

Immune Function

Changes in immune function may also mediate the relationship between physical activity and breast cancer risk and prognosis.[5] The immune system is thought to play a role in protecting against breast cancer by recognizing and eliminating abnormal cells. A growing literature of small exercise intervention studies shows that physical activity improves immune function, both functionally and numerically.[5] Physical activity appears to enhance proliferation of lymphocytes, increases the number of natural killer cells, and increases lymphokine-activated killer cell activity.

Other Biological Mechanisms and Intermediate Endpoints

Other intermediate endpoints have been proposed, such as mammographic density,[5,8] adipocytokines (e.g., tumor necrosis factor [TNF]-α, leptin, and adiponectin),[5] and oxidative stress.[5] Strong evidence exists that the characteristics of breast tissue as seen on a mammogram, measured as mammographic density, provide information about breast cancer risk. Women with high levels of mammographic density have four to six times the risk of developing breast cancer than women with lower levels of mammographic density; thus, mammographic density is a stronger predictor of breast cancer risk than most traditional risk factors. Mammographic density reflects proliferation of the breast epithelium and stroma, in response to growth factors induced by current and past circulating sex hormone levels. Mammographic density may vary throughout one's lifetime, with the pattern reflecting the accumulated breast cancer risk at the time the mammogram was obtained. Factors that change mammographic density may also change breast cancer risk. Physical activity may influence mammographic density by favorably changing certain hormones associated with mammographic density and breast cancer risk. Both mammographic dense area and percent density have been found to be inversely related to physical activity in obese postmenopausal women.[5,8]

Adipocytokines exhibit strong associations with body mass index, abdominal fat mass, and hyperinsulinemia. In addition, several adipocytokines, including interleukin-6 (IL-6), TNF-α, and leptin, promote angiogenesis, which is essential for breast cancer development and progression, and can stimulate estrogen biosynthesis by the induction of aromatase activity. C-reactive Protein (CRP) is not an adipocytokine *per se*, but its production is promoted by TNF-α and IL-6. C-reactive protein is a well-known systemic marker for inflammation that is produced by the liver and is present only during episodes of chronic inflammation. So far, varying effects of physical activity for the different adipocytokines have been observed.[5] For postmenopausal women, the evidence most strongly supports physical activity decreasing circulating leptin, IL-6, and CRP. The evidence is mixed on TNF-α, and no studies have yet found an association between exercise and adiponectin.

STRATEGIES FOR INCREASING PHYSICAL ACTIVITY AFTER A CANCER DIAGNOSIS

Becoming physically active is a difficult challenge for healthy adults and is likely to be even more difficult after a cancer diagnosis and during medical treatments. In reviewing papers that examined predictors of physical activity adoption and maintenance in healthy men and women and cancer survivors, a physician's recommendation to exercise has been shown to be a strong predictor. Survey studies have also shown that cancer survivors want to receive information about physical activity. Oncologists should become aware of the benefits of exercise, assist their patients by endorsing existing physical activity guidelines and refer their patients to certified cancer exercise trainers.

Most recently, working together, the American Cancer Society and the American College of Sports Medicine developed a certification called "the certified cancer exercise trainer" for personal trainers, physical therapists, nurse practitioners, or other health professionals to become certified in counseling and training cancer survivors in how to exercise safely and at recommended levels. These "Certified Cancer Exercise Trainers" are knowledgeable of the potential physical limitations associated with surgery and treatment, and have the skills and abilities to help cancer survivors overcome some of the recent and late effects of surgery and treatment (go to www.acsm.org for more information).

With regard to when to initiate an exercise program after diagnosis, some scientists and oncologists feel the timing of physical activity programs may be critically important because the teachable moment may best be capitalized on if programs are offered soon after diagnosis.[16] Certainly issues such as concurrent demands of treatment are key concerns in the timing of programs, and therefore appropriate balance is necessary in determining the optimal time at which the patient is both physically and psychologically ready to undertake behavior change.

SUMMARY

One of the most common questions cancer survivors ask is: "What can I do to improve my survival?" Physical activity is a modifiable behavior with a multitude of health benefits. A growing number of publications show a strong relationship between physical activity and breast cancer prevention and improved survival. Numerous observational studies have also demonstrated that obesity and weight gain adversely affect breast cancer risk and prognosis, adding further evidence to the hypothesis that physical activity, one of the critical components of obesity and weight gain, influences breast cancer risk and survival.

Furthermore, many existing cancer therapies are costly and have significant side effects that can result in long-term morbidity. Therefore, non-pharmacologic methods, such as participating in physical activity to lower the risk of cancer mortality, especially methods that are also associated with improvements in quality of life and other chronic diseases, may offer an attractive addition to the currently available treatment options. Oncologists and primary care physicians should be encouraged to counsel their patients proactively about physical activity. The simplest, evidence-based recommendation at present would be to undertake 30 minutes of moderate-intensity recreational physical activity, such as brisk walking, five times per week. Because a majority of cancer survivors are not currently participating in recommended levels of physical activity, resulting in greater disease risk and health-care costs, this therapy has the potential to benefit a large number of cancer survivors.

REFERENCES

1. American Cancer Society (ACS). *Cancer Facts and Figures 2005*. Atlanta: American Cancer Society, Inc; 2005.
2. Friedenreich C, Orenstein M. Physical activity and cancer prevention: etiologic evidence and biological mechanisms. *J Nutr.* 2002;132(11): 3456S–3464S.
3. Holmes MD, Chen WY, Feskanich D, et al. Physical activity and survival after breast cancer diagnosis. *JAMA.* 2005;293(20):2479–2486.

4. Irwin ML. Influence of pre- and post-diagnosis physical activity on survival in breast cancer survivors: the Health, Eating, Activity, and Lifestyle (HEAL) Study. *J Clin Oncol.* 2008;26(24):1–7.

5. Irwin ML. Randomized controlled trials of physical activity and breast cancer prevention. *Exerc. Sport Sci Rev.* 2006;24(4):182–93. PMID: 17031257

6. Prentice RL, Caan B, Chlebowski R, et al. Low-fat dietary pattern and risk of invasive breast cancer: the Women's Health Initiative Randomized Controlled Dietary Modification Trial. *JAMA.* 2006;295(6):629–642.

7. Copeland T, Grosvenor M, Mitchell DC, et al. Designing a quality assurance system for dietary data in a multicenter clinical trial: Women's Intervention Nutrition Study. *J Am Diet Assoc.* 2000;100:1186–1190.

8. Pierce JP, Faerber S, Wright FA, et al. A randomized trial of the effect of a plant-based dietary pattern on additional breast cancer events and survival: the Women's Healthy Eating and Living (WHEL) Study. *Control Clin Trials.* 2002;23:728–756.

9. Irwin ML, McTiernan A, Baumgartner R, et al. Changes in body fat and weight after a breast cancer diagnosis: influence of demographic, prognostic and lifestyle factors. *J Clin Oncol.* 2005;23(4):774–782.

10. Irwin ML, Yasui Y, Ulrich C, et al. Effect of moderate- to vigorous-intensity exercise on total and intra-abdominal body fat in postmenopausal women: a one-year randomized controlled trial. *JAMA.* 2003;289:323–330.

11. Goodwin PJ, Ennis M, Pritchard KI, et al. Fasting insulin and outcome in early stage breast cancer: results of a prospective cohort study. *J Clin Oncol.* 2002;20:42–51.

12. Ligibel JA, Campbell N, Partridge A, et al. Impact of a mixed strength and endurance exercise intervention on insulin levels in breast cancer survivors. *J Clin Oncol.* 2008;26(6):907–912.

13. Irwin ML, Varma K, Alvarez-Reeves, et al. Randomized controlled exercise trial on insulin and IGFs in breast cancer survivors: The Yale Exercise and Survivorship Study. *Cancer Epidemiol Biomarkers Prev.* 2009;18(1): 306–313.

14. Endogenous Hormones and Breast Cancer Collaborative Group. Endogenous sex hormones and breast cancer in postmenopausal women: reanalysis of nine prospective studies. *J Natl Cancer Inst.* 2002;94:606–616.

15. McTiernan A, Tworoger SS, Ulrich CM, et al. Effect of exercise on serum estrogens in postmenopausal women: a 12-month randomized clinical trial. *Cancer Res.* 2004;64:2923–2928.

16. Demark-Wahnefried W, Rock CL, Patrick K, Byers T. Lifestyle interventions to reduce cancer risk and improve outcomes. *Am Fam Physician.* 2008;77(11):1573–1578.

14

Nutrition and Prevention in Cancer Survivors

Susan T. Mayne, PhD

&

Stephanie M. George, MPH, MA

ABSTRACT

The role of nutrition in cancer survivorship is increasingly of interest to cancer patients, who may use their diagnosis as a stimulus for health behavior change. Although there has been extensive research looking at diet and nutrient supplement use in the prevention of first cancers, there is more limited evidence regarding the impact of diet and nutrient supplement use on cancer prognosis. This chapter reviews recent nutrition guidelines for cancer survivors, highlighting key research studies that serve as the basis for current dietary guidelines. The goal is to provide health professionals with both a summary and key articles so they can best advise patients as to appropriate dietary approaches for cancer prevention and survivorship.

INTRODUCTION

Cancer survivorship is a continuum ranging from treatment, to recovery, to living after recovery, to living with advanced cancer. Nutritional needs of cancer survivors vary, depending upon their stage in the continuum. Many factors can impact cancer survivors' nutritional status (e.g., reduced appetite, alterations in taste due to chemotherapy), and dietary strategies are available to help cancer patients through the treatment and recovery process. While nutritional needs are evident across the continuum, most nutrition research in the area of cancer survivorship has addressed the topic of nutrition while living after recovery, and this chapter will focus mostly on that area. There has been limited scientific evidence evaluating what happens when cancer patients take supplements, herbals, or botanicals during the actual treatment process. At this point, sufficient data are not available to determine whether supplementation is going to be helpful or harmful; the prudent approach in the absence of solid data is to avoid high-dose nutrient supplements during treatment or in the short-term recovery process. Cancer patients should certainly consult a registered dietitian for specialized nutrition counseling during the treatment phase of the cancer process.

With the increasing number of cancer survivors today, evidence-based guidance on effective health promotion interventions targeted to survivors is needed. To address this need, the American Cancer Society (ACS) recently convened an advisory committee to review the scientific evidence looking at nutrition, physical activity, and cancer survivorship. This evidence is summarized in a 30-page publication highlighting specific guidelines for each of the major cancer sites, as summarized in Table 14.1 (please refer to the ACS publication for further information).[1] Although there has been extensive research looking at diet in the prevention of first cancers, which is also true for physical activity research, there is more limited evidence regarding the role of diet in secondary cancer prevention.

Thus, the ACS guidelines for general cancer prevention are currently recommended for cancer survivors. This ACS publication serves as a helpful and timely resource for cancer survivors and covers the gamut of topics on nutrition, physical activity, and cancer status. This brief chapter uses these guidelines as a foundation for considering recommended diet and nutrient supplementation for survivors after recovery.

DIET AND ACTIVITY GUIDELINES

Diet and activity guidelines focus on the following areas: (1) maintaining a healthy weight; (2) adopting a physically active lifestyle; (3) limiting intake of high-fat foods, particularly from animal sources (not an

TABLE 14.1 Summary of American Cancer Society (ACS) Guidelines on Nutrition and Physical Activity for Cancer Prevention

---

Maintain a healthy weight throughout life.

- Balance calorie intake with physical activity.
- Avoid excessive weight gain throughout life.
- Achieve and maintain a healthy weight if currently overweight or obese.

Adopt a physically active lifestyle.

- *Adults:* Engage in at least 30 minutes of moderate to vigorous physical activity, above usual activities, on 5 or more days of the week; 45 to 60 minutes of intentional physical activity are preferable.
- *Children and adolescents:* Engage in at least 60 minutes per day of moderate to vigorous physical activity at least 5 days per week.

Eat a healthy diet, with an emphasis on plant sources.

- Choose foods and drinks in amounts that help achieve and maintain a healthy weight.
- Eat five or more servings of a variety of vegetables and fruits each day.
- Choose whole grains over processed (refined) grains.
- Limit intake of processed and red meats.

If you drink alcoholic beverages, limit your intake.

- Drink no more than one drink per day for women or two per day for men.

Source: Adapted from information from the American Cancer Society.

official ACS guideline but a topic of recent research and lay interest); (4) emphasizing consumption of plant food sources, specifically 5 or more servings of vegetables and fruits every day; (5) choosing whole grain products instead of refined grains; (6) limiting consumption of processed and red meats; and (7) limiting alcohol consumption (for those who choose to drink alcoholic beverages). This chapter reviews the guidelines and briefly discusses the scientific evidence underlying them, mentioning high-impact studies where appropriate.

Maintain a Healthy Weight

Recent evidence indicates that obesity increases the risk of many more cancers than has been previously recognized. As an example, in the ACS Cancer Prevention Study II, a longitudinal cohort study, obesity was shown to increase the risk of dying due to numerous cancers.[2] This study confirmed the known relationship of obesity to risk of dying of various cancers, like colon and prostate, as has been found in previous studies, but the analysis revealed some surprising findings as well. Of particular interest, there was a 52% increase (Relative Risk [RR]: 1.52) in the risk of all cancer death for men who were severely obese (body mass index [BMI] of ≥ 40) as compared to men who were normal body weight (BMI of 18.5–24.9).[2] The data for women revealed an increased risk of breast cancer death (RR: 2.12), which has been seen in many studies, but a more extensive effect was also observed, with obese women having a greater risk of dying due to a variety of different cancers compared to women who were normal body weight (BMI of 18.5–24.9).[2] Women who were severely obese (BMI of ≥ 40) were 88% more likely to die from cancer (RR: 1.88). Because surviving cancer is not just about treating the primary cancer but also about preventing any second cancers for which patients are at risk, striving to prevent obesity is critically important for cancer survivors.

Adopt a Physically Active Lifestyle

This guideline will not be reviewed here. Please refer to Chapter 13 for a detailed discussion of the relationship between physical activity and cancer (breast cancer, in particular).

Limit Intake of High-Fat Foods, Particularly from Animal Sources

This older ACS guideline[3] is not included in the 2006 report but is mentioned here given the continuing interest by survivors and researchers about dietary fat content in relation to cancer risk. The Women's Intervention Nutrition Study was the first randomized clinical trial of a dietary intervention in breast cancer survivors.[4] In this study, 2000 women who had postmenopausal breast cancer were randomized into an intervention consisting of a low-fat diet (33 g total fat/day) or into a usual diet (averaging 51.3 g total fat/day). Participants were followed for 5 years to see if the low-fat diet reduced the risk of second breast cancer. Initial results of the trial, published in 2006, showed that the relative risk of second breast cancer in the women who were randomized to the low-fat diet was 0.76 (95% CI, 0.60–1.00; $P = .03$), translating to a 24% statistically significant reduction in risk.[4] Of particular interest, when the results were stratified by the estrogen receptor (ER) status (positive vs negative) of the women's first breast cancer, a more substantial benefit was observed in women who had ER-negative breast cancer (RR: 0.58; 95% CI, 0.37–0.91).[4] Women with ER-positive breast cancer who were randomized to the low-fat diet also had fewer second breast cancers, but the result was not statistically significant (RR: 0.85; 95% CI, 0.63–1.14). Of note, this more modest benefit was observed above and beyond the normal preventive approaches that women with ER-positive breast cancer had available (e.g., tamoxifen).[4] Additional follow-up of the women in this trial is ongoing.

While these data look promising for cancer survivors, a large body of literature suggests that the type of fat consumed may be more important than total fat intake when considering general health promotion recommendations for cancer survivors. Dietary guidelines for health promotion emphasize restricting saturated and trans fats, but not necessarily restricting mono- and polyunsaturated oils, the latter of which are considered heart-healthy fats.[5] Moreover, there is compelling evidence that omega-3 fatty acids (fish oils) have cardiovascular disease-preventive benefits, as well as other health benefits.[6] Consequently, the ACS has not made current recommendations about total fat consumption for survivors. From a practical point of view, limiting intake of high-fat foods from animal sources will result in lower intake of saturated fats, which will reduce cardiovascular disease risk and may reduce future cancer risk.

Consume Five or More Servings of Vegetables and Fruits Each Day

The American Cancer Society guidelines recommended consumption of at least five daily servings of a variety of fruits and vegetables. The amount of fruits and vegetables each person needs depends on caloric needs, which vary by age, gender and physical activity level. For example, intake of four and one-half cups of fruits and vegetables (nine servings) daily are now recommended for the reference 2,000 calorie level as shown in the current Dietary Guidelines for Americans (*www.health.gov/Dietary Guidelines*). Survivors can learn more about personalized diet recommendations at *www.mypyramid.gov* in preparation for talking with their providers. Recently, the World Cancer Research Fund and the American Institute for Cancer Research completed a comprehensive review of the literature on diet and cancer prevention, including fruits and vegetables.[7] The panel concluded that there was *probable* evidence that intake of plant foods (including nonstarchy vegetables and fruits) was associated with reduced risk of various cancers, with strongest effects noted for oral, pharynx, larynx, esophageal, and stomach cancers and fruit intake was associated with reduced risk of lung cancer. This panel's conclusion is highly concordant with that of another panel convened by the World Health Organization and the Food and Agriculture Organization, which concluded there was a probable link between higher intake of fruits and vegetables and reduced risk of certain cancers, especially oral, esophageal, gastric, and colorectal.[8]

Most of the evidence supporting a protective effect of fruit and vegetable intake comes from observational studies, because randomized intervention trials with cancer endpoints as primary outcomes are lacking, with the following exception. The Women's Healthy Eating and Living Study (WHEL) was a randomized clinical trial in which a low-fat diet high in fruits and vegetables was compared to a normal diet in breast cancer survivors.[9] This trial demonstrated that women randomized to a high fruit and vegetable diet increased consumption of fruits and vegetables, as supported by marked increases in plasma carotenoids, which are biomarkers of fruit and vegetable intake.[10] Despite this apparent adherence, rates of second breast cancer were similar in the two dietary arms of this trial.[11] The women in the non-intervention arm of this study were consuming 3.8 servings of vegetables and 3.4 servings of fruit at baseline; therefore, this trial was evaluating incremental benefits in cancer risk reduction for consuming very high intakes versus high intakes. The observational evidence commonly suggests that the incremental benefits are largest when intervening in populations with low intakes, so the results of this trial should be interpreted in their proper context (no additional benefit to consuming beyond five-a-day).

While the dietary intervention in WHEL did not show significant improvement in outcomes, a recent observational analysis of the non-intervention arm of the WHEL study suggested that the combination of fruit and vegetable intake with physical activity was beneficial. More specifically, breast cancer survivors who consumed more than five daily servings of fruits and vegetables and who exercised an amount equivalent to walking 30 minutes 6 days each week had a significant survival advantage.[12] This outcome was not seen in women who engaged in only 1 of the 2 behaviors (either diet or physical activity); rather, the combined influence of diet and physical activity was associated with risk reduction. Notably, only a minority of breast cancer survivors engaged in both health-promoting behaviors, suggesting obvious opportunities for survivorship interventions.

Choose Whole Grains over Refined Grains

Whole grains contain many micronutrients (e.g., vitamin E) and macronutrients (e.g., dietary fiber) in comparison to refined grains. From observational research, we know that people who have a higher intake of whole grains and fiber have a lower risk for many different cancers, especially colorectal cancer. As an example, in 2003, the fiber–colorectal cancer findings were published from a large, prospective cohort study, the European Prospective Investigation Into Cancer and Nutrition (EPIC). Bingham and colleagues found that as fiber intake increased in this multinational cohort, the relative risk for colorectal cancer decreased substantially (by about 40% for the highest intake group).[13] While not all observational studies of fiber demonstrate this same benefit, it should be noted that other studies may be compromised by limitations, such as a narrow range of fiber intake within a particular population. (Of note, the observational data suggesting benefits for cancer prevention reflect intake of fiber-rich foods rather than fiber supplements.)

Fiber or whole grain intervention trials with colon cancer endpoints have yet to be done. Some short-term intervention trials using intermediate endpoints have been performed, with the endpoint used most often being adenomatous polyps. One such randomized trial was the Polyp Prevention Trial. In this trial, men and women who had an adenomatous polyp removed were randomized to a high-fiber diet or not and followed for 3 years to see if the intervention affected risk of recurrence of adenomatous polyps.[14] The risk ratios for number, location, size, and stage adenomatous polyps hovered around 1, suggesting no benefit of fiber intake with this 3-year intervention; however, there was also no evidence of harm.[14]

Definitive findings indicating that whole grain foods reduce cancer risk are lacking; however, evidence suggests many other health benefits to higher fiber intake—and cancer survivors are interested in promoting optimal health, not just preventing second cancers. In the Nurses Health Study, the women who consumed more whole grains and more fiber consistently weighed less than women who consumed less ($P_{trend} <$ .0001).[15] Women with the greatest increase in fiber intake longitudinally gained an average of 1.52 kg less than women with the smallest increase in fiber intake ($P_{trend} < .0001$), independent of age, body weight at baseline, and other covariates. Women in the highest quintile of whole grain intake were 0.51 times as likely to gain major weight as compared with women in the lowest quintile.[15] Women in the lowest quintile of fiber intake weighed more at the start and over time, and women in the lowest quintile of refined grain intake weighed less at the start and over time.[15] Because prevention of weight gain is a key strategy for cancer prevention, selecting whole grain foods and increasing fiber intake follow logically as prudent approaches for cancer prevention.

Just as all fats are not the same, all carbohydrates are not the same. Long-term strategies for weight control in cancer survivors include a diet rich in fiber. Fibers are carbohydrates; therefore, recommendations to patients should avoid stigmatizing carbohydrates. Carbohydrates are important for weight control, if they are the right type.

In measuring diet, we often are not measuring just fat or fiber alone, but rather dietary patterns. One study examined the relative risk of excess weight in young and middle-aged US adults as a function of their dietary pattern. The study found that those at the greatest risk of excess weight were the low-fiber, high-fat group.[16]

Limit Consumption of Processed and Red Meats

A large body of evidence indicates that intake of red and processed meat increases the risk of colon cancers. The recent World Cancer Research Fund/American Institute for Cancer Research report evaluated the links among red meat and processed meat intake and colorectal cancer risk as "convincing."[7] An example of the data underlying this conclusion can be found in the EPIC cohort study. This large-scale prospective cohort study across Europe has been able to capture great dietary diversity and found that the lowest risk for colon cancer is found in the group that has low consumption of red and processed meat and high consumption of fiber.[17] There is limited evidence for associations of red meat with cancers of the esophagus, lung, pancreas, and endometrium, and of processed meat with cancers of the esophagus, lung, stomach, and prostate.[7] The data are the most compelling at this point, however, for colorectal cancer.

Limit Alcohol Consumption, If You Drink at All

A large body of evidence clearly demonstrates a synergistic interaction between alcohol consumption and tobacco use in raising the risk of many epithelial cancers, including oral cavity, pharynx, larynx, and esophageal squamous cell carcinoma.[18] Alcohol consumption also increases the risk of hepatocellular carcinoma (liver cancer). The doses at which these risks are observed tend to be relatively high doses of ethanol, frequently exceeding two to three drinks per day. However, there are data suggesting that even moderate drinking (defined as one drink/ day) is associated with an increase in the risk of breast cancer.[18] Because moderate drinking appears to reduce the risk of cardiovascular disease, breast cancer survivors in particular have to make difficult choices regarding alcohol consumption. Survivors need to be informed of potential health benefits and risks associated with alcohol consumption. While moderate drinking appears to be cardioprotective, higher levels of drinking do not appear to convey any additional protection and dramatically increase the risk of several cancers, which explains the emphasis on drinking in moderation, if one drinks at all.

SUPPLEMENTAL NUTRIENTS

Among cancer survivors, there has been much interest in nutrient supplementation for cancer prevention. Results are now available both from trials looking at primary prevention of cancer incidence within healthy populations as well as secondary prevention of cancer recurrence in cancer survivors. The clinical trial evidence supporting cancer preventive effects for nutrient supplements is inconsistent, with some trials showing benefit, some showing mixed results, and others showing harm.

Beginning with findings of benefit, a randomized trial involving nutrient supplements for cancer prevention in a micronutrient-deficient population in China observed a statistically significant reduction in gastric cancer incidence for those participants receiving antioxidant nutrient supplementation.[19] This trial was one of the first micronutrient cancer prevention trials completed, and the results strongly supported the concept of cancer prevention with micronutrient supplements. More recently, the Calcium Polyp Prevention Study found a significant reduction in recurrent adenomatous polyps in the group randomized to receive supplemental calcium.[20]

In contrast to these promising findings, many trials have had mixed results. Some trials have failed to find that supplemental nutrients reduced the incidence of their primary endpoint but unexpectedly observed a reduction in a different cancer endpoint than the trial was designed to evaluate. For example, the Alpha-Tocopherol Beta-Carotene (ATBC) Cancer Prevention Trial was designed to look at differences in lung cancer incidence among male smokers who received either supplemental vitamin E, beta-carotene, both supplements, or placebo.[21] No reduction in lung cancer risk was observed for participants receiving supplemental vitamin E (433 new lung cancer diagnoses in the vitamin E group vs 443 in the placebo), but unexpectedly a 30% to 40% decrease in prostate cancer incidence was found in the men who were randomized to receive supplemental vitamin E (99 new prostate cancer diagnoses in the vitamin E group vs 151 in the placebo).[21] The beta-carotene results are discussed in the following paragraph. Likewise, in a trial evaluating selenium supplementation for the prevention of second skin cancers among a sample of 1,312 people from low-selenium regions,[22] the investigators observed an adverse effect on skin cancers (the primary endpoint) but an unexpected statistically significant decrease in cancers of the prostate (13 in selenium group vs 35 in placebo; $P = .002$), lung (17 in selenium group vs 31 placebo; $P = .04$), and colon/rectum (8 in selenium group vs 19 in placebo; $P = .03$). Based on the small sample size, a cautious interpretation of the findings is warranted. Nutritional status, smoking, and drinking have also been shown to modify the efficacy of chemoprevention. For example, when evidence from the selenium trial was looked at more closely, the benefit on total cancer incidence was only evident in people who were in the lowest levels of plasma selenium at entry.[23] For those in the lowest third, of plasma selenium at entry, risk for total cancer was reduced by 50% with supplements of selenium, whereas in the middle third, there was a 30% reduction in risk, and in the highest third there was a 19% increase in risk of total cancers.[23] Similarly, in the Antioxidant Polyp Prevention Trial, beta-carotene supplementation resulted in a 50% reduction in recurrent adenomas among nonsmokers and nondrinkers, but the risk of adenomas doubled among heavy smokers and heavy drinkers who received beta-carotene.[24] These examples illustrate that whether supplements will be of benefit or harm is a function of many factors that we really do not fully understand at this time.

Some key trials have reported adverse effects of micronutrients on primary endpoints. Beta-carotene supplementation was found to have adverse effects on lung cancer incidence among smokers in the ATBC trial,[21] with the group that received beta-carotene supplements having a statistically significant excess of lung cancer (474 new lung cancer diagnoses in the beta-carotene group vs. 402 in placebo). This finding was replicated in the Carotene and Retinol Efficacy Trial (CARET).[25] In CARET, the active-treatment group received supplemental beta-carotene in combination with retinol (vitamin A) and had a relative risk of lung cancer of 1.28 (95% CI: 1.04–1.57; P = 0.02) as compared with the placebo group.

Designed to follow-up on the unexpected reductions in prostate cancer incidence observed with vitamin E in ATBC, and with selenium in the skin cancer prevention trial, the Selenium and Vitamin E Chemoprevention Trial (SELECT) randomized 35,000 males into vitamin E, selenium, combination, or placebo groups.[26] The trial was terminated early in 2008 per the recommendation of the Data Safety Monitoring Committee due to evidence of lack of benefit, and the evidence also showed two trends of concern. There was a nonsignificant increase in the risk of prostate cancer in the vitamin E group, and a nonsignificant increase in type II diabetes in the selenium group.[26] Another recent randomized, placebo-controlled, double-blinded trial, the Physicians' Health Study II (PHS), found that among 14,641 male U.S. physicians initially aged 50 years or older (with 1,307 men with a history of prior cancer), there were no significant effects of vitamin E or vitamin C on prostate, total, colorectal, lung or site-specific cancers over 8 years of follow-up.[27] The lack of consistent evidence of cancer preventive efficacy for micronutrient supplementation shows that the science is not supporting original expectations.

There are other nutrient supplements that are of current interest for cancer prevention, such as vitamin D.[28] However, the enthusiasm surrounding this particular nutrient is quite reminiscent of similar enthusiasm surrounding many other nutrients that have failed the test of time and well-designed clinical research trials. The hypothesis that nutrient supplements might be of benefit, and certainly cannot cause harm, has been rejected over the past two decades. However, supplement use is widespread among cancer survivors and physicians are generally unaware of supplement use among their patients.[29] This suggests that increased communication is needed to assist survivors in making well-informed decisions.

CONCLUSION

Cancer survivorship research remains a relatively young field, and the evidence base demonstrating that nutritional interventions can improve outcomes in cancer survivors remains limited. Thus, heavy reliance is placed on a larger body of literature that describes dietary patterns that may reduce the risk of cancer in general and have been proven to reduce the risk of many other chronic diseases. Adherence to the dietary recommendations, specifically emphasizing plant food sources and whole grains while limiting consumption of processed and red meats, should be a goal for all survivors. This goal, along with maintaining a healthy weight and adopting a physically active lifestyle, remains the best strategy for survivors.

REFERENCES

1. Doyle C, Kushi LH, Byers T, et al. Nutrition and physical activity during and after cancer treatment: an American Cancer Society guide for informed choices. *CA Cancer J Clin.* 2006;56:323–353.
2. Calle EE, Rodriguez C, Walker-Thurmond K, et al. Overweight, obesity, and mortality from cancer in a prospectively studied cohort of U.S. adults. *N Engl J Med.* 2003;348:1625–1638.

3. Brown J, Byers T, Thompson K, et al. Nutrition during and after cancer treatment: a guide for informed choices by cancer survivors. *CA Cancer J Clin.* 2001;51:153–181.

4. Chlebowski RT, Blackburn GL, Thomson CA, et al. Dietary fat reduction and breast cancer outcome: interim efficacy results from the Women's Intervention Nutrition Study. *J Natl Cancer Inst.* 2006;98:1767–1776.

5. Know Your Fats. American Heart Association Web site. http://www.americanheart.org/presenter.jhtml?identifier=532. Published November 22, 2008. Updated July 17, 2008. Accessed November 22, 2008.

6. Committee on Nutrient Relationships in Seafood: Selections to Balance Benefits and Risks. Seafood choices: balancing benefits and risks. Washington, DC: Institute of Medicine, National Academies Press; 2007.

7. World Cancer Research Fund, American Institution for Cancer Research. Food, nutrition, physical activity, and the prevention of cancer: a global perspective. Washington, DC: AICR; 2007.

8. Joint WHO/FAO Expert Consultation on Diet, Nutriton and the Prevention of Chronic Diseases. Diet, nutrition and the prevention of chronic diseases: report of a joint WHO/FAO expert consultation. Geneva: World Health Organization, 2003).

9. Pierce JP, Faerber S, Wright FA, et al. A randomized trial of the effect of a plant-based dietary pattern on additional breast cancer events and survival: the Women's Healthy Eating and Living (WHEL) Study. *Control Clin Trials.* 2002;23:728–756.

10. Pierce JP, Natarajan L, Sun S, et al. Increases in plasma carotenoid concentrations in response to a major dietary change in the women's healthy eating and living study. *Cancer Epidemiol Biomarkers Prev.* 2006;15:1886–1892.

11. Pierce JP, Natarajan L, Caan BJ, et al. Influence of a diet very high in vegetables, fruit, and fiber and low in fat on prognosis following treatment for breast cancer: the Women's Healthy Eating and Living (WHEL) randomized trial. *JAMA.* 2007;298:289–298.

12. Pierce JP, Stefanick ML, Flatt SW, et al. Greater survival after breast cancer in physically active women with high vegetable-fruit intake regardless of obesity. *J Clin Oncol.* 2007;25:2345–2351.

13. Bingham SA, Day NE, Luben R, et al. Dietary fibre in food and protection against colorectal cancer in the European Prospective Investigation into Cancer and Nutrition (EPIC): an observational study. *Lancet.* 2003;361:1496–1501.

14. Schatzkin A, Lanza E, Corle D, et al. Lack of effect of a low-fat, high-fiber diet on the recurrence of colorectal adenomas. Polyp Prevention Trial Study Group. *N Engl J Med.* 2000;342:1149–1155.

15. Liu S, Willett WC, Manson JE, et al. Relation between changes in intakes of dietary fiber and grain products and changes in weight and development of obesity among middle-aged women. *Am J Clin Nutr.* 2003;78:920–927.

16. Howarth NC, Huang TT, Roberts SB, et al. Dietary fiber and fat are associated with excess weight in young and middle-aged US adults. *J Am Diet Assoc.* 2005;105:1365–1372.

17. Norat T, Bingham S, Ferrari P, et al. Meat, fish, and colorectal cancer risk: the European Prospective Investigation into Cancer and Nutrition. *J Natl Cancer Inst.* 2005;97:906–916.

18. Longnecker MP. Alcohol consumption and risk of cancer in humans: an overview. *Alcohol.* 1995;12:87–96.

19. Blot WJ, Li JY, Taylor PR, et al. Nutrition intervention trials in Linxian, China: supplementation with specific vitamin/mineral combinations, cancer incidence, and disease-specific mortality in the general population. *J Natl Cancer Inst.* 1993;85:1483–1492.

20. Baron JA, Beach M, Mandel JS, et al. Calcium supplements for the prevention of colorectal adenomas. Calcium Polyp Prevention Study Group. *N Engl J Med.* 1999;340:101–107.

21. The Alpha-Tocopherol Beta-Carotene Cancer Prevention Study Group. The effect of vitamin E and beta carotene on the incidence of lung cancer and other cancers in male smokers. *N Engl J Med.* 1994;330:1029–1035.

22. Clark LC, Combs GF Jr, Turnbull BW, et al. Effects of selenium supplementation for cancer prevention in patients with carcinoma of the skin. A randomized controlled trial. Nutritional Prevention of Cancer Study Group. *JAMA.* 1996;276:1957–1963.

23. Duffield-Lillico AJ, Reid ME, Turnbull BW, et al. Baseline characteristics and the effect of selenium supplementation on cancer incidence in a randomized clinical trial: a summary report of the nutritional prevention of cancer trial. *Cancer Epidemiol Biomark Prev.* 2002;11:630–639.

24. Baron JA, Cole BF, Mott L, et al. Neoplastic and antineoplastic effects of beta-carotene on colorectal adenoma recurrence: results of a randomized trial. *J Natl Cancer Inst.* 2003;95:717–722.

25. Omenn GS, Goodman GE, Thornquist MD, et al. Effects of a combination of beta carotene and vitamin A on lung cancer and cardiovascular disease. *N Engl J Med.* 1996;334:1150–1155.

26. Lippman SL, Klein EA, Goodman PJ, et al. Effect of selenium and vitamin E on risk of prostate cancer and other cancers: the Selenium and Vitamin E Cancer Prevention Trial (SELECT). *JAMA.* 2008; published online December 9, 2008.

27. Gaziano, JM, Glynn, RJ, Christen, WG, et al. Vitamins E and C in the prevention of prostate and total cancer in men: the Physicians' Health Study II randomized controlled trial. *JAMA.* 2009; 301:52–62.

28. Holick MF. Vitamin D: its role in cancer prevention and treatment. *Prog Biophys Mol Biol.* 2006;92:49–59.

29. Velicer CM and Ulrich CM. Vitamin and mineral supplement use among US adults after cancer diagnosis: a systematic review. *J. Clin. Oncol.* 2008;26:665–673.

15

The Epidemiology of Second Primary Cancers

Andrea K. Ng, MD, MPH

&

Lois B. Travis, MD, ScD

ABSTRACT

Significant improvements in cancer detection, supportive care, and therapeutic advances in the past few decades have resulted in increasing numbers of cancer survivors. In the United States alone, there were an estimated 10.8 million cancer survivors in 2004, with an overall 5-year relative survival rate of almost 66%. Given the major strides in survival rates for increasing numbers of patients, identification and characterization of the late sequelae of cancer and its treatment have become critical. The diagnosis of a new cancer represents one of the most serious events experienced by cancer survivors. The number of patients who develop second or higher order cancers is increasing, with these diagnoses now comprising about one of every six (16%) cancer incidents reported to the National Cancer Institute's (NCI's) Surveillance, Epidemiology, and End Results (SEER) Program in 2004. Moreover, solid tumors are an important cause of mortality among a number of groups of long-term survivors, in particular, patients with Hodgkin disease (HD). This chapter focuses on second primary cancers in survivors of selected adult cancers.

INTRODUCTION

Significant improvements in cancer detection, supportive care, and therapeutic advances in the past few decades have resulted in increasing numbers of cancer survivors. In the United States alone, there were an estimated 10.8 million cancer survivors in 2004, with an overall 5-year relative survival rate of almost 66%.[1] This number represents more than a tripling of the estimated 3 million survivors in the early 1970s. In view of the prolonged survival in increasing numbers of patients,[2] the identification and quantification of the late effects of cancer and its therapy have moved to the forefront.

The diagnosis of a new cancer represents one of the most devastating events experienced by cancer survivors. The number of survivors with second or higher order cancers is increasing rapidly; these independent malignancies comprised about one of every six (16%) cancer incidents reported to the NCI's SEER program in 2004.[1] Moreover, solid tumors are a leading cause of death among several groups of long-term survivors, in particular, patients with HD.[3] Second cancers can reflect the late effects of therapy, the impact of lifestyle choices (e.g., alcohol or tobacco use), host factors, environmental determinants, and the operation of joint effects, including gene-environment and gene-gene interactions.[4] Travis and colleagues recently grouped second primary cancers into three major categories according to dominant etiologic factors: therapy-related, syndromic, and those due to shared etiologic influences.[5] Examples of etiologic influences in each of these categories are provided in Table 15.1. In their categorization, these authors emphasized the nonexclusivity of these groups.[5]

This chapter focuses on malignancies in survivors of selected adult cancers, especially those for which a relatively large amount of information has been generated. Second tumors among childhood cancer survivors were recently described by Bhatia and colleagues.[6] The reader is referred elsewhere for comprehensive reviews of multiple primary cancers[7,8] and discussions of possible underlying genetic mechanisms.[5,9]

TABLE 15.1 Dominant Etiologic Factors for the Development of Second Malignancies

Dominant Etiologic Factors	Examples
Prior Therapy Exposures	• Radiation Therapy • Chemotherapy • Hormonal Therapy (Tamoxifen)
Cancer Syndromes	• Bloom Syndrome • BRCA-1 and/or BRCA-2· Related Cancers • Cowden Disease • Fanconi Anemia • Hereditary Nonpolyposis Colorectal Cancer • Li Fraumeni Syndrome • Xeroderma Pigmentosum
Shared Etiologic Influences	• Tobacco • Alcohol • Sun Exposure • Diet/Nutrition • Immune Dysfunction • Infectious Causes • Genetic Predisposition (other than familial syndromes)

Source: Modified from Travis et al. *J Natl Cancer Inst.* 2006;98:15–25.

SECOND MALIGNANCIES AMONG SURVIVORS OF SELECTED ADULT CANCERS

Hodgkin Disease

A large number of studies have addressed the risk of subsequent malignancies among survivors of HD, given the high curability of the disease and the typically young age at diagnosis, which together result in a lifetime for the manifestation of the late effects of treatment. The increased risk of therapy-related leukemias in HD patients is highest in the first 10 years after treatment,[10] with the first reports dating back to the early 1970s.[11] The elevated risk is largely due to alkylating agent chemotherapy, with the existence of a strong dose–response relationship.[12,13] Although splenectomy and the addition of radiation therapy to chemotherapy have been postulated as additional risk factors, data are conflicting.[14,15]

The prognosis of HD patients with secondary leukemia is extremely poor, with a median survival of less than 1 year.[16] Given the replacement of mustargen, oncovin, procarbazine, and prednisone (MOPP) by adriamycin, bleomycin, vinblastine, and dacarbazine (ABVD), the risk of leukemia has been substantially reduced. Possibly leukemogenic agents, however, are still used in the context of salvage therapy and are often included in several newer regimens, such as bleomycin, etoposide, adriamycin, cyclophosphamide, procarbazine, and prednisone (BEA-COPP).[17] Thus, an elevated risk of secondary leukemia may eventually become manifest in subgroups of HD patients given selected types of modern therapy.

Although an increased risk of non-Hodgkin lymphoma (NHL) after HD has been reported,[10] the relationship with prior therapy is unclear. Patients with history of lymphocyte predominant HD have been shown to be at higher risk for developing NHL than those with other histologic types. The prognosis of NHL after HD appears to be comparable to patients with de novo advanced-stage NHL.[18]

Solid tumors have now emerged as the major type of second malignancy after HD, accounting for up to 75% to 80% of all cases.[19] Radiotherapy-associated solid tumors usually develop after a considerably longer latency period (at least 5–9 years) as measured from primary therapy of HD, with elevated risks persisting for at least 3 decades.[19] The majority of these solid tumors arise within or at the edges of prior HD radiotherapy fields, supporting the case for antecedent radiation contributing to tumor occurrence. Recent studies have also documented a significant relationship with radiation dose for HD to the site of second tumor occurrence for selected solid cancers. In a large international case-control investigation of women treated for HD before 30 years of age who developed breast cancer (105 cases; 266 matched controls), radiation dose to the area of the breast where the tumor developed in the case (and a comparable area in matched controls) was estimated for each case-control set.[20] Breast cancer risk increased significantly with increasing radiation dose to reach 8-fold for the highest category (median dose 42 Gy) compared to the lowest dose group (< 4 Gy; $P < .001$).

In a separate Dutch study of women treated for HD before 40 years of age,[21] similar results were found, with most of the latter patients also included in the international investigation.[20] In both studies, women who received both chemotherapy and radiation therapy had a significantly diminished risk (about 50%) compared to women given radiation therapy alone[20,21]; moreover, the radiation-associated risks were reduced by therapy with alkylating agents and/or a radiation dose of 5 Gy or more to the ovaries. In particular, the Dutch study clearly showed that the marked risk reduction associated with chemotherapy was secondary to the high number of women who developed premature menopause. Findings in both investigations indicated that ovarian hormones are a critical influence in promoting tumorigenesis once an initiating event has been produced by radiation.[20,21]

A highly significant dose–response relationship with radiation has similarly been shown for the occurrence of lung cancer after HD. In an international investigation by Travis and colleagues, lung cancer risk increased with increasing radiation dose to the area of the lung in which cancer developed, even among HD patients who received 40 or more Gy ($P < .001$); risk reached 7- to 9-fold at doses of 30 or more Gy. All risks were calculated in relation to patients who received < 5 Gy to the area of the lung in which cancer developed.

It should be noted that the data on solid tumors after radiotherapy for HD were based on patients treated in an era during which large treatment fields and very high radiation doses were used. In contrast, radiation treatment fields are significantly smaller with the current standard of involved-field radiation therapy given as part of combined modality therapy. Moreover, current studies are also exploring the effect of further reductions in radiation treatment dose for HD, and a trend exists toward the application of involved-node radiation therapy. Both of these factors will result in additional reductions in the exposure of normal tissue to radiation.[23] Therefore, it is likely that HD patients who receive radiotherapy in the modern treatment era will incur a lower risk of solid tumors.

Given the historically important role of radiation therapy in the cure of HD, there is a dearth of long-term data on late effects in HD patients treated with chemotherapy alone. In a British survey of 1,693 HD patients given chemotherapy only, the relative risk (RR) of lung cancer was significantly increased 3-fold (RR: 3.3; 95% CI, 2.2–4.7).[24] The elevated risk of lung cancer was comparable in magnitude to HD patients who received either radiation therapy alone (RR: 2.9; 95% CI, 1.9–4.1) or combined modality therapy (RR: 4.3; 95% CI, 2.9–6.2). Most HD patients in this study were treated with alkylating agent-based chemotherapy. The important role of alkylating agents given for HD in the subsequent occurrence of lung cancer was confirmed in a case-control study by the same British collaboration group,[25] and in the NCI international case-control study described previously.[22] Both investigations demonstrated a significant dose–response relationship between cumulative amount of alkylating agent chemotherapy and lung cancer risk.

Age also appears to be an important factor in modifying the risk of selected treatment-related second cancers after HD. Young age at mantle irradiation has consistently been associated with a significantly increased risk of breast cancer in women.[16,19,20,26] In a recent population-based cohort study by Hodgson and colleagues, the absolute risks of breast cancer in women diagnosed with HD at 15 to 25 years of age were 34 to 47 per 10,000 person years at 10 years, which was higher than the absolute risks of women in the general population between 50 and 54 years of age, a standard age when mammography screening is recommended.[19]

The increasing awareness of the sizable risk of breast cancer after therapy for HD at a young age has generated a need for informed counseling. Estimates of the cumulative absolute risk of breast cancer among young women treated for HD aged 30 years or younger, however, have been inconsistent, ranging from 4.2% to 34% at 20 to 25 years after therapy.[6,24,27,28] Most estimates have not taken into account the impact of alkylating agent therapy, which can reduce breast cancer risk,[20,21] or the effect of competing causes of mortality.[29] Accurate projections of breast cancer risk, as generated for women in the general population,[30] are important to predict the disease burden among the growing population of HD survivors treated with past regimens and to enable the development of risk-adapted long-term follow-up recommendations.

Estimates of the cumulative absolute risk of breast cancer for women treated for HD aged 30 years or younger were recently provided in terms of measures of radiation dose and chemotherapy that exist in medical records.[8] The estimates also factored in the influence of age and calendar year of HD diagnosis, age at counseling, baseline breast cancer incidence rates, and competing causes of mortality. For instance, for an HD survivor treated at 25 years of age with a chest radiation dose of at least 40 Gy without alkylating agents, estimated cumulative absolute risks of breast cancer by age 35, 45, and 55 years were 1.4%, 11.1%, and 29.0%, respectively. Cumulative absolute risks were predictably lower in women also treated with alkylating agents of the past, which frequently resulted in ovarian failure. In comparison, in the general population, the absolute risks of breast cancer in white women from 20 years of age to 30, 40, 50, and 60 years of age are, respectively, 0.04%, 0.5%, 2.0%, and 4.3%. Travis and colleagues emphasized that the risk estimates are most relevant for HD survivors treated with past regimens and should be used with considerable caution in patients treated with more recent approaches,[8] including limited-field radiotherapy and/or ovary-sparing chemotherapy.

Tobacco use is another important factor that can modify the risk of treatment-related lung cancer among HD survivors. In the NCI international case-control study of lung cancer,[22] in which the reference (comparison) group was comprised of HD patients with minimal radiation exposure who were nonsmokers or light smokers, those patients given either alkylating agent chemotherapy alone or 5 or more Gy of radiation therapy alone to the region of the lung in which cancer developed later experienced 4.3-fold and 7.2-fold increased risks of lung cancer, respectively. These RRs increased to 16.8-fold and 20.2-fold, respectively, among those HD patients who also smoked at least one pack of cigarettes per day. For those cigarette smokers (at least one pack per day) also given alkylating agent chemotherapy and 5 or more Gy of radiation therapy to the area of the lung in which cancer developed, the RR of subsequent lung cancer was 49.1, consistent with a multiplicative effect of smoking on the risk of treatment-related lung cancer.

As information on second malignancy risk after HD therapy has accrued, there has been increasing research and clinical efforts directed toward the development of programs for early detection and prevention of a new malignancy and for risk factor modification (e.g., smoking cessation) as well as treatment refinements (as described in this section).[31] These iterative efforts may provide a useful model for managing survivors of other primary cancers for whom long-term data on excess second malignancies are only now emerging.

Testicular Cancer

Similar to HD, testicular cancer is highly curable and largely affects young patients, whose 5-year relative survival rate after treatment completion is currently 95%. Past treatments for testicular cancer also included the use of relatively large radiotherapy fields, and second malignancies are an important cause of death among survivors of testicular cancer.[4,32]

Increased risks for secondary leukemias have been reported in survivors of testicular cancer, as well as excess solid tumors, including malignant mesothelioma and cancers of the lung, thyroid, esophagus, stomach, pancreas, colon, rectum, kidney, bladder, and connective tissue.[33] Excess contralateral testicular cancers have also been observed, which are likely due to underlying predisposition rather than treatment. In a large population-based study of 29,515 U.S. testicular cancer survivors, the 15-year cumulative risk of contralateral testicular cancer was 1.9% and was 12.4 times higher than that expected in the general population.[34]

Many solid tumors that follow testicular cancer, depending on site, are likely due in part to the historical use of para-aortic and pelvic radiation therapy for testicular cancer; through the 1970s, mediastinal radiation was also given. In the largest, international population-based study of testicular cancer survivors to date, Travis and colleagues described site-specific solid tumor risk among 40,576 testicular cancer survivors who were followed for an average of 11.8 years.[33] The RRs of developing a solid tumor were significantly increased after both radiation therapy alone and chemotherapy alone (RR: 2.0 and 1.8, respectively). Although the RR was somewhat higher among patients who received both chemotherapy and radiation therapy (RR: 2.9), the risk did not differ significantly from those patients treated with single-modality therapy. For the group with infradiaphragmatic solid tumors that were likely related to prior radiation treatment (based on anatomic site of development), the RRs increased with increasing follow-up time.

The risk of leukemia after testicular cancer is related to both chemotherapy and radiation therapy.[32,35–37] Chemotherapeutic agents that have been associated with the development of leukemia include cisplatin and etoposide.[35–37] A population-based study by Travis and colleagues explored treatment-associated leukemia in 18,567 men with testicular cancer who had survived at least 1 year. The risk of leukemia increased significantly with increasing radiation field size, which was reflected in total dose to active bone marrow. Further, after taking into account the dose of radiation to active bone marrow, the risk of leukemia was also significantly associated with cumulative amount of cisplatin,[35] with too few patients exposed to etoposide to reliably evaluate risk.

Breast Cancer

Women with breast cancer account for about 20% of all cancer survivors. The largest amount of data with regard to second primary cancers among these patients exist for contralateral breast cancer, which is related in large part to preexisting breast cancer risk factors.[38–40] Prior radiation therapy may also contribute to the risk, especially among women who received treatment at a young age. Another second malignancy that is related to both shared risk factors and breast cancer therapy, in particular tamoxifen therapy, is endometrial cancer. Lung cancer and sarcoma are other solid tumors that have been reported in breast cancer survivors, with risks largely related to radiotherapy exposure. An increased risk of leukemia after breast cancer has been associated with antecedent chemotherapy and radiation therapy.

The risk of contralateral breast cancer is increased 2- to 5-fold among breast cancer survivors.[39] Conflicting data exist on the contribution of radiation therapy to the excess risk.[38–42] In a case-control study by Boice and colleagues, the overall RR of contralateral breast cancer was not significantly increased after radiation therapy (RR: 1.19; 95% CI, 0.94–1.15).[39] Among women who were under 45 years of age at the time of irradiation, however, the RR was significantly elevated (RR: 1.59; 95% CI, 1.07–2.36). In contrast, in a large Danish case-control study, there was no significant difference in the risk of contralateral breast cancer in women who did and did not receive radiation therapy, regardless of age at treatment.[40] In the latter investigation, contralateral tumors were uniformly distributed in the medial, lateral, and central portions of the breast, which was also not consistent with a causal role of radiotherapy.

In a report from the Early Breast Cancer Trialists' Collaborative Group, a significantly increased risk of contralateral breast cancer was found after radiotherapy, primarily during the period 5 to 14 years after randomization (RR: 1.43; $P = .00001$), a latency pattern that is not consistent with the typical late effects of radiotherapy; excess risks after irradiation were significant even among women aged 50 years or older when randomized (RR: 1.25; p $= .002$).[43] A recent large-scale survey of

13,472 breast cancer patients treated at the Institut Curie in Paris did not demonstrate an increased overall risk of contralateral tumors among women who received radiation therapy compared to those who did not receive radiation (RR: 1.1; 95% CI, 0.96–1.27); however, analyses by patient age were not performed.[38]

Tamoxifen, which is given to many breast cancer patients with estrogen receptor-positive tumors as adjuvant therapy, has been shown to reduce the risk of contralateral tumors by 30% to 40%.[44] Nonetheless, a number of large investigations have clearly demonstrated a 2- to 4-fold increased risk of endometrial cancer after tamoxifen therapy.[45,46] Whereas earlier studies indicated that endometrial cancer after tamoxifen therapy might have a more favorable prognosis compared with de novo tumors, more recent data have suggested that tamoxifen-related endometrial cancers may demonstrate more aggressive behavior.[47–49] It should be noted, however, that most cases of secondary endometrial cancer are detected at an early stage, and can therefore be surgically resected.[49] Consequently, endometrial cancer after tamoxifen therapy does not appear to be associated with poorer endometrial cancer-specific survival.

Radiation therapy is an important modality in the treatment of breast cancer, either as part of breast-conserving therapy or as post-mastectomy radiation therapy. Other solid tumors have also been linked to radiotherapy for breast cancer, including lung cancer, soft tissue sarcoma, and esophageal cancer. In a number of studies, women who received radiation therapy have been shown to be 1.5 to 3 times more likely to develop lung cancer than women who did not receive radiation therapy.[38,50,51] The increased risk appeared to be more clearly related to post-mastectomy radiation therapy, in which the target volume often also includes the supraclavicular, axillary, and/or internal mammary nodal region, thus exposing a larger volume of underlying lung tissue to radiation; the existence of any increased risk after post-lumpectomy radiation therapy is less certain.[52,53] The observation that lung cancer after breast cancer therapy is more frequently found in the ipsilateral lung also supports a contributing role of radiation therapy to the elevated risk.[52] Several studies showed an even greater increase in lung cancer risk among smokers given breast radiation,[54,55] although any interaction between tobacco exposure and prior radiation therapy on subsequent lung cancer risk is not as well delineated as in HD survivors.

The 15-year cumulative incidence of sarcoma after breast cancer is low (< 0.5%), although the RR has been estimated to be as high as 7-fold, given the low background incidence in the general population.[38,56–58] In an Italian study of breast cancer survivors, all subsequent sarcomas were either localized to the previously irradiated fields or to the upper extremity of the arm ipsilateral to the treated breast among women initially given radiotherapy.[59] By estimating the initial radiation dose to the site of sarcoma development, using a dose of ≤14 Gy as reference, women who received 14 to 44 Gy had a 1.6-fold increased risk of sarcoma while those who received ≥ 45 Gy to the site had a 30.6-fold increased risk ($P < .001$). Angiosarcoma after breast cancer was initially shown to be associated with chronic lymphedema following radical mastectomy.[60] Given the increasing use of radiotherapy with breast-conserving surgery, a growing number of reports document the occurrence of cutaneous angiosarcoma of the breast arising in the radiation field.[58,61–63] Dissimilar to other radiation-related soft tissue sarcomas, breast angiosarcoma has a short latency, with diagnoses documented in the first 5 years after therapy.

Excess leukemias following breast cancer are related to prior chemotherapy and radiation therapy.[39,64–66] In a population-based, nested case-control study of women treated for breast cancer between 1973 and 1985, Curtis and colleagues showed that compared to women who did not receive alkylating chemotherapy or radiation therapy, the RR of acute myelogenous leukemia after radiation therapy alone, alkylating chemotherapy alone, and both chemotherapy and radiation therapy were 2.4, 10.0, and 17.4, respectively.[64] A significant dose–response relation was observed for either cumulative dose of melphalan, cyclophosphamide, or radiation to the active bone marrow, and subsequent leukemia risk. This study, however, was conducted in a period when higher cumulative doses of chemotherapy and larger field radiation therapy were used than what are presently used. Moreover, melphalan-containing regimens are no longer used in the treatment of breast cancer. Recent data demonstrate that the risk of secondary acute leukemia is more significantly related to the dose-intensity of cyclophosphamide than with cumulative dose,[67] an observation that is noteworthy in view of the increasing trend toward the use of dose-intensified regimens for breast cancer. Even as evolutions in systemic chemotherapy for breast cancer may eventually affect the risk of second malignancies, recent advances in radiation therapy, including the use of intensity-modulated radiation therapy (IMRT)and the growing interest in partial breast irradiation,[68] may also influence the risk profile. The degree to which second cancer risk will be affected by these newer radiation therapy approaches and techniques will have to be established through long-term follow-up of sufficiently large cohorts of breast cancer survivors, which will enable sufficient statistical power for the detection of increased site-specific risks.

Prostate Cancer

Given the large number of prostate cancer survivors, the late effects of this cancer and its treatment have become critically important. In recent years, increasing reports have described the risk of second malignancies after radiation therapy for prostate cancer.[10] In an early report by Neugut and colleagues, the risk of second cancers following radiotherapy for prostate carcinoma was evaluated among patients reported to the population-based registries that comprise the NCI's SEER program (1973–1990).[69] Patients treated with radiation therapy had significant excesses of bladder cancer after a latent period of 8 years (RR: 1.5; 95% CI, 1.1–2.0), while excesses were not apparent among men who did not receive radiation therapy. In a more recent survey, utilizing the Mayo Clinic Cancer Registry, the overall relative risk of bladder cancer after radiation therapy was not significantly increased.[70] However, among those men given adjuvant radiation therapy after a radical prostatectomy, the RR of bladder cancer was five times higher than expected ($P = .05$), which may reflect the larger volume of bladder tissue exposed to radiation in the postoperative setting.

In an updated study of prostate cancer patients reported to the SEER Program (1973–1993), second cancer risks among men who were initially given radiation therapy were compared with those observed after surgery alone.[71] Men given radiotherapy demonstrated significant excesses of sarcoma and cancers of the lung, bladder, and rectum. The elevated risks of lung cancer were hypothesized to reflect low scatter doses of radiation to the lungs. This finding may be more relevant to men given cobalt radiation to the whole pelvis, although the SEER program does not collect data on type of radiotherapy. A more recent investigation using the linked SEER-Medicare database studied a larger group of prostate cancer patients, including those treated in the more recent era.[72] Men given external beam radiotherapy demonstrated significantly increased risks of malignant melanoma and cancers of the bladder, rectum, colon, brain, stomach, and lung, with odds ratios ranging from 1.25 to 1.85 when compared with men who did not receive external beam radiation therapy. Patients who received radioactive implants with or without external beam radiation therapy, however, did not show significant excesses of second cancers when compared with those who did not receive radiation.

Another survey of prostate cancer patients reported to the SEER program (1973–2001) focused on the risk of rectal cancer following irradiation.[73] Unlike previous studies, a significant association between radiation therapy and subsequent excesses of rectal cancer was not reported. Results of Cox proportional hazards analysis (with prostate radiation, prostate surgery, and age at diagnosis entered as covariates) showed that only increasing age was associated with an increased risk of subsequent rectal cancer.

In a study of prostate cancer patients treated with radiotherapy and reported to the British Columbia Tumor Registry, significantly increased risks of sarcoma (RR: 1.7; $P < .05$), colorectal cancer (RR: 1.21; $P < .01$), and pleural cancer (RR: 2.28; $P < .01$) were observed.[74] Although significant bladder cancer excesses were not apparent in the radiotherapy cohort, risks for both bladder cancer (RR: 1.32; $P < .01$) and testicular cancer (RR: 2.82; $P < .05$) were significantly increased in the non-irradiation cohort, which were attributed to heightened surveillance.

Most of the investigations to date that evaluate the risk of malignancies among prostate cancer survivors are based on data reported to population-based tumor registries. The conflicting observations with regard to the contribution of radiotherapy to various second malignancies after prostate cancer may reflect a number of factors, including the practice of most registries to gather data only on initial course of therapy, the incomplete registration of initial treatment, and misclassification. Moreover, selection bias may determine whether patients are given surgery or radiation therapy, and the limited data available in most population-based registries do not allow for the identification of confounding factors. Patients with significant comorbid illnesses and/or a history of heavy tobacco use may not be treated with surgery and may be more likely to receive radiation therapy. Further, among prostate cancer patients given radiation therapy, treatment-related sequelae such as cystitis, hematuria, proctitis, and rectal bleeding may lead to additional cystoscopies or colonoscopies, which can then result in an apparent increased incidence of urologic and colorectal cancers.

In those studies that show significant excesses of cancers after radiotherapy for prostate cancer, the overall risk appears to be low. In the investigation by Brenner and colleagues, which included prostate cancer patients given larger field cobalt radiation, the risk of developing a second malignancy was estimated at 1 in 290.[71] In the last few years, IMRT has been increasingly utilized to treat prostate cancer in order to permit more conformal dose distribution and dose escalation.[75] Depending on treatment energy, IMRT is associated with three to five times the number of monitor units as compared with conventional treatment. Applying risk coefficients from the National Council of Radiation Protection and Measurements for specific anatomic sites to this configuration, the risks of second malignancy using IMRT techniques have been estimated to be two to three times higher than after conventional radiation therapy.[76] These preliminary estimates remain to be confirmed in epidemiologic studies that include large numbers of patients given IMRT who have been followed for sufficient periods of time to permit detection of any increased radiotherapy-associated risk.

CONCLUSION

In view of the increasing number of cancer survivors, the development of second cancer malignancies has emerged as a significant problem that can affect quality of life and long-term survival. It is critical to continue to describe and quantify the risks of second malignancies. Moreover, the evolving patterns have important implications for patient counseling and the recommendation of behavioral changes, cancer screening, and prevention strategies. Where efficacious screening methods (e.g., mammography) are available, these modalities should be included in patient follow-up, as indicated, including women treated for HD at a young age with the wide-field, high-dose chest radiotherapy treatments of the past. Preventive approaches (e.g., smoking cessation, avoidance of ultraviolet light) may also decrease the risk of selected second cancers, and cancer survivors should be strongly advised to implement practices consistent with a healthy lifestyle. An improved recognition and understanding of therapy-related second malignancies can inform modifications in regimens to minimize exposure to cytoxic agents. Key strategies to reduce the negative impact of second malignancies on cancer survivors are summarized in Table 15.2.

Modification or reduction of current treatments that have established efficacy, however, should not be undertaken outside the context of clinical trials. Further, it is important to remember that second malignancies, although a serious issue, are actually a problem of success and are not observed unless a patient survives a cancer diagnosis; thus, the survival benefits provided by many cancer treatments greatly outweigh the risk of developing a second primary cancer. Moreover, as reviewed in this chapter, second cancers can reflect not only the late effects of therapy but the impact of lifestyle choices (e.g., alcohol or tobacco

TABLE 15.2 ∼ Key Strategies to Reduce the Impact of Second Malignancy on Cancer Survivors

Strategies	Examples
Patient Education	• Increase patient awareness of risks • Promote healthy lifestyle and health practices (smoking cessation, sun safety awareness, adherence to screening guidelines for the general population)
Screening	• Early detection of selected second cancers (mammography, breast magnetic resonance imaging, colonoscopy, routine screening skin examination)
Prevention	• Smoking cessation • Sun safety practices • Prophylactic surgeries
Survivorship Research	• Documentation of long-term second cancer risks with newer treatments • Prospective evaluation of screening and prevention strategies
Treatment Modifications	• Trials evaluating reduction/modification of upfront treatment in selected primary cancers

use), host factors, environmental determinants, and the operation of joint effects, including gene-environment and gene-gene interactions.[5]

REFERENCES

1. Ries L, Melbert D, Krapcho M, et al. SEER Cancer Statistics Review, 1975–2004. Bethesda: National Cancer Institute; 2007.
2. Anonymous. Cancer survivors: living longer, and now, better. *Lancet.* 2004;364:2153–2154.
3. Dores G, Schonfeld S, Chen J, et al. Long-term cause-specific mortality among 41,146 one-year survivors of Hodgkin lymphoma (HL). *Proc Am Soc Clin Oncol.* 2005;23:562S.
4. Schairer C, Hisada M, Chen BE, et al. Comparative mortality for 621 second cancers in 29356 testicular cancer survivors and 12420 matched first cancers. *J Natl Cancer Inst.* 2007;99(16):1248–1256.
5. Travis L, Rabkin C, Brown L, et al. Cancer survivorship—genetic susceptibility and second primary cancers: research strategies and recommendations. *J Natl Cancer Inst.* 2006;98:15–25.
6. Bhatia S, Yasui Y, Robison LL, et al. High risk of subsequent neoplasms continues with extended follow-up of childhood Hodgkin's disease: report from the Late Effects Study Group. *J Clin Oncol.* 2003;21(23):4386–4394.
7. Travis L. Therapy-associated solid tumors. *Acta Oncol.* 2002;41:323–333.
8. Travis LB, Hill D, Dores GM, et al. Cumulative absolute breast cancer risk for young women treated for Hodgkin lymphoma. *J Natl Cancer Inst.* 2005;97(19):1428–1437.
9. Allan J, Travis L. Mechanism of therapy-related carcinogenesis. *Nat Rev Cancer.* 2005;5:943–955.
10. van Leeuwen F, Travis L. Second cancers. In: DeVita VT Jr, et al, eds. *Cancer: Principals and Practice of Oncology.* 7th ed. Philadelphia: Lippincott Williams & Wilkins; 2005:2575–2602.
11. Arseneau JC, Sponzo RW, Levin DL, et al. Nonlymphomatous malignant tumors complicating Hodgkin's disease. Possible association with intensive therapy. *N Engl J Med.* 1972;287(22):1119–1122.
12. Kaldor JM, Day NE, Clarke EA, et al. Leukemia following Hodgkin's disease. *N Engl J Med.* 1990;322(1):7–13.
13. van Leeuwen FE, Chorus AM, van den Belt-Dusebout AW, et al. Leukemia risk following Hodgkin's disease: relation to cumulative dose of alkylating agents, treatment with teniposide combinations, number of episodes of chemotherapy, and bone marrow damage. *J Clin Oncol.* 1994;12(5):1063–1073.

14. Henry-Amar M. Second cancer after the treatment for Hodgkin's disease: a report from the International Database on Hodgkin's Disease. *Ann Oncol.* 1992;3(suppl 4):117–128.

15. Andrieu JM, Ifrah N, Payen C, et al. Increased risk of secondary acute nonlymphocytic leukemia after extended-field radiation therapy combined with MOPP chemotherapy for Hodgkin's disease. *J Clin Oncol.* 1990;8(7): 1148–1154.

16. Ng AK, Bernardo MV, Weller E, et al. Second malignancy after Hodgkin disease treated with radiation therapy with or without chemotherapy: long-term risks and risk factors. *Blood.* 2002;100(6):1989–1996.

17. Diehl V, Franklin J, Pfreundschuh M, et al. Standard and increased-dose BEACOPP chemotherapy compared with COPP-ABVD for advanced Hodgkin's disease. *N Engl J Med.* 2003;348(24):2386–2395.

18. Rueffer U, Josting A, Franklin J, et al. Non-Hodgkin's lymphoma after primary Hodgkin's disease in the German Hodgkin's Lymphoma Study Group: incidence, treatment, and prognosis. *J Clin Oncol.* 2001;19(7): 2026–2032.

19. Hodgson DC, Gilbert ES, Dores GM, et al. Long-term solid cancer risk among 5-year survivors of Hodgkin's lymphoma. *J Clin Oncol.* 2007; 25(12):1489–1497.

20. Travis LB, Hill DA, Dores GM, et al. Breast cancer following radiotherapy and chemotherapy among young women with Hodgkin disease. *JAMA.* 2003;290(4):465–475.

21. van Leeuwen FE, Klokman WJ, Stovall M, et al. Roles of radiation dose, chemotherapy, and hormonal factors in breast cancer following Hodgkin's disease. *J Natl Cancer Inst.* 2003;95(13):971–980.

22. Travis LB, Gospodarowicz M, Curtis RE, et al. Lung cancer following chemotherapy and radiotherapy for Hodgkin's disease. *J Natl Cancer Inst.* 2002;94(3):182–192.

23. Girinsky T, van der Maazen R, Specht L, et al. Involved-node radiotherapy (INRT) in patients with early Hodgkin lymphoma: concepts and guidelines. *Radiother Oncol.* 2006;79(3):270–277.

24. Swerdlow AJ, Barber JA, Hudson GV, et al. Risk of second malignancy after Hodgkin's disease in a collaborative British cohort: the relation to age at treatment. *J Clin Oncol.* 2000;18(3):498–509.

25. Swerdlow AJ, Schoemaker MJ, Allerton R, et al. Lung cancer after Hodgkin's disease: a nested case-control study of the relation to treatment. *J Clin Oncol.* 2001;19(6):1610–1618.

26. van Leeuwen FE, Klokman WJ, Veer MB, et al. Long-term risk of second malignancy in survivors of Hodgkin's disease treated during adolescence or young adulthood. *J Clin Oncol.* 2000;18(3):487–497.

27. Aisenberg AC, Finkelstein DM, Doppke KP, Koerner FC, Boivin JF, Willett CG. High risk of breast carcinoma after irradiation of young women with Hodgkin's disease. *Cancer*. 1997;79(6):1203–1210.

28. Sankila R, Garwicz S, Olsen JH, et al. Risk of subsequent malignant neoplasms among 1,641 Hodgkin's disease patients diagnosed in childhood and adolescence: a population-based cohort study in the five Nordic countries. Association of the Nordic Cancer Registries and the Nordic Society of Pediatric Hematology and Oncology. *J Clin Oncol*. 1996;14(5):1442–1446.

29. Gooley TA, Leisenring W, Crowley J, Storer BE. Estimation of failure probabilities in the presence of competing risks: new representations of old estimators. *Stat Med*. 1999;18(6):695–706.

30. Gail MH, Brinton LA, Byar DP, et al. Projecting individualized probabilities of developing breast cancer for white females who are being examined annually. *J Natl Cancer Inst*. 1989;81(24):1879–1886.

31. Mauch P, Ng A, Aleman B, et al. Report from the Rockefeller Foundation Sponsored International Workshop on reducing mortality and improving quality of life in long-term survivors of Hodgkin's disease: July 9–16, 2003, Bellagio, Italy. *Eur J Haematol Suppl*. 2005(66):68–76.

32. van den Belt-Dusebout AW, de Wit R, Gietema JA, et al. Treatment-specific risks of second malignancies and cardiovascular disease in 5-year survivors of testicular cancer. *J Clin Oncol*. 2007;25(28):4370–4378.

33. Travis LB, Fossa SD, Schonfeld SJ, et al. Second cancers among 40,576 testicular cancer patients: focus on long-term survivors. *J Natl Cancer Inst*. 2005;97(18):1354–1365.

34. Fossa SD, Chen J, Schonfeld SJ, et al. Risk of contralateral testicular cancer: a population-based study of 29,515 U.S. men. *J Natl Cancer Inst*. 2005; 97(14):1056–1066.

35. Travis LB, Andersson M, Gospodarowicz M, et al. Treatment-associated leukemia following testicular cancer. *J Natl Cancer Inst*. 2000;92(14): 1165–1171.

36. Pedersen-Bjergaard J, Daugaard G, Hansen SW, Philip P, Larsen SO, Rorth M. Increased risk of myelodysplasia and leukaemia after etoposide, cisplatin, and bleomycin for germ-cell tumours. *Lancet*. 1991;338(8763): 359–363.

37. Kollmannsberger C, Hartmann JT, Kanz L, Bokemeyer C. Therapy-related malignancies following treatment of germ cell cancer. *Int J Cancer*. 1999;83(6):860–863.

38. Kirova YM, Gambotti L, De Rycke Y, Vilcoq JR, Asselain B, Fourquet A. Risk of second malignancies after adjuvant radiotherapy for breast can-

cer: a large-scale, single-institution review. *Int J Radiat Oncol Biol Phys.* 2007;68(2):359–363.

39. Boice JD Jr, Harvey EB, Blettner M, Stovall M, Flannery JT. Cancer in the contralateral breast after radiotherapy for breast cancer. *N Engl J Med.* 1992;326(12):781–785.

40. Storm HH, Andersson M, Boice JD, Jr., et al. Adjuvant radiotherapy and risk of contralateral breast cancer. *J Natl Cancer Inst.* 1992;84(16): 1245–1250.

41. Gao X, Fisher SG, Emami B. Risk of second primary cancer in the contralateral breast in women treated for early-stage breast cancer: a population-based study. *Int J Radiat Oncol Biol Phys.* 2003;56(4): 1038–1045.

42. Hill-Kayser CE, Harris EE, Hwang WT, et al. Twenty-year incidence and patterns of contralateral breast cancer after breast conservation treatment with radiation. *Int J Radiat Oncol Biol Phys.* 2006;66(5):1313–1319.

43. Clarke M, Collins R, Darby S, et al. Effects of radiotherapy and of differences in the extent of surgery for early breast cancer on local recurrence and 15-year survival: an overview of the randomised trials. *Lancet.* 2005; 366(9503):2087–2106.

44. Effects of chemotherapy and hormonal therapy for early breast cancer on recurrence and 15-year survival: an overview of the randomised trials. *Lancet.* 2005;365(9472):1687–1717.

45. Fisher B, Costantino JP, Redmond CK, et al. Endometrial cancer in tamoxifen-treated breast cancer patients: findings from the National Surgical Adjuvant Breast and Bowel Project (NSABP) B-14. *J Natl Cancer Inst.* 1994;86(7):527–537.

46. Fisher B, Costantino JP, Wickerham DL, et al. Tamoxifen for prevention of breast cancer: report of the National Surgical Adjuvant Breast and Bowel Project P-1 Study. *J Natl Cancer Inst.* 1998;90(18):1371–1388.

47. Magriples U, Naftolin F, Schwartz PE, et al. High-grade endometrial carcinoma in tamoxifen-treated breast cancer patients. *J Clin Oncol.* 1993;11(3):485–490.

48. Bergman L, Beelen ML, Gallee MP, et al. Risk and prognosis of endometrial cancer after tamoxifen for breast cancer. Comprehensive Cancer Centres' ALERT Group. Assessment of liver and endometrial cancer risk following tamoxifen. *Lancet.* 2000;356(9233):881–887.

49. Saadat M, Truong PT, Kader HA, et al. Outcomes in patients with primary breast cancer and a subsequent diagnosis of endometrial cancer: comparison of cohorts treated with and without tamoxifen. *Cancer.* 2007;110(1):31–37.

50. Roychoudhuri R, Evans H, Robinson D, et al. Radiation-induced malignancies following radiotherapy for breast cancer. *Br J Cancer*. 2004;91(5): 868–872.

51. Neugut AI, Robinson E, Lee WC, et al. Lung cancer after radiation therapy for breast cancer. *Cancer*. 1993;71(10):3054–3057.

52. Zablotska LB, Neugut AI. Lung carcinoma after radiation therapy in women treated with lumpectomy or mastectomy for primary breast carcinoma. *Cancer*. 2003;97(6):1404–1411.

53. Deutsch M, Land SR, Begovic M, et al. The incidence of lung carcinoma after surgery for breast carcinoma with and without postoperative radiotherapy. Results of National Surgical Adjuvant Breast and Bowel Project (NSABP) clinical trials B-04 and B-06. *Cancer*. 2003; 98(7):1362–1368.

54. Neugut AI, Murray T, Santos J, et al. Increased risk of lung cancer after breast cancer radiation therapy in cigarette smokers. *Cancer*. 1994;73(6): 1615–1620.

55. Ford MB, Sigurdson AJ, Petrulis ES, et al. Effects of smoking and radiotherapy on lung carcinoma in breast carcinoma survivors. *Cancer*. 2003; 98(7):1457–1464.

56. Huang J, Mackillop WJ. Increased risk of soft tissue sarcoma after radiotherapy in women with breast carcinoma. *Cancer*. 2001;92(1):172–180.

57. Karlsson P, Holmberg E, Samuelsson A, et al. Soft tissue sarcoma after treatment for breast cancer—a Swedish population-based study. *Eur J Cancer*. 1998;34(13):2068–2075.

58. Kirova YM, Vilcoq JR, Asselain B, et al. Radiation-induced sarcomas after radiotherapy for breast carcinoma: a large-scale single-institution review. *Cancer*. 2005;104(4):856–863.

59. Rubino C, de Vathaire F, Shamsaldin A, et al. Radiation dose, chemotherapy, hormonal treatment and risk of second cancer after breast cancer treatment. *Br J Cancer*. 2003;89(5):840–846.

60. Jessner M, Zak FG, Rein CR. Angiosarcoma in postmastectomy lymphedema (Stewart-Treves syndrome). *AMA Arch Derm Syphilol*. 1952; 65(2):123–129.

61. Esler-Brauer L, Jaggernauth W, Zeitouni NC. Angiosarcoma developing after conservative treatment for breast carcinoma: case report with review of the current literature. *Dermatol Surg*. 2007;33(6):749–755.

62. Virtanen A, Pukkala E, Auvinen A. Angiosarcoma after radiotherapy: a cohort study of 332,163 Finnish cancer patients. *Br J Cancer*. 2007;97(1): 115–117.

63. Simonart T, Heenen M. Radiation-induced angiosarcomas. *Dermatol*. 2004;209(3):175–176.

64. Curtis RE, Boice JD Jr, Stovall M, et al. Risk of leukemia after chemotherapy and radiation treatment for breast cancer. *N Engl J Med.* 1992;326(26): 1745–1751.

65. Praga C, Bergh J, Bliss J, et al. Risk of acute myeloid leukemia and myelodysplastic syndrome in trials of adjuvant epirubicin for early breast cancer: correlation with doses of epirubicin and cyclophosphamide. *J Clin Oncol.* 2005;23(18):4179–4191.

66. Campone M, Roche H, Kerbrat P, et al. Secondary leukemia after epirubicin-based adjuvant chemotherapy in operable breast cancer patients: 16 years experience of the French Adjuvant Study Group. *Ann Oncol.* 2005; 16(8):1343–1351.

67. Smith RE, Bryant J, DeCillis A, et al. Acute myeloid leukemia and myelodysplastic syndrome after doxorubicin-cyclophosphamide adjuvant therapy for operable breast cancer: the National Surgical Adjuvant Breast and Bowel Project Experience. *J Clin Oncol.* 2003;21(7):1195–1204.

68. Chen PY, Vicini FA. Partial breast irradiation. Patient selection, guidelines for treatment, and current results. *Front Radiat Ther Oncol.* 2007; 40:253–271.

69. Neugut AI, Ahsan H, Robinson E, et al. Bladder carcinoma and other second malignancies after radiotherapy for prostate carcinoma. *Cancer.* 1997;79(8):1600–1604.

70. Chrouser K, Leibovich B, Bergstralh E, et al. Bladder cancer risk following primary and adjuvant external beam radiation for prostate cancer. *J Urol.* 2005;174(1):107–110;(discussion)110–111.

71. Brenner DJ, Curtis RE, Hall EJ, et al. Second malignancies in prostate carcinoma patients after radiotherapy compared with surgery. *Cancer.* 2000;88(2):398–406.

72. Moon K, Stukenborg GJ, Keim J, et al. Cancer incidence after localized therapy for prostate cancer. *Cancer.* 2006;107(5):991–998.

73. Kendal WS, Eapen L, Macrae R, et al. Prostatic irradiation is not associated with any measurable increase in the risk of subsequent rectal cancer. *Int J Radiat Oncol Biol Phys.* 2006;65(3):661–668.

74. Pickles T, Phillips N. The risk of second malignancy in men with prostate cancer treated with or without radiation in British Columbia, 1984–2000. *Radiother Oncol.* 2002;65(3):145–151.

75. Guckenberger M, Flentje M. Intensity-modulated radiotherapy (IMRT) of localized prostate cancer: a review and future perspectives. *Strahlenther Onkol.* 2007;183(2):57–62.

76. Kry SF, Salehpour M, Followill DS, et al. The calculated risk of fatal secondary malignancies from intensity-modulated radiation therapy. *Int J Radiat Oncol Biol Phys.* 2005;62(4):1195–1203.

Radiation-Associated Malignancies

Rachel Blitzblau, MD, PhD

&

Kenneth B. Roberts, MD

ABSTRACT

Cancer survivors treated with radiation therapy are at risk for treatment-associated malignances later in life. Much of the clinical data on this uncommon, but devastating long-term complication comes from Hodgkin disease (HD) patients. The advent of the use of radiation therapy, and later chemotherapy, to treat HD dramatically improved survival, which in turn highlighted late treatment effects. The study of this patient population has revealed factors that influence the development of radiation-associated cancers and has led to significant changes in the therapeutic use of ionizing radiation, which appears to be effectively decreasing the risk for radiation-associated malignancies.

> ∿ Case Example 16.1
>
> In 1981, a 24-year-old woman was treated with subtotal nodal irradiation (STNI) for stage II HD. A mantle field, the standard treatment at the time, received a total dose of 3625 cGy with an additional 600 cGy boost to her mediastinal lymph nodes. The total dose in that region was therefore 4225 cGy. She was cured and did well until 2003, when she was

(continues)

Case Example 16.1 (*continued*)
found to have stage II left-sided breast cancer located in the upper, inner quadrant of the breast and involving 4/7 axillary lymph nodes. Calculations from her previous treatment estimated the dose to her medial breast at 3650 cGy. The left axillary dose was estimated at 3625 cGy. It was felt that this was likely a radiation-associated malignancy. Given her prior radiation exposure, she underwent a mastectomy rather than breast-conserving therapy of lumpectomy and breast radiation.

INTRODUCTION

For a second malignancy to be considered radiation associated, certain criteria should be met.[1] First, the cancer should arise in a tissue that received radiation, though it does not have to be in a full-dose area. Second, the second cancer must be a different histology than the first. Third, there should be an appropriate latency period from the exposure to radiation, measured in years. Fourth, the second cancer cannot have been present at the time of the radiation exposure. Finally, patients with cancer-predisposing factors such as retinoblastoma-1 mutation or Li-Fraumeni syndrome should be considered separately.

Case Example 16.1 fits all of these criteria and highlights several important factors that influence the risk for development of a radiation-associated malignancy. These factors include age at exposure to radiation, total dose received, tissue exposed, length of time prior to the development of the second cancer, and gender. Other factors such as concurrent treatments, genetics, and lifestyle/environment also impact risk. This case also highlights how prior radiation therapy may impact treatment decisions for second cancers.

In this chapter, we will discuss all these issues, primarily using studies of HD patients, the source of many clinical studies on secondary cancers. Other significant sources of data, which cannot be included to any great extent, include long-term follow-up of other curable cancers occurring in younger patients (e.g., testicular cancer and pediatric cancers) and outcomes of people exposed to radiation during accidents or the World War II atomic bombings. Data obtained from cell culture and animal studies, though considerable and another source of information about the risk of secondary cancers and mutagenesis, are difficult to correlate with clinical experience at this time.

HISTORICAL TREATMENT OF HODGKIN DISEASE

While HD is a relatively rare hematologic malignancy, with 7,500 cases diagnosed each year in the United States, its importance to the field of oncology has been profound. First described in 1832 by Thomas Hodgkin,[2] this cancer largely remained incurable until the development of megavoltage radiotherapy. Building on the earlier work of Vera Peters in Toronto in the 1950s,[3,4] who first determined the radiosensitive nature of HD and the need to treat regions of adjacent lymph nodes to prevent recurrence, Henry Kaplan at Stanford University was able to cure appreciable numbers of patients.[5,6] He developed diagnostic tools to stage this lymphoma; then in the 1960s, he developed extended field radiotherapy using the new therapeutic x-ray machine called the linear accelerator, which has since become the workhorse of radiation oncology departments worldwide.

Over the decades, the diagnostic tools of lymphangiography and staging laporotomy with lymph node, liver, and bone marrow biopsies and splenectomy have been replaced by the modern studies of high resolution computed tomography, magnetic resonance imaging (MRI), and positron emission tomography (PET), as well as pathologic immunophenotyping and flow cytometry. In addition, the traditional physical examination; laboratory testing of serum, blood, and marrow; and symptomatic manifestations are used to diagnose patients with HD and classify them into prognostic groups. Staging of HD still uses the Ann Arbor stages I to IV with lymph node regions that correspond to areas to be treated with radiotherapy. An A or B designation implies the absence or presence of fevers, sweats, or weight loss due to the underlying lymphoma.

The principles of extended field radiotherapy alone for curing early stage HD represented an old standard of care dating from the 1960s until the early 1990s. Hodgkin disease was recognized to require treatment of generous lymph node regions. As one of the early malignancies to be cured by radiotherapy (along with cervical cancer, which emphasized in the decades earlier, from the 1920s to the present, the development of brachytherapy or implanted radiation), much of the oncology field owes its development to understanding the late effects of successful cancer therapy, with HD serving as a model. With more patients being cured, decades of follow-up led to an appreciation of the long-term effects of external beam radiotherapy, and tolerance of various normal organs and tissues became appreciated. Extended field radiotherapy (total irradiation or STNI) for HD evolved and was refined over several decades as the effects of radiation fractionation and organ and normal tissue tolerance were better understood.

As in the case example, STNI aimed to irradiate large volumes of nodal tissues to 30 to 45 Gy. For a typical presentation as in this case with lymphadenopathy in the neck and mediastinum, daily weekday treatments to the supradiaphragmatic regions generally took 4 to 5 weeks. Using a so-called mantle field, the regions of the neck, mediastinum, and axilla would be treated in continuity using anterior and posterior radiation fields. Blocking patterns were developed to optimize dose distributions that reduced the acute and subacute toxicity of the heart, lungs, and spinal cord. Figure 16.1 shows a typical blocking pattern of a mantle field with the coronary arteries superimposed to emphasize which cardiopulmonary tissues would be exposed to therapeutic radiation. After a 1-month rest period for hematologic recovery, the subdiaphragmatic regions would be treated, entailing radiation directed at the para-aortic lymph nodes as well as the spleen, if that organ had not been surgically removed as part of the original staging procedures.

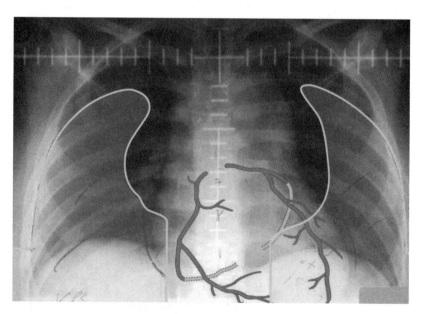

FIGURE 16.1   A typical blocking pattern of a mantle field.

While the doses required were hotly debated at the time, regions of microscopic burden generally required only 30 Gy, while grossly detectable disease would be treated with 36 to 44 Gy, with higher doses to bulkier sites of disease.[7,8] Periodically, the radiation fields would be planned to shrink to take into account normal tissue tolerances and to boost gross lymphoma. This STNI for the common presentations of lymphoma in the neck, chest, or axilla produced high cure rates, in the 70% to 80% range for early-stage disease. Some investigators had advocated treating only a mantle field in this situation, because the incremental improvement in cure rates from the abdominal fields added only an additional 5% to 10% in disease-free survival.[9] Pelvic or inguinal nodes would be included in total lymphoid irradiation, when lymphoma presented at diagnosis in the abdomen or pelvis. The additional price in toxicity for pelvic radiotherapy included infertility and other gonadal effects.

With the success of full-dose extended field irradiation for HD, there were thousands of patients being observed over decades without evidence of recurrence. The management of pediatric HD adopted the use of chemotherapy and low doses of radiotherapy in the mid-1980s in order to reduce the effects of radiation on musculoskeletal development, eliminating scoliosis, short stature, and other boney deformities as a consequence of radiotherapy. This move was prescient, because the management of adults with HD was recognized to need a change in strategy when the Stanford group first recognized other major late effects of extended field radiotherapy, particularly secondary cancers and cardiac complications. After 15 years of follow-up after curative radiotherapy for early-stage HD, the overall mortality rate from causes other than HD begins to exceed that seen from HD.[10–13] Moreover, in comparison to a matched control population, these long-term survivors are seen to have a significantly worse survival rate.[10,11] Specifically, the long-term observed survival was 29%, versus 81% HD-specific survival and 79% expected survival. Analysis of the project actuarial causes of death showed that for the first 15 years following treatment, death due to HD predominated. In patients followed for more than 15 years after treatment, however, intercurrent illnesses became the leading cause of death rather than HD itself—64% vs. 19% at 35 years (Figure 16.2).

Of these other causes of death, one of the most common was second cancers, both hematologic and solid tumors, which were thought

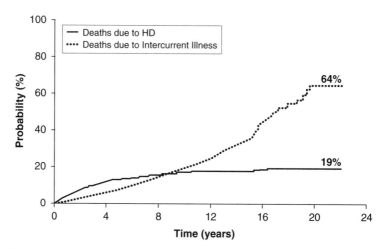

FIGURE 16.2   Risk of death due to HD versus death due to incurrent illness.[10]

to be related to treatment with chemotherapy and radiation therapy. A Boston study of 794 patients further illustrates the prevalence of second cancers in HD survivors: Of 124 deaths at a mean follow-up of 11 years, 56 were from HD, 36 were from second malignancies, 15 were from cardiac disease, and 8 were from other causes.[12] The actuarial risk of death from competing causes in this study is graphically shown in Figure 16.3. Deaths from HD primarily occurred in the first 5 to 10 years, while deaths after 10 years are principally from second malignancies that continue to occur at a steady rate over time. The estimated excess risk of mortality was approximately 1% per year over the first 20 years, in agreement with other observations.[14] It is particularly worrisome that the relative risk of solid tumors has continued to increase with further follow-up.[15,16]

At the same time that radiotherapy for HD was being refined in the 1960s to 1980s, combination chemotherapy was likewise being developed and studied for lymphomas. Drs. Vincent DeVita and Emil Frei developed MOPP (mustargen, oncovin, procarbazine and prednisone) chemotherapy in the mid-1960s as effective therapy in relapsed or advanced-stage HD.[17–19] Over time, MOPP and MOPP-like regimens were found to be a major cause of myelodysplasia and acute myeloge-

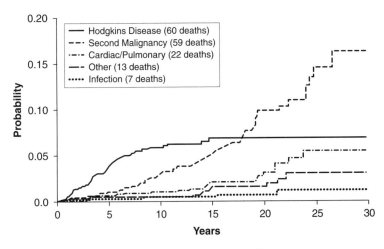

FIGURE 16.3   Risk of death due to various causes.[12]

nous leukemia, although several pieces of indirect evidence continued to suggest that higher doses of radiation were the most important factor in the development of solid tumors. For example, two studies have shown that the addition of chemotherapy to standard-dose radiation did not result in an increase in solid tumors compared to patients treated with radiation alone.[10,11,20] Data from the International Database on HD showed that treatment with radiation alone or radiation followed by chemotherapy alone was associated with the highest risk of second cancers but that chemotherapy alone or chemotherapy plus localized radiation was not associated with a significant risk of solid tumors.[21] As a result of the problems with alkylating agent-induced myeloid disease, other chemotherapy combinations for HD have been perfected. Developed by Gianni Bonadona in Italy in the 1970s, ABVD (adriamycin, bleomycin, vinblastine, and dacarbazine) is now considered a standard in the United States.[22] Aside from a negligible risk for myelodysplasia and acute myeloid leukemia, this combination has significantly less effects on fertility than MOPP regimens, which are associated with considerable problems with gonadal dysfunction.

MODERN TREATMENT OF HODGKIN DISEASE

Using clinical risk factors, patients are now further stratified into risk groups: favorable, intermediate or early stage with unfavorable features, and advanced. Unfavorable risk factors include higher stage, older age, bulky disease, extranodal involvement, elevated sedimentation rates, and presence of B symptoms.[23–25] Currently, treatment algorithms are based on groupings in which favorable patients generally present with stage I to IIA disease without risk factors, advanced patients present with stage IIIB to IVB, and the intermediate group have some constellation of poor prognostic factors. Nevertheless, with modern therapy, cure rates are 90% to 99% for favorable patients, 85% to 95% for intermediate patients, and 70% to 85% for advanced patients. How rapidly the lymphoma responds to chemotherapy as assessed by PET scanning is also emerging as a prognostic factor.[26] Clinical trials are underway to see if this information may be used to tailor therapy, in some instances even testing the deletion of radiotherapy if there is a rapid early response to chemotherapy.

But as a general rule, patients are now treated with combined-modality therapy emphasizing initial adriamycin-based chemotherapy programs to produce an initial good response. Radiotherapy is no longer the primary treatment modality but is instead an adjuvant to chemotherapy to eliminate any residual microscopic disease and allow for fewer cycles of chemotherapy to be used compared to a strategy of chemotherapy alone. Thus, radiotherapy using full-dose extended fields is rarely used anymore. The current standard is for radiotherapy to be delivered at lower doses than used historically and to an involved region, where HD would be predicated to recur if chemotherapy were the sole treatment modality. Figure 16.4 depicts this change in the management of early-stage HD from large-volume, full-dose radiotherapy alone to chemotherapy plus low-dose involved-field radiotherapy (IFRT).

Thus, it is important to point out that the radiotherapy techniques associated with a substantial risk of secondary cancers and cardiac sequela are no longer being used. Instead of large volumes of lymphatic tissues and accompanying normal organs being exposed to 30 to 45 Gy, the role of radiotherapy has been reduced to being an adjuvant therapy to primary chemotherapy, where original sites of disease that have responded to chemotherapy are treated with lower radiation doses along

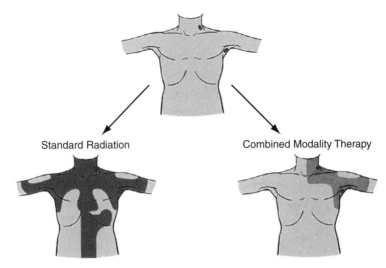

FIGURE 16.4 Schematic of subtotal nodal irradiation versus low-dose involved field radiotherapy fields for stage IIa Hodgkin disease.

with a reduction in the volume of radiotherapy. One cannot extrapolate the risks of older techniques to the newer treatment paradigms. With the switch to combined-modality therapy using low-dose IFRT, one cannot use the old estimates of risk for second cancers. In a similar manner, this strategy as initially applied to children has largely eliminated the problems of developmental toxicity such as musculoskeletal hypoplasia. While cure rates of HD have improved as therapy has been refined, the hope is that these changes will also result in a marked reduction in secondary malignancies and cardiac sequela. There has not been enough follow-up as yet to define that risk. One recent theoretical analysis suggests that the volume and dose reduction from shifting from 35 Gy to a mantle field to 20 Gy to an involved field has the potential to reduce the incidence of secondary breast and lung cancers by 77% and 57%, respectively.[27]

In adults with early stage HD, the shift to combined-modality therapy using low-dose IFRT has also come about in a circuitous series of clinical trials. A trial by the Southwest Oncology Group (trial #9133) showed that the addition of three cycles of adriamycin and vinblastine chemotherapy to STNI to full doses improved the 3-year disease-free survival rate from 81% to 94%, and also suggested that staging laparotomy was not needed.[28] Long-term results from an Italian trial comparing ABVD with STNI versus ABVD with IFRT using 40 Gy ("full dose") had an equivalent 12-year survival of roughly 95%. Of interest, in the IFRT group with a median follow-up of 9 years, there were no second malignancies, suggesting the importance of a reduction in the volume of radiation in reducing the risk of secondary cancers.[29] A trial by the European Organization for Research and Treatment of Cancer (EORTC H7F trial) further showed that EBVP chemotherapy (epirubicin, bleomycin, vinblastine, prednisone) with full-dose IFRT had a superior 10-year disease-free survival compared to STNI (88% vs 78%) but with equivalent survival of 92%, pointing out the ability to frequently salvage relapses after radiotherapy.[30]

The German Hodgkin's Lymphoma Study Group (GHSG) performed two consecutive trials between 1984 and 1992 in which surgically staged patients with one or more adverse features were given four cycles of chemotherapy followed by radiotherapy. In the first study, patients were given either 20, 30, or 40 Gy irradiation to nonbulky sites of disease; in the second trial, a similar cohort of patients received 30 Gy to nonbulky sites of disease. There was no significant difference in relapse in the patients who were given lower doses of radiation.[31] Two additional randomized trials have since shown that adult early stage HD may be effectively managed with reduced radiation doses to involved fields after chemotherapy. In the GHSG HD10 trial for favorable patients, two cycles versus four cycles of ABVD have been further compared to 20 Gy or 30 Gy IFRT in a double randomization schema. After a fourth interim analysis, all four arms have equivalent disease-free and overall survival.[32] In the EORTC H9F trial, patients were treated with six cycles of EBVP alone or the same chemotherapy followed by different doses of IFRT, either 20 Gy or 36 Gy. The overall survival at 4 years is the same, at 98%.[33] Disease-free survival shows that the chemotherapy alone was inferior to either of the combined-modality arms (70% vs 84% vs 87%). These trials and several others beyond the scope of this chapter have collectively documented that in early stage HD patients, chemotherapy in conjunction with IFRT has a superior disease-free survival compared to radiotherapy or chemotherapy alone.

Cooperative group trials have notorious difficulty analyzing long-term outcomes, particularly late effects including secondary cancer. A single-institution retrospective study from Duke University is of note, given a bias toward using lower radiation doses for both STNI as well as IFRT. Koontz and colleagues compared 111 patients with favorable HD who were treated with STNI to 70 similar patients who were treated with combined-modality therapy using low-dose (25.5 Gy) IFRT at two different time periods, reflecting the change in standards of care occurring in the mid 1990s.[34] The combined-modality patients had an improved survival rate at 20 years follow-up (83% vs 70%), although the findings were not statistically significant. The differences in incidence of second tumors were striking. The radiotherapy alone group had a 16% actuarial risk of second cancers at 20 years, in line with observations from other groups. Within the combined-modality therapy group, no second cancers were observed, with a median follow-up of 8.1 years (Figure 16.5). While very preliminary, this type of data is suggestive of a reduction in second cancers from radiotherapy by both a reduction in volume and dose.

Radiation dose and the incidence of subsequent solid tumors have been analyzed in detail in only a few other series. Salloum and colleagues compared the incidence of solid tumors after chemotherapy plus low-dose radiation versus standard-dose extended field radiation.[35] The patients who were treated with combined-modality therapy had advanced disease, while standard-dose radiation was given to early-stage patients. The analysis was limited to patients who did not relapse in order to avoid the confounding effect of subsequent treatment and because patients

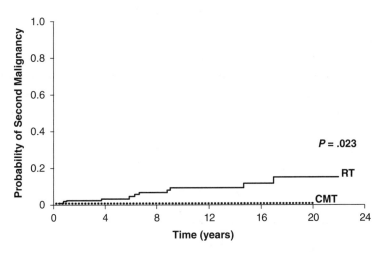

FIGURE 16.5 Probability of second malignancy over time.

with advanced disease were more likely to die from HD and therefore not live long enough to be at risk for a solid tumor. Similarly, because of the latency period of solid tumors, the study was restricted to patients who had a potential follow-up of more than 9 years. The relative risk of solid tumors was not significantly increased in the combined-modality group (low-dose radiation group), and no cases of breast or lung cancer were observed despite nearly all patients receiving mediastinal radiotherapy. In contrast, the relative risk of solid tumors was 3.3 in the group that received standard-dose radiation therapy, and the relative risk of lung cancer was 10.7. Importantly, the increase in the relative risk of solid tumors first became significant after more than 10 years of follow-up in the radiation arm.

In a study of children treated at Stanford University Medical Center between 1960 and 1995, solid tumors were highly correlated with radiation field and dose, with 43 of 48 tumors within or at the margin of a treatment field and 93% of tumors occurring in areas that had been irradiated to at least 35 Gy.[36] In agreement with the Salloum study, there were no cases of breast cancer in patients who received less than 40 Gy. In contrast, the relative risk of breast cancer was markedly increased in patients who received higher doses,[37] a finding corroborated by the Late Effects Study Group.[38,39]

BREAST CANCER RISK AFTER RADIOTHERAPY FOR HODGKIN DISEASE

Young women with HD undergoing primary radiotherapy are at particular risk for secondary breast cancer. The Stanford group was the first to report this problem after observing 25 invasive breast cancers and one case of multi-focal ductal carcinoma in situ in a cohort of 885 female patients treated with radiotherapy followed for an average of 10 years.[37] Compared to the general population, this represented 4.4 relative risk, but what was particularly striking was the age at treatment in determining the future risk of secondary breast cancer. Radiotherapy before age 15 had a relative risk for future breast cancer of 136. If treated at an age over 30 years, however, the relative risk was 0.7. The risk of secondary breast cancer increases with length of follow-up as well. While the Stanford group found that MOPP chemotherapy increased the risk of radiation-induced breast cancer, other groups have observed an opposite effect of chemotherapy.[40]

Radiation dose has been found to be an important factor in the development of secondary breast cancer as well. Van Leeuwen and colleagues demonstrated that the breast cancer risk is a direct function of radiation dose delivered, with a relative risk observed of 4.5 if the prescribed dose was over 38.5 Gy.[40] Chemotherapy was speculated to deter breast cancer progression by indirect hormonal effects, because menopause before 36 years of age was strongly protective and had a relative risk of 0.06. A matched case-control study of women diagnosed with HD younger than 30 years of age from six international registries showed an increased risk for the development of breast cancer.[41] In this study, performed by the National Cancer Institute (NCI), the median age at diagnosis was 22, and almost 20% of patients were less than 18 years old. The outcome studied was development of breast cancer after radiation, alkylating chemotherapy, or combined-modality treatment. In patients treated with radiation therapy alone, the relative risk of developing a breast cancer was 3.2. The relative risk with alkylating-agent treatment alone was 0.6, and relative risk was 1.4 with combined-modality treatment. Patients with menopause induced by chemotherapy or radiation to the ovaries had a decreased risk as well, suggesting that the protective effects of alkylating agents may be due to decreased estrogen exposure.

A second study from the NCI looked at cumulative risk of developing breast cancer after radiation in the same population of women. In this study, patients were divided into groups of no radiation, low-dose radiation, or higher-dose radiation, all plus and minus alkylating agents.[42] The data showed that the risk of developing breast cancer was increased by higher doses of radiation given at younger ages. This risk was reduced when radiation and an alkylating agent were used together. The data also showed that the cumulative risk of developing breast cancer continued to increase, even at 30 years follow-up (Table 16.1).

The age of female patients with HD at the time of treatment is an important determinant of subsequent risk. Data clearly show that younger age at radiation exposure increases the risk for a second cancer. This finding is likely due to both greater sensitivity of younger breast tissue and more years at risk. Hodgson reported on this phenomenon in

TABLE 16.1 Cumulative Absolute Risk of Developing Breast Cancer Related to Radiation Dose[42]

Treatment for HL[†]		Cumulative absolute risk, % (95% CI)											
		Age 15 years at HL diagnosis			Age 20 years at HL diagnosis			Age 25 years at HL diagnosis			Age 30 years at HL diagnosis		
mRT	AA	10-y F	20-y F	30-y F	10-y F	20-y F	30-y F	10-y F	20-y F	30-y F	10-y F	20-y F	30-y F
None	Yes	0 (0 to 0)	0.1 (0.0 to 0.4)	0.8 (0.3 to 2.7)	0 (0 to 0.1)	0.4 (0.1 to 0.3)	1.6 (0.5 to 5.3)	0.1 (0.1 to 0.4)	0.9 (0.3 to 2.9)	2.6 (0.9 to 8.5)	0.4 (0.2 to 1.0)	1.8 (0.7 to 5.5)	4.0 (1.4 to 12.4)
20-<40 Gy	Yes	0 (0 to 0)	0.7 (0.4 to 1.0)	4.1 (2.6 to 5.9)	0.2 (0.1 to 0.2)	1.9 (1.2 to 2.8)	7.9 (5.0 to 11.4)	0.6 (0.4 to 0.8)	4.4 (2.8 to 6.4)	12.5 (8.0 to 17.8)	1.5 (1.0 to 2.1)	8.2 (5.2 to 11.8)	18.1 (11.8 to 25.3)
≥40 Gy	Yes	0 (0 to 0)	0.8 (0.5 to 1.2)	5.0 (3.0 to 7.5)	0.2 (0.1 to 0.3)	2.3 (1.4 to 3.5)	9.5 (5.8 to 11.3)	0.7 (0.4 to 1.0)	5.3 (3.2 to 8.1)	15.0 (9.3 to 22.1)	1.8 (1.1 to 2.6)	9.9 (6.1 to 14.8)	21.6 (13.6 to 30.9)
None	No	0 (0 to 0)	0.3 (0.1 to 0.8)	1.7 (0.6 to 5.3)	0.1 (0 to 0.2)	0.8 (0.3 to 2.5)	3.4 (1.3 to 10.1)	0.3 (0.1 to 0.7)	1.9 (0.7 to 5.7)	5.5 (2.1 to 15.9)	0.7 (0.3 to 1.9)	3.6 (1.4 to 10.5)	8.2 (3.2 to 22.7)
20-<40 Gy	No	0 (0 to 0.1)	1.4 (0.9 to 2.1)	8.5 (5.5 to 12.7)	0.3 (0.2 to 0.5)	4.0 (2.6 to 6.1)	16.0 (10.5 to 23.3)	1.1 (0.7 to 1.7)	9.1 (5.9 to 13.7)	24.6 (16.6 to 34.8)	3.0 (1.9 to 4.5)	16.6 (10.9 to 24.2)	34.1 (23.6 to 46.5)
≥40 Gy	No	0.1 (0 to 0.1)	1.7 (1.1 to 2.6)	10.3 (6.8 to 15.2)	0.4 (0.3 to 0.6)	4.9 (3.2 to 7.4)	19.1 (13.0 to 27.4)	1.4 (0.9 to 2.1)	11.1 (7.4 to 16.3)	29.0 (20.2 to 40.1)	3.6 (2.4 to 5.4)	19.8 (13.5 to 28.5)	39.6 (28.4 to 52.6)

a larger epidemiologic study of 13 international tumor registries.[43] For instance, a patient diagnosed at age 30 with HD who survived to 40 years of age or older had a relative risk of breast cancer of 6.1 over the general population. In comparison, a patient diagnosed at age 20 who survived at least 10 years had a relative risk of breast cancer of 29. Another implication of this risk is that such a patient should be undergoing breast cancer screening at an age 10 years before that which is recommended for the general population.

Absolute risk increases over time and, based on atomic bomb survivor data, may continue to increase over the entire remaining lifetime of the person exposed to radiation. The atomic bomb data also demonstrate a link between dose and risk.[44] This relationship appears to be roughly linear. No clear minimum dose has been established, and it is commonly felt that there is some risk, albeit smaller, with even low-dose exposures. Thus, while the experience following the introduction of low-dose IFRT is relatively short (roughly 10 years in adults and 15–20 years in children with HD), it is anticipated that there will be some increase in relative risk for secondary breast cancers. The magnitude will need to be determined in future studies but is hoped to be a clinically small risk.

Hormonal, genetic, and environmental effects are felt to modify the risk of a secondary breast cancer. One finding that supports this belief comes from the NCI studies of the development of breast cancer after radiation, chemotherapy, or combined-modality therapy. In these patients, there was a decreased risk of developing breast cancer in women treated with alkylating agents or radiation to the ovaries, supporting the idea that estrogen exposure following treatment influenced breast cancer development, a known correlation in women without prior cancers. Genetics may play a role as well. In particular, this relationship has been shown in retinoblastoma patients with *Rb* gene mutations and in patients with Li-Fraumeni syndrome. In pediatric patients, certain primary cancers also appear to be inherently associated with an increased frequency of second cancers, in particular HD and sarcomas. Thus, the presence of mutations in DNA repair genes such as *BRCA1* or *BRCA2* may potentially have increased risks for HD patients. In one very preliminary study, a polymorphism in *MLH1*, a mismatch repair gene, was found to correlate with secondary breast cancers after HD.[45] Additional modifying risk factors include smoking, alcohol use, and diet. In fact, young HD patients who smoke during radiation treatment are at a much increased risk for a second cancer.

IMPACT ON THE USE OF RADIATION

In response to the data from HD survivors, we have significantly changed the way we use radiation therapy in the treatment of this cancer. Previously we treated large fields in almost all patients, often using STNI that exposed much of the body to radiation. With modern combination chemotherapy, we now treat very few patients with radiation therapy alone. Standard of care has shifted to combined-modality therapy in which radiotherapy when applied uses both substantially smaller volumes (e.g., smaller fields) and lower total radiation doses. The data on the risk of second cancers do not apply to current management, but patients treated with older radiation techniques do need to be monitored closely for late effects such as secondary malignancies. These principles have been applied to the use of radiation therapy in other situations. Many newer technologies in radiation therapy focus on delivering high doses to tumors while minimizing dose to surrounding normal tissues.

These newer techniques include intensity-modulated radiation therapy, stereotactic radiosurgery, and gating and image-guided therapy. Additionally, the use of proton radiotherapy, a modality with no exit dose, is now becoming more widely utilized as the technology is better studied and more available. Finally, there is much research focused on drugs that may sensitize tumor cells to radiation allowing the use of lower doses to greater effect and on drugs that protect normal tissues, decreasing the toxicity of radiation treatment. Given the lag in development of second cancers after radiation treatment, it will undoubtedly be many years before we can fully quantify the effects of these changes in utilization of radiation therapy.

PRACTICAL CONSIDERATIONS

Because HD is highly curable, it is estimated that there are now 120,000 patients in the United States who are survivors of this disease and need to be followed for risks of secondary cancer and other late effects.[46] Counseling patients regarding the risk for a second malignancy is a critical aspect of pretreatment discussion, particularly for patients under the age of 30. Patients should be advised to avoid tobacco use and to quit if they already smoke. Additionally, it is important that these patients undergo close lifelong surveillance and cancer screening. Given their potentially increased risk for certain cancers, it may be appropriate that screening should begin at an earlier age and/or occur on a more frequent basis.[47] The use of additional screening modalities may also be appropriate, such as MRI screening for breast cancer. With cure rates continuing to improve, there are ever-larger numbers of cancer survivors for whom these considerations will be very important. Finally, patients who do develop a second cancer may well have limited or altered treatment options, given their prior treatments.[48] For example, as demonstrated in the case at the start of this chapter, breast conserving therapy may not be an option for a woman who develops breast cancer after already having radiation to her chest.

REFERENCES

1. Cahan W, Woodard H, Higinbotham N, Stewart F, Coley B. Sarcoma arising in irradiated bone: report of eleven cases. *Cancer.* 1948;1(1):3–29.
2. Hodgkin T. On some morbid appearances of the absorbent glands and spleen. *Medico-Chirurgical Trans.* 1832;17:68.
3. Peters MV. A study of survivals in Hodgkin's disease treated radiologically. *Am J Roentgenol Radium Ther.* 1950;63:299–311.
4. Peters MV. Prophylactic treatment of adjacent areas in Hodgkin's disease. *Cancer Res.* 1966;26(6):1232–1243.
5. Kaplan HS. Long-term results of palliative and radical radiotherapy of Hodgkin's disease. *Cancer Res.* 1966;26(6):1250–1253.
6. Kaplan HS, Rosenberg SA. The treatment of Hodgkin's disease. *Med Clin North Am.* 1966;50(6):1591–1610.
7. Kaplan HS. Evidence for a tumoricidal dose level in the radiotherapy of Hodgkin's disease. *Cancer Res.* 1966;26(6):1221–1224.
8. Vijayakumar S, Myrianthopoulos LC. An updated dose-response analysis in Hodgkin's disease. *Radiother Oncol.* 1992;24(1):1–13.
9. Wirth A, Chao M, Corry J, et al. Mantle irradiation alone for clinical stage I-II Hodgkin's disease: long-term follow-up and analysis of prognostic factors in 261 patients. *J Clin Oncol.* 1999;17(1):230–240.
10. Hancock SL, Cox RS, Rosenberg SA. Correction: deaths after treatment of Hodgkin's disease. *Ann Intern Med.* 1991;114:810.

11. Hancock SL, Hoppe RT, Horning SJ, Rosenberg SA. Intercurrent death after Hodgkin disease therapy in radiotherapy and adjuvant MOPP trials. *Ann Intern Med.* 1988;109(3):183–189.

12. Ng AK, Bernardo MP, Weller E, et al. Long-term survival and competing causes of death in patients with early-stage Hodgkin's disease treated at age 50 or younger. *J Clin Oncol.* 2002;20(8):2101–2108.

13. Ng AK, Bernardo MV, Weller E, et al. Second malignancy after Hodgkin disease treated with radiation therapy with or without chemotherapy: long-term risks and risk factors. *Blood.* 2002;100(6):1989–1996.

14. Tucker MA. Solid second cancers following Hodgkin's disease. *Hematol Oncol Clin North Am.* 1993;7(2):389–400.

15. Hoppe RT. Hodgkin's disease: complications of therapy and excess mortality. *Ann Oncol.* 1997;8(suppl 1):115–118.

16. Mauch PM, Kalish LA, Marcus KC, et al. Long-term survival in Hodgkin's disease. *Cancer J Sci Am.* 1995;1(1):33.

17. Devita VT Jr, Serpick AA, Carbone PP. Combination chemotherapy in the treatment of advanced Hodgkin's disease. *Ann Intern Med.* 1970;73(6):881–895.

18. DeVita VT Jr, Simon RM, Hubbard SM, et al. Curability of advanced Hodgkin's disease with chemotherapy. Long-term follow-up of MOPP-treated patients at the National Cancer Institute. *Ann Intern Med.* 1980;92(5):587–595.

19. Frei E III, DeVita VT, Moxley JH III, Carbone PP. Approaches to improving the chemotherapy of Hodgkin's disease. *Cancer Res.* 1966;26(6):1284–1289.

20. van Leeuwen FE, Klokman WJ, Hagenbeek A, et al. Second cancer risk following Hodgkin's disease: a 20-year follow-up study. *J Clin Oncol.* 1994;12(2):312–325.

21. Henry-Amar M. Second cancer after the treatment for Hodgkin's disease: a report from the International Database on Hodgkin's Disease. *Ann Oncol.* 1992;3(suppl 4):117–128.

22. Bonadonna G, Zucali R, Monfardini S, De Lena M, Uslenghi C. Combination chemotherapy of Hodgkin's disease with adriamycin, bleomycin, vinblastine, and imidazole carboxamide versus MOPP. *Cancer.* 1975;36(1):252–259.

23. Specht L. Prognostic factors in Hodgkin's disease. *Semin Radiat Oncol.* 1996;6(3):146–161.

24. Sutcliffe SB, Gospodarowicz MK, Bergsagel DE, et al. Prognostic groups for management of localized Hodgkin's disease. *J Clin Oncol.* 1985;3(3):393–401.

25. Hasenclever D, Diehl V. A prognostic score for advanced Hodgkin's disease. International Prognostic Factors Project on Advanced Hodgkin's Disease. *N Engl J Med.* 1998;339(21):1506–1514.

26. Gallamini A, Hutchings M, Rigacci L, et al. Early interim 2-[18F]fluoro-2-deoxy-D-glucose positron emission tomography is prognostically superior to international prognostic score in advanced-stage Hodgkin's lymphoma: a report from a joint Italian-Danish study. *J Clin Oncol.* 2007; 25(24):3746–3752.

27. Hodgson DC, Koh ES, Tran TH, et al. Individualized estimates of second cancer risks after contemporary radiation therapy for Hodgkin lymphoma. *Cancer.* 2007;110(11):2576–2586.

28. Press OW, LeBlanc M, Lichter AS, et al. Phase III randomized intergroup trial of subtotal lymphoid irradiation versus doxorubicin, vinblastine, and subtotal lymphoid irradiation for stage IA to IIA Hodgkin's disease. *J Clin Oncol.* 2001 2001;19(22):4238–4244.

29. Bonadonna G, Bonfante V, Viviani S, Di Russo A, Villani F, Valagussa P. ABVD plus subtotal nodal versus involved-field radiotherapy in early-stage Hodgkin's disease: long-term results. *J Clin Oncol.* 2004;22(14): 2835–2841.

30. Noordijk EM, Carde P, Dupouy N, et al. Combined-modality therapy for clinical stage I or II Hodgkin's lymphoma: long-term results of the European Organisation for Research and Treatment of Cancer H7 randomized controlled trials. *J Clin Oncol.* 2006;24(19):3128–3135.

31. Loeffler M, Diehl V, Pfreundschuh M, et al. Dose-response relationship of complementary radiotherapy following four cycles of combination chemotherapy in intermediate-stage Hodgkin's disease. *J Clin Oncol.* 1997; 15(6):2275–2287.

32. Fuchs M, Diehl V, Re D. Current strategies and new approaches in the treatment of Hodgkin's lymphoma. *Pathobiology.* 2006;73(3):126–140.

33. Noordijk E, Thomas J, Ferme C, van 't Veer M. First results of the EORTC-GELA H9 randomized trials: H9-F trial (comparing 3 radiation dose levels) and H9-U trial (comparing 3 chemotherapy schemes) in patients with favorable or unfavorable early stage Hodgkin's lymphoma (HL). *J Clin Oncol.* 2005;23:6505a.

34. Koontz BF, Kirkpatrick JP, Clough RW, et al. Combined-modality therapy versus radiotherapy alone for treatment of early-stage Hodgkin's disease: cure balanced against complications. *J Clin Oncol.* 2006;24(4):605–611.

35. Salloum E, Doria R, Schubert W, et al. Second solid tumors in patients with Hodgkin's disease cured after radiation or chemotherapy plus adjuvant low-dose radiation. *J Clin Oncol.* 1996;14(9):2435–2443.

36. Wolden SL, Lamborn KR, Cleary SF, Tate DJ, Donaldson SS. Second cancers following pediatric Hodgkin's disease. *J Clin Oncol.* 1998;16(2): 536–544.
37. Hancock SL, Tucker MA, Hoppe RT. Breast cancer after treatment of Hodgkin's disease. *J Natl Cancer Inst.* 1993;85(1):25–31.
38. Bhatia S, Robison LL, Oberlin O, et al. Breast cancer and other second neoplasms after childhood Hodgkin's disease. *N Engl J Med.* 1996;334(12): 745–751.
39. Bhatia S, Yasui Y, Robison LL, et al. High risk of subsequent neoplasms continues with extended follow-up of childhood Hodgkin's disease: report from the Late Effects Study Group. *J Clin Oncol.* 2003;21(23):4386–4394.
40. van Leeuwen FE, Klokman WJ, Stovall M, et al. Roles of radiation dose, chemotherapy, and hormonal factors in breast cancer following Hodgkin's disease. *J Natl Cancer Inst.* 2003;95(13):971–980.
41. Travis LB, Hill DA, Dores GM, et al. Breast cancer following radiotherapy and chemotherapy among young women with Hodgkin disease. *JAMA.* 2003;290(4):465–475.
42. Travis LB, Hill D, Dores GM, et al. Cumulative absolute breast cancer risk for young women treated for Hodgkin lymphoma. *J Natl Cancer Inst.* 2005;97(19):1428–1437.
43. Hodgson DC, Gilbert ES, Dores GM, et al. Long-term solid cancer risk among 5-year survivors of Hodgkin's lymphoma. *J Clin Oncol.* 2007; 25(12):1489–1497.
44. Pierce DA, Preston DL. Radiation-related cancer risks at low doses among atomic bomb survivors. *Radiat Res.* 2000;154(2):178–186.
45. Worrillow LJ, Smith AG, Scott K, et al. Polymorphic MLH1 and risk of cancer after methylating chemotherapy for Hodgkin lymphoma. *J Med Genet.* 2008;45(3):142–146.
46. Travis LB. Evaluation of the risk of therapy-associated complications in survivors of Hodgkin lymphoma. *Hematology Am Soc Hematol Educ Program.* 2007;2007:192–196.
47. Cutuli B, Borel C, Dhermain F, et al. Breast cancer occurred after treatment for Hodgkin's disease: analysis of 133 cases. *Radiother Oncol.* 2001;59(3): 247–255.
48. Wolden SL, Hancock SL, Carlson RW, Goffinet DR, Jeffrey SS, Hoppe RT. Management of breast cancer after Hodgkin's disease. *J Clin Oncol.* 2000;18(4):765–772.

Therapy-Related Cancers After Chemotherapy: Leukemia, Non-Hodgkin Lymphoma, and Solid Tumors

Peter W. Marks, MD, PhD

ABSTRACT

Cancers that occur after cytotoxic chemotherapy administered for another malignancy are most appropriately categorized as therapy-related cancers. The most well-studied therapy-related cancers are leukemia, non-Hodgkin lymphoma, and solid tumors. Alkylating agents and topoisomerase II inhibitors are the chemotherapies most commonly associated with these therapy-related cancers. Individuals treated with radiation therapy in addition to chemotherapy appear to have a higher risk of therapy-related cancers than those treated with chemotherapy alone. The relative risk of acute leukemia is generally greatest during the first 5 years after chemotherapy, whereas the risk of solid tumors generally continues to grow over time. Persons treated at a younger age have the highest increase in relative risk over time. Overall, the risk of chemotherapy-related cancer is modest in patients treated with current standard therapies compared with the risk of dying from the presenting disease. Ongoing clinical research efforts are focusing on the administration of chemotherapy drug combinations and schedules that minimize the risk of therapy-related malignancy.

◯◡ Case Example 17.1

A 50-year-old woman presented with a right breast mass and was found to have a node-negative 2 cm infiltrating ductal carcinoma that was estrogen receptor and progesterone receptor negative but HER2 positive. She was treated with lumpectomy and radiation therapy as well as adjuvant chemotherapy. The chemotherapy consisted of four cycles of doxorubicin and cyclophosphamide administered every 2 weeks with growth factor support followed by 1 year of trastuzumab. About 1 year after completing chemotherapy, she was found, upon routine complete blood count, to have a white blood cell count of 65 000/(μL with 85% blasts. Further evaluation revealed that she had acute myeloid leukemia of the M5 subtype with a cytogenetic rearrangement involving the multi-lineage leukemia gene (*MLL* gene) locus on chromosome 11q23. Based on the appropriate temporal and cytogenetic association with the administration of a drug having topoisomerase II activity (doxorubicin), she was diagnosed with a therapy-related leukemia. Treatment consisted of induction chemotherapy for leukemia with idarubicin and cytarabine followed by hematopoietic stem cell transplantation from a sibling donor.

INTRODUCTION

Therapy-related cancers are malignancies that arise after the treatment of another disorder with chemotherapy and/or radiation therapy (Table 17.1). Although these disorders are sometimes called secondary cancers, they can also be referred to as therapy-related cancers because it distinguishes malignancies that are related to prior therapy (e.g., therapy-related acute myeloid leukemia) from those that have evolved as part of the natural history of a preexisting disorder (e.g., acute myeloid leukemia secondary to a preexisting myelodysplastic syndrome).[1] Although a wide variety of therapy-related cancers and myelodysplastic syndromes may be observed after chemotherapy, the most well described are leukemias and solid tumors.

The chemotherapeutic agents most well associated with therapy-related cancers are the alkylating agents and topoisomerase II inhibitors.

TABLE 17.1 Agents and Therapy-Related Cancers

Agent	Example of Cancer Type
Radiation Therapy	Solid tumors
Alkylating Agents	Acute myeloid leukemia
Topoisomerase II Inhibitors	Acute myeloid leukemia
Immunosuppressive Agents	Non-Hodgkin lymphoma

The development of acute myeloid leukemia associated with treatment with these agents is well described and illustrates the pathogenesis of these disorders.[2] Acute lymphoid leukemia has also been associated with the use of topoisomerase II inhibitors.[3]

Alkylating agents such as cyclophosphamide and melphalan are associated to varying extents (cyclophosphamide less than melphalan) with the development of leukemia with a latency of about 3 to 8 years following treatment. Chromosomal abnormalities described in the leukemia cells include deletions of all or part of chromosome 5 and/or chromosome 7.

Agents with topoisomerase II activity such as doxorubicin and etoposide are associated with the development of leukemia with a latency of about 2 to 3 years following treatment. Chromosomal abnormalities involve deletions and translocations of the 11q23 locus. Therapy-related acute leukemia may appear de novo or may be preceded by cytopenias and the development of a myelodysplastic syndrome that rapidly progresses.[4] The prognosis for therapy-related leukemia is generally poor with conventional chemotherapy, although hematopoietic stem cell transplantation offers the chance for cure.

In addition to chemotherapy, immunosuppressive agents have also been associated with therapy-related cancers. Agents such as azathioprine and cyclosporine that are administered in the setting of hematopoietic stem cell transplantation or solid organ transplantation have been associated with the development of cancers—in particular, non-Hodgkin lymphoma. These disorders, which may be associated with Epstein-Barr viral infection, sometimes resolve with reduction or withdrawal of immunosuppression.[5] However, this is not always feasible or effective, and chemotherapy is sometimes required.

Finally, data indicate that there are important interactions and potential synergistic effects between the administration of chemotherapy and radiation therapy. This interaction of the two modalities is illustrated in the treatment of several different malignancies. To illustrate the effects of chemotherapy alone or when combined with radiation therapy, three examples (using Hodgkin disease (HD), testicular cancer, and breast cancer) are provided below, with citations regarding some of the available evidence.

HODGKIN DISEASE

Hodgkin disease represents a success story in the modern history of cancer treatment. It is a highly treatable malignancy with a 5-year survival rate in excess of 80%.[6] Depending in part on the stage of the disease at presentation, treatment regimens have incorporated radiation therapy alone, chemotherapy alone, or combined-modality therapy using radiation therapy and chemotherapy. The cytotoxic medications that have been utilized include alkylating agents, such as mechlorethamine and procarbazine (incorporated into the older MOPP regimen of), as well as those with topoisomerase II activity, such as doxorubicin (incorporated into the more recently employed ABVD regimen).

The success in the improvement of 5-year survival has come in part at the cost of developing therapy-related malignancies. The association of radiation therapy alone with therapy-related cancers is well described and is covered elsewhere in this book. Chemotherapy, when combined with radiation therapy, potentially has a synergistic effect in promoting the development of these malignancies. Overall, with treatment regimens used for HD in pediatric patients from the 1980s to the mid-1990s, therapy-related malignancies are the leading cause of excess mortality. In a cohort of individuals treated at Stanford, by 20 years after initial treatment, about 10% of males and 17% of females had developed a therapy-related cancer.[7]

As a more specific example, in one cohort of 1,319 patients with stage I through stage IV HD treated between April 1969 and December 1997 with either radiation therapy alone or radiation therapy with chemotherapy, the risk of a therapy-related malignancy increased over time, with a risk reaching 4% per year 20 years out from primary therapy.[8] Although solid tumors were the most common types of cancer observed, with an absolute risk of 59.1 per 10,000 patient years, the relative risk was relatively modest (3.5) because such tumors are also more common in the aging population. In contrast, although the absolute risk of acute leukemia was more modest (14.3 per 10,000 patient years), the relative risk was markedly elevated (82.5), because leukemia is a less common disease in the general population. Whereas the relative risk of solid tumors increased with time, the relative risk of acute leukemia was highest during the first 5 years after HD therapy. In this cohort of patients, one of the most notable findings was that the development of acute leukemia was associated with a very poor 5-year survival of about 5% and a median survival of less than 6 months.

Newer treatment strategies for HD use chemotherapy agents associated with a lower risk of therapy-related malignancies and avoid the concomitant use of chemotherapy and radiation therapy unless specific indications are met. Hopefully, studies performed on these cohorts of individuals will demonstrate a marked reduction in the incidence of therapy-related cancers, and data are emerging that this may indeed be the case.[9]

TESTICULAR CANCER

Testicular cancer is similar to HD, in that it represents another success story in the treatment of cancer, with a 5-year survival rate in excess of 95%. In addition to surgical resection, depending on the stage of disease present, treatment regimens include radiation therapy alone, chemotherapy alone using regimens that contain a topoisomerase II inhibitor (etoposide), and combined-modality therapy.

In the case of testicular cancer, cardiovascular toxicity and therapy-related cancers are the two leading causes of excess mortality in those treated.[10] The increased risk of therapy-related cancers appears to persist for at least 40 years after diagnosis. Interestingly, the relative risk appears to be highest in younger individuals receiving treatment, being more than five times higher for individuals diagnosed in their 20s than for individuals diagnosed in their 50s.

In data from one study obtained from tumor registries between the years 1943 and 2001, of 40,576 long-term survivors living in North

America and Europe (and representing more than 458,383 person years of follow-up), there were 2,285 therapy-related solid tumors reported.[11] Of note, those treated with chemotherapy alone or radiation therapy alone had relative risks of 1.8 and 2.0, respectively. However, combined therapy was associated with a higher relative risk of 2.9.

The chemotherapy agent potentially of greatest concern in the treatment of testicular cancer is etoposide. High doses of this agent have been clearly associated with a modestly increased risk of therapy-related acute leukemia, often, but not invariably, associated with cytogenetic abnormalities involving the MLL gene locus at the 11q23 chromosome.[12] These leukemias appear to develop in between 1% and 2% of treated individuals. Because such high-dose etoposide is used in the setting of salvage chemotherapy, this risk is considered to be acceptable.

Aside from high-dose treatment strategies, the incidence of therapy-related cancers, though clearly increased above the general population, is relatively modest in testicular cancer, particularly when compared to HD. Radiation therapy and chemotherapy appear to have similar risks, but the combination of the two modalities has a somewhat increased risk over either modality alone.

BREAST CANCER

The treatment of breast cancer is dependent on stage at diagnosis. Therapies include surgery, radiation therapy, hormonal therapy, chemotherapy, and various combinations. Unlike with HD and testicular cancer, widespread metastatic disease is generally considered incurable and is usually treated with hormonal therapy or chemotherapy.

In patients with localized breast cancer treated with standard therapy, the incidence of therapy-related solid tumors and leukemia appears to be relatively modest in comparison to the potential survival benefit. The therapy-related solid tumor risk appears to be most directly related to the administration of radiation therapy, although chemotherapy may increase this risk somewhat as well. The risk of therapy-related leukemia appears to be most closely linked to the use of systemic chemotherapy, and data suggest that the link is strongest for its use at high intensity or over prolonged periods.

One study that provides some insight into both solid tumor and leukemia risk examined 376,825 1-year survivors of breast cancer in Sweden, Denmark, Norway, and Finland from the years 1943 through

2002.[13,14] The overall risk of potentially radiation-therapy associated cancers, such as those of the esophagus, lung, and thyroid, was 1.34 times that expected based on population rates. Of note, in those individuals who were followed for at least 30 years from diagnosis, this rate was 2.19 times that based on population rates. For solid tumors associated with chemotherapy and not potentially associated with radiation or hormonal therapy, the rate of occurrence was 1.09 times that expected based on population rates. In those who were followed for at least 30 years from diagnosis, this rate increased to only 1.21 times that expected based on population rates. For cancers of the body of the uterus, potentially related to hormonal therapies, this rate was 1.41 times that expected based on population rates.

The increased risk of leukemia in this same cohort was relatively modest, at 1.79 times that expected based on population rates. Of note, rates of acute myeloid leukemia, acute lymphoid leukemia, and chronic myeloid leukemia were all increased. Patients with distant disease were at highest risk for the development of leukemia, most likely related to the chemotherapy that these individuals received. Even in this population of patients with distant disease, however, the absolute excess risk was relatively small, at about 25 per 100,000.

The above described study in the Nordic population did note a trend toward decreased leukemia risk in later calendar years, likely reflecting changes in treatments administered. This finding is important to recognize, because more modern chemotherapy regimens may reduce the risk of therapy-related leukemia. Because the rate of solid tumors potentially related to chemotherapy is already small, additional risk reduction will require further analysis. The increased risk of cancers of the body of the uterus likely linked to hormonal therapies may be reduced by the introduction of agents such as the aromatase inhibitors, which appear to have a lower incidence of this complication.

LESSONS LEARNED

The experience with HD has provided significant insight into factors placing individuals at risk for the development of therapy-related cancers. Recent changes in the practice of radiation therapy and chemotherapy likely will result in a reduction in the occurrence in therapy-related cancers both for patients with HD and other tumor types.

In addition, although only a small portion of the available literature on therapy-related cancers due to chemotherapy was reviewed in this chapter, several key principles can be derived from these and other studies. These principles both help guide the current management of patients and point toward the further risk reduction that may be possible.

The incidence of therapy-related cancers differs depending on the primary presenting tumor type. These differences are likely at least in part related to the treatment modalities utilized. The risk appears to be greatest for those treated with chemotherapy plus radiation therapy, somewhat less for those treated only with radiation therapy, and still lower for those treated with chemotherapy only. Whether this risk will change with newer radiation therapy techniques and chemotherapy agents remains to be seen.

In general, the risk of therapy-related solid cancers appears to continue to increase over time after initial treatment, particularly for patients treated at a younger age. These patients experience the highest increase in relative risk over time, which may in part be related to the latency period required for the development of solid tumors in patients treated with potentially genotoxic therapy, including chemotherapy and radiation therapy. For leukemia, there are some conflicting data in the literature. However, overall, it appears that the increase in relative risk is greatest during the first 5 years after initial treatment and is primarily related to the administration of chemotherapy.

Future directions in risk reduction will likely include decreased use of alkylating agents, particularly those that are associated with the highest risk such as mechlorethamine and melphalan. The combination of chemotherapy with radiation therapy appears to have synergy in producing an increased risk of therapy-related cancers (Table 17.2). Therefore, the use of combined-modality therapy employing both chemotherapy and radiation therapy only when absolutely indicated should also help in this regard. Additionally, exploration of chemotherapy drug combinations and schedules that minimize the risk of therapy-related cancers may prove beneficial.

PRACTICAL CONSIDERATIONS

Although specific screening for therapy-related malignancies may be appropriate under certain circumstances for patients judged to be at

TABLE 17.2   Relative Risk of Therapy-Related Cancers

Modality	Risk
Chemotherapy Alone	Lowest
Radiation Therapy Alone	Intermediate
Chemotherapy and Radiation Therapy	Highest

high risk, for the majority of patients treated with adjuvant chemotherapy, the absolute risk of therapy-related cancer is too small to justify specific screening measures.[15] However, an important aspect of the management of such patients who have been previously treated for cancer is the performance of recommended age-appropriate preventative studies such as mammography and colorectal screening. These studies can sometimes be overlooked when the focus is on following up with the primary malignancy.

Individuals who appear to be at high risk for therapy-related cancers include hematopoietic stem cell transplant recipients, in addition to long-term survivors of HD. A significantly increased risk of a variety of solid tumors, including malignant melanoma and cancers of the buccal mucosa, liver, central nervous system, thyroid, and connective tissue, has been described in hematopoietic transplant recipients.[16] Heightened surveillance to detect precursor lesions and early cancers has been suggested. In addition, it has been recommended that these patients avoid additional carcinogenic exposures that might further increase the risk of solid tumors. This practical recommendation might well be extended to any patient treated for cancer.

Finally, because the absolute increased risk for therapy-related cancers in most patients is relatively small, one of the most important messages to communicate to patients is that the benefit of appropriate disease management according to the current standards of care outweighs the risk of therapy-related malignancies. Even with high-dose chemotherapy approaches used for diseases such as relapsed non-Hodgkin lymphoma or metastatic testicular cancer, the potential survival benefit of treatment greatly outweighs the risk of therapy-related malignancy.

REFERENCES

1. Larson RA. Is secondary leukemia an independent poor prognostic factor in acute myeloid leukemia? *Best Pract Res Clin Haematol.* 2007;20:29–37.
2. Leone G, Voso MT, Sica S, et al. Therapy related leukemias: susceptability, prevention and treatment. *Leuk Lymphoma.* 2001;41:255–276.
3. Andersen MK, Christiansen DH, Jensen BA, et al. Therapy-related acute lymphoblastic leukaemia with *MLL* rearrangements following DNA topoisomerase II inhibitors, an increasing problem: report on two new cases and review of the literature since 1992. *Br J Haematol.* 2001;114: 539–543.
4. Smith SM, Le Beau MM, Huo D, et al. Clinical-cytogenetic associations in 306 patients with therapy-related myelodysplasia and myeloid leukemia: the University of Chicago series. *Blood.* 2003;102:43–52.
5. Loren AW, Porter DL, Stadtmauer EA, Tsai DE. Post-transplant lymphoproliferative disorder: a review. *Bone Marrow Transplant.* 2003;31: 145–155.
6. Aleman BM, van Leeuwen FE. Are we improving the long-term burden of Hodgkin's lymphoma patients with modern treatment? *Hematol Oncol Clin North Am.* 2007;21:961–975.
7. Wolden SL, Lamborn KR, Cleary SF, et al. Second cancers following pediatric Hodgkin's disease. *J Clin Oncol.* 1998;16:536–544.
8. Ng AK, Bernardo MV, Weller E, et al. Second malignancy after Hodgkin disease treated with radiation therapy with or without chemotherapy: long-term risks and risk factors. *Blood.* 2002;100:1989–1996.
9. Hoppe RT. Hodgkin's disease: complications of therapy and excess mortality. *Ann Oncol.* 1997;8(suppl 1):115–118.
10. Chaudhary UB, Haldas JR. Long-term complications of chemotherapy for germ cell tumours. *Drugs.* 2003;63:1565–1577.
11. Travis LB, Fosså SD, Schonfeld SJ, et al. Second cancers among 40576 testicular cancer patients: focus on long-term survivors. *J Natl Cancer Inst.* 2005;97:1354–1365.
12. Kollmannsburger C, Beyer J, Droz JP, et al. Secondary leukemia following high cumulative doses of etoposide in patients treated for advanced germ cell tumors. *J Clin Oncol.* 1998;16:3386–3391.
13. Brown LM, Chen BE, Pfeiffer RM, et al. Risk of second non-hematological malignancies among 376,825 breast cancer survivors. *Breast Cancer Res Treatment.* 2007;106:439–451.
14. Howard RA, Gilbert ES, Chen BE, et al. Leukemia following breast cancer: an international population-based study of 376,825 women. *Breast Cancer Res Treatment.* 2007;105:359–368.

15. Hayes DF. Follow-up of patients with early breast cancer. *N Engl J Med.* 2007;356:2505–2513.

16. Curtis RE, Rowlings PA, Deeg HJ, et al. Solid cancers after bone marrow transplantation. *N Engl J Med.* 1997;336:897–904.

18

Health Issues for Adult Survivors of Childhood Cancer

Debra L. Friedman, MD

ABSTRACT

With improvements in therapy for childhood cancer, the expectation that most patients will survive and enter adulthood is now a reality. However, adult survivors of childhood cancer face unique challenges. They are at risk for chronic health conditions, yet may not have access to healthcare providers with expertise in the very long-term complications of childhood cancer. In addition, adult survivors must undergo a successful transition from acute to follow-up care together with transition from the pediatric to the adult healthcare systems. Because the long-term effects of cancer and its therapy are described in detail elsewhere, this chapter will focus on the healthcare challenges faced by childhood cancer survivors when they reach adulthood.

RISK OF CHRONIC HEALTH CONDITIONS

Cancer and its treatments place survivors at increased risk for long-term adverse physiological and psychological sequelae, many of which do not manifest until the adult years. These sequelae include organ dysfunction, second malignant neoplasms, early mortality, impaired fertility, and psychosocial effects.[1–10] This increased risk associated with cancer treatment has been most extensively studied in the Childhood Cancer Survivor Study (CCSS), a retrospective cohort study of more than 14 000 childhood cancer survivors treated between 1970 and 1986 (additional information on the CCSS can be found at www.stjude.org/ccss).[11] Within the CCSS, Oeffinger and colleagues examined chronic health conditions in 10,397 adult survivors and compared these individuals with 3,034 sibling controls. At a mean age of 26.6 years (ranging from 18–48 years of age) for the survivors, and 29.2 years (18–56 years of age) for the siblings, 62.3% of the survivors had reported at least one chronic health condition, compared with only 36.8% of siblings reporting a chronic health condition. The adjusted relative risk of a chronic health condition in a survivor, compared with siblings, was 3.3; for grade 3 (severe) or 4 (life threatening) conditions, the relative risk was 8.2. Chronic conditions included major joint replacement, congestive heart failure, second malignant neoplasms, severe cognitive dysfunction, coronary artery disease, cerebrovascular accident, renal failure, hearing loss, legal blindness, and ovarian failure. Risk was elevated for all childhood cancer diagnoses, and cumulative incidence increased with ongoing time since diagnosis, with an overall cumulative incidence of 73.4% at 30 years.[2]

SURVIVORS' KNOWLEDGE OF THEIR THERAPY AND HEALTHCARE NEEDS

Despite the significant incidence of chronic health conditions in adult survivors, many survivors are not familiar with their childhood cancer therapy and do not appreciate the potential health risks associated with the therapy.[12,13] In a study from the CCSS, Kadan-Lottick and colleagues surveyed 635 adult participants and found that only 72% accurately reported their diagnosis, only 30% recalled receiving daunorubicin and 52% doxorubicin (both associated with risk of cardiomyopathy), and only 70% were able to accurately state the site of their radiotherapy. Perhaps most concerning was that only 35% thought their cancer therapy could be associated with adverse long-term health problems.[13] This lack of past treatment awareness illustrates the need to examine healthcare practices among adult survivors and consider models of care that will meet their ongoing healthcare needs.

HEALTHCARE UTILIZATION

While the majority of adult survivors of childhood cancer have access to health care, many are not receiving care targeted toward monitoring for adverse long-term effects of therapy. In a CCSS analysis of 9,434 adult survivors, healthcare practices over a 2-year period were assessed. Eighty-seven percent of survivors reported a general medical contact, 71.4% a general physical examination, 41.9% a cancer-related visit, and 19.2% a visit to a cancer center. Risk factors for lack of healthcare were lack of health insurance, lack of concern for future health, male sex, and age over 30 years.[14] Delphi panels of young adult survivors and healthcare policy experts both identified the major barriers to appropriate follow-up to be a lack of knowledge about survivors' needs on the part of both survivors and physicians.[15,16] It is therefore clear that there exists a significant need to educate survivors and primary healthcare providers about the unique needs of adult survivors of childhood cancer.

HEALTH INSURANCE AND EMPLOYMENT

The financial challenges of obtaining health insurance and appropriate employment are of paramount importance for the long-term survivor entering young adulthood. In the United States, where most health insurance is private and employer-based, the two challenges are intertwined. Approximately 10% to 30% of young adult survivors face insurance and/or job discrimination; employment rates are lower overall in survivors, compared with control. In addition, survivors, compared with peers, have significantly greater worries about getting or changing jobs and obtaining medical or life insurance.[17–26] Strategies have been published to assist survivors in gaining access to health insurance coverage[27,28] and in obtaining work and dealing with discrimination in the workplace.[27,29] Younger age at childhood cancer diagnosis; lower level of attained education; lower income; being widowed, divorced, or separated; or having been treated with cranial radiotherapy are risk factors for unemployment and/or lack of insurance.[25,26]

MODELS OF CARE

The need to develop systematic follow-up and dedicated care for childhood cancer survivors has been acknowledged for several decades.

Models of care for long-term survivors of childhood cancer must be flexible to meet the needs of young children, adolescents, and young and older adults, and must be sensitive to change throughout the life cycle. In addition, they must accommodate patients with a wide range of treatment exposures and risks for adverse long-term sequelae.[30]

To date, there are no uniformly effective long-term follow-up plans for childhood cancer survivors as they enter adulthood, as evidenced by published research over the past decade that documents a significant lost-to-follow-up rate, lack of knowledge on the part of survivors about their past treatment and potential for adverse health sequelae, inadequate provisions of follow-up care, and poor utilization of available health services.[13–15,31–36] Various national bodies have addressed the problem by developing long-term follow-up guidelines, which provide a foundation for how follow-up care should be delivered. However, they are not completely consistent with one another, and there is a lack of sufficient resources committed to ensure their implementation.[37–41] Therefore, ongoing research is required to develop a uniform set of "best practice" guidelines that can serve as an integral part of a care model for childhood cancer survivors.

Childhood cancer is unlike most chronic diseases of childhood (e.g., cystic fibrosis and congenital heart disease) where ongoing, organ-directed treatment is usually required, and it is obvious which specialty should take overall charge throughout the lifespan, including the transition to adult care. In contrast, most childhood cancer survivors do not require anti-neoplastic therapy or other acute care services traditionally provided by pediatric or medical oncologists. Instead, survivors must be provided with expertise from various specialties to manage long-term complications of prior cancer treatment.

While many childhood cancer centers follow their long-term survivors during the childhood and adolescent years, only a minority of institutions have programs focused on the care of adult survivors or input from adult-focused healthcare providers.[35] To better understand this lack of appropriate care available to childhood cancer survivors, one needs to understand the models of care that have evolved over time. Specific programs vary according to the resources they require and the exact services they can provide; each has advantages and disadvantages.[42]

The most common model of care for survivors of childhood cancer, including adult survivors, is cancer center-based. Follow-up can be coordinated by the primary oncology team in the oncology clinic, by a dedicated late-effects team in the oncology clinic, or by a dedicated late-effects team outside of the oncology clinic. While these models are the ones most commonly employed, those with a dedicated survivorship team apparently exist in only 50% of childhood cancer treatment centers in the United States and the United Kingdom. Furthermore, survivors do not necessarily avail themselves of the services.[14,35,36,42]

Cancer center-based survivor clinics, regardless of the staff or space details, generally provide comprehensive and systematic follow-up, which can benefit survivors in a multitude of ways, as described in the following list[43–45]:

▷ Centers offer continuity of care from the acute phase to the follow-up phase of the illness.
▷ Centers can support medical training of professionals who will be providing care to the survivors in the community at a later date.
▷ Patients develop a sense of the survivor community.
▷ Health education is a focus of the comprehensive care delivered.
▷ Physiological and psychosocial needs can be more easily addressed in an integrated fashion.
▷ Survivors have ready access to clinical research studies.

However, the impact of cancer center models is of consequence to patients. Many survivors do not want to return indefinitely to the cancer center once they have achieved cure because of negative emotional associations, a desire to "move on" with their lives, and geographical obstacles, especially in the mobile population of young adults. The cancer center may also provide an artificially protected environment for survivors and not allow them (or their parents) to develop the skills eventually needed to successfully navigate complex healthcare systems as self-sufficient adults.

For adult survivors in particular, unless there is a specific program and a focus on transition from the pediatric setting to adult health care, such a cancer center-based program is unlikely to be adequate or, in some situations, appropriate.[35,46,47] With increasing information on late effects of childhood cancer being published in general pediatric, nursing, and family practice literature,[1,4,48,49] as well as availability of long-term follow-up guidelines by the Children's Oncology Group, the foundation has been laid for community-based primary care providers to follow adult survivors of childhood cancer in their practices. The clear advantage of a community-based model is that there is coordination between the risk-adapted follow-up that the survivor requires and the general primary care that promotes independence for survivors and their families. However, even with the growing number of childhood cancer survivors entering the general population, it is unlikely that any one community healthcare practice will care for any significant number of survivors, resulting in an inadequate knowledge of the depth and breadth of the issues that face long-term survivors. In addition, monitoring and management of the complex physiological and psychological needs of the childhood cancer survivor are time-consuming and often cannot be easily integrated into a busy community practice. Such practices may not be able to provide coordination between primary and multiple subspecialty care, and may not have easy access to complex diagnostic testing. Health education may be less rigorously provided, and psychosocial support may be less available.

A combination of the cancer center and community models appears to be the most ideal for adult survivors of childhood cancer, but they require effort on the part of the survivor, the oncology team, and the primary healthcare provider.

In this scenario, follow-up in the cancer center model for a specified time period transfers into follow-up with a community-based primary care practice, with variable levels of continued involvement from the survivorship team. However, prior to transfer, both the survivor and the primary care physician would have the appropriate knowledge required for optimal care. This knowledge would include, but would not be limited to a Survivorship Care Plan that summarizes the cancer treatment, real and potential adverse long-term effects, and recommendations for monitoring and screening.

The time of transfer could be designed based on a combination of factors, including risk for developing adverse late effects, complexity of those late effects, psychosocial and developmental issues, and the knowledge demonstrated by the survivors or their family.

Involvement of the cancer center clinic could be advised by the primary care provider. Alternatively, the survivorship team at the cancer center could provide ongoing guidance with respect to monitoring and management of late effects using specified guidelines. Under such a model, there would be defined phone, mail, or electronic contact on at least an annual basis between the survivor and the community health-care provider. This contact would help break down the barriers to appropriate community-based care noted in the Delphi panel analyses from the CCSS.[15,16]

The success of this model is highly dependent on the interaction between the cancer center, the community physician, and the survivor. It is unlikely to be successful in situations where one or more of these parties have significant competing priorities. Thus, it is essential for primary care providers to become more knowledgeable about the health risks faced by childhood cancer survivors as they enter and progress through adulthood. Significant efforts are still required to train primary care physicians in the unique needs of childhood cancer survivors. Such training could be done through publications, professional society meetings, continuing medical education courses, and Web-based learning.

ᖾ Case Example 18.1

Jackie, a 30-year-old woman who was treated for Hodgkin disease at age 15 in the nearby academic medical center, tells her community healthcare provider that she is concerned about a breast lump. She has no family history of breast or ovarian cancer. Jackie is also attempting to get pregnant but is concerned about her ability to have children and is now worried she might have another cancer. She has also been wheezing lately and is worried that she may have asthma.

To approach the care of Jackie, the single most important question is "how was she treated for her Hodgkin disease?" If she does not recall details of her treatment and the community physician is unable to get such details from the cancer center, necessary screening may be omitted or unnecessary tests may be undertaken. However, if Jackie instead presents to the primary care physician after a systematic transfer from the cancer center, the healthcare delivery can be appropriately targeted. Assuming the latter situation, the primary healthcare provider finds the Survivorship Care Plan and transfer documents from the cancer center. The provider learns that Jackie was treated for stage IVB Hodgkin disease

(continues)

Case Example 18.1 (*continued*)

with eight cycles of escalated bleomycin, etoposide, doxorubicin, cyclcophosphamide, vincristine, prednisone, and procarbazine and 30 Gy involved field radiation, with modified mantle and periaortic fields. The Survivorship Care Plan outlines the pertinent exposures and risks.

In this scenario, Jackie is at increased risk of breast cancer, and dedicated breast cancer screening with mammography and/or breast magnetic resonance imaging (MRI) is indicated. Due to high doses of alkylating agents (e.g., cyclophosphamide and procarbazine), together with potential scatter from the periaortic radiotherapy to the ovaries, Jackie is at risk of premature menopause and impaired fertility. In addition, due to the thoracic radiotherapy and the doxorubicin exposure, she is at risk for cardiomyopathy, which could manifest with wheezing. Furthermore, should she become pregnant, there is an increased risk of sudden onset of congestive heart failure during the last trimester of pregnancy and particularly during labor and delivery. Jackie is also at risk for pulmonary fibrosis and diffusion abnormalities due to the thoracic radiotherapy and the bleomycin exposure. Thus, in addition to the history and physical that the primary care provider would perform with any patient, the provider also would:

1) Perform a careful breast examination and obtain imaging studies to rule out secondary breast cancer
2) Refer Jackie to a reproductive medicine specialist to assess fertility
3) Obtain a baseline echocardiogram and electrocardiogram and recommend close follow-up during pregnancy, should Jackie so proceed
4) Obtain pulmonary function tests
5) Evaluate for any other long-term adverse effects of treatment for Hodgkin disease, using the Survivorship Care Plan and the Children's Oncology Group Long-Term Follow-up Guidelines (www.survivorshipguidelines.org)
6) Take the opportunity to educate Jackie about the need for continued healthcare follow-up and specific long-term health-related risks of therapy
7) Consult back with the survivorship program for any questions and also to update them on her current status

This scenario would have indeed been different had Jackie not had a Survivorship Care Plan and a systematic transition from the survivorship program. In addition, if Jackie had been unemployed and/or had no health insurance, she might not have sought care for these concerns or would have utilized public health resources where her cancer history may or may not have been considered.

CONCLUSION

There is a growing number of adult survivors of childhood cancer whose healthcare concerns are currently not being adequately met. Adult survivors are at increased risk of psychosocial and medical adverse long-term effects and chronic health conditions. Most childhood cancer centers do not have the appropriate resources to follow their adult patients, and unemployment and lack of health insurance further complicate availability of follow-up for adult survivors.

While most survivors do receive some healthcare follow-up from primary care, many providers are unfamiliar with the risks of this growing population. In addition, survivors will need to be diligent and advocate for their needs, while navigating a progressively more complex healthcare system. This area clearly requires systematic research. Different models of care should be compared and assessed. In addition, different models of educating primary healthcare providers must also be assessed. Screening recommendations must be constantly reviewed, updated, and, whenever possible, based on evidence, as opposed to consensus. Healthcare policy research should identify barriers to adequate care, on the part of the survivor, the healthcare providers, and the healthcare system. Observational studies will still be required to assess the incidence, prevalence, and severity of risk factors for adverse long-term health-related outcomes in this population in the face of constantly changing therapeutic exposures. Lastly, interventions should be designed to prevent, ameliorate, and manage adverse long-term outcomes.

REFERENCES

1. Oeffinger KC, Hudson MM. Long-term complications following childhood and adolescent cancer: foundations for providing risk-based health care for survivors. *CA Cancer J Clin.* 2004;54(4):208–236.
2. Oeffinger KC, Mertens AC, Sklar CA, et al. Chronic health conditions in adult survivors of childhood cancer. *N Engl J Med.* 2006;355(15):1 572–1582.
3. Barakat LP, Alderfer MA, Kazak AE. Posttraumatic growth in adolescent survivors of cancer and their mothers and fathers. *J Pediatr Psychol.* 2006;31(4):413–419.
4. Friedman DL, Meadows AT. Late effects of childhood cancer therapy. *Pediatr Clin North Am.* 2002;49(5):1083–1106, x.

5. Green DM. Late effects of treatment for cancer during childhood and adolescence. *Curr Probl Cancer.* 2003;27(3):127–142.

6. Hobbie WL, Stuber M, Meeske K, et al. Symptoms of posttraumatic stress in young adult survivors of childhood cancer. *J Clin Oncol.* 2000;18(24): 4060–4066.

7. Hudson MM, Mertens AC, Yasui Y, Hobbie, et al. Health status of adult long-term survivors of childhood cancer: a report from the Childhood Cancer Survivor Study. *JAMA.* 2003;290(12):1583–1592.

8. Kazak AE. Evidence-based interventions for survivors of childhood cancer and their families. *J Pediatr Psychol.* 2005;30(1):29–39.

9. Meacham L. Endocrine late effects of childhood cancer therapy. *Curr Probl Pediatr Adolesc Health Care.* 2003;33(7):217–242.

10. Neglia JP, Friedman DL, Yasui Y, et al. Second malignant neoplasms in five-year survivors of childhood cancer: childhood cancer survivor study. *J Natl Cancer Inst.* 2001;93(8):618–629.

11. Robison LL, Mertens AC, Boice JD, et al. Study design and cohort characteristics of the Childhood Cancer Survivor Study: a multi-institutional collaborative project. *Med Pediatr Oncol.* 2002;38(4):229–239.

12. Caprino D, Wiley TJ, Massimo L. Childhood cancer survivors in the dark. *J Clin Oncol.* 2004;22(13):2748–2750.

13. Kadan-Lottick NS, Robison LL, Gurney JG, et al. Childhood cancer survivors' knowledge about their past diagnosis and treatment: Childhood Cancer Survivor Study. *JAMA.* 2002;287(14):1832–1839.

14. Oeffinger KC, Mertens AC, Hudson MM, et al. Health care of young adult survivors of childhood cancer: a report from the Childhood Cancer Survivor Study. *Ann Fam Med.* 2004;2(1):61–70.

15. Mertens AC, Cotter KL, Foster BM, et al. Improving health care for adult survivors of childhood cancer: recommendations from a Delphi panel of health policy experts. *Health Policy.* 2004;69(2):169–178.

16. Zebrack BJ, Eshelman DA, Hudson MM, et al. Health care for childhood cancer survivors: insights and perspectives from a Delphi panel of young adult survivors of childhood cancer. *Cancer.* 2004;100(4):843–850.

17. Weiner SL, Simone JV, Hewitt M, eds. *Childhood Cancer Survivorship: Improving Care and Quality of Life.* National Cancer Policy Board; Institute of Medicine and National Research Council. Washington, DC: National Academies Press; 2004.

18. Green DM, Zevon MA, Hall B. Achievement of life goals by adult survivors of modern treatment for childhood cancer. *Cancer.* 1991;67(1):206–213.

19. Hewitt M, Breen N, Devesa S. Cancer prevalence and survivorship issues: analyses of the 1992 National Health Interview Survey. *J Natl Cancer Inst.* 1999;91(17):1480–1486.

20. Langeveld NE, Stam H, Grootenhuis MA, Last BF. Quality of life in young adult survivors of childhood cancer. *Support Care Cancer*. 2002;10(8): 579–600.

21. Langeveld NE, Ubbink MC, Last BF, Grootenhuis MA, Voute PA, De Haan RJ. Educational achievement, employment and living situation in long-term young adult survivors of childhood cancer in the Netherlands. *Psycho-Oncol*. 2003;12(3):213–225.

22. Nagarajan R, Neglia JP, Clohisy DR, et al. Education, employment, insurance, and marital status among 694 survivors of pediatric lower extremity bone tumors: a report from the childhood cancer survivor study. *Cancer*. 2003;97(10):2554–2564.

23. Pui CH, Cheng C, Leung W, et al. Extended follow-up of long-term survivors of childhood acute lymphoblastic leukemia. *N Engl J Med*. 2003; 349(7):640–649.

24. Zeltzer LK, Chen E, Weiss R, et al. Comparison of psychologic outcome in adult survivors of childhood acute lymphoblastic leukemia versus sibling controls: a cooperative Children's Cancer Group and National Institutes of Health study. *J Clin Oncol*. 1997;15(2):547–556.

25. Pang JW, Friedman DL, Whitton JA, et al. Employment status among adult survivors in the Childhood Cancer Survivor Study. *Pediatr Blood Cancer*. 2008;50(1):104–110.

26. Park ER, Li FP, Liu Y, et al. Health insurance coverage in survivors of childhood cancer: the Childhood Cancer Survivor Study. *J Clin Oncol*. 2005;23(36):9187–9197.

27. Hoffman B. Cancer survivors' employment and insurance rights: a primer for oncologists. *Oncol* (Huntingt). 1999;13(6):841–846, (discussion)846, 849, 852.

28. Monaco GP, Fiduccia D, Smith G. Legal and societal issues facing survivors of childhood cancer. *Pediatr Clin North Am*. 1997;44(4):1043–1058.

29. Parsons SK. Financial issues in pediatric cancer. In: Pizzo PA, Poplack DG, eds. *Principles and Practice of Pediatric Oncology*. Lippincott, Williams & Wilkins: Philadelphia; 2002.

30. Friedman DL, Freyer DR, Levitt GA. Models of care for survivors of childhood cancer. *Pediatr Blood Cancer*. 2006;46(2):159–168.

31. Blacklay A, Eiser C, Ellis A. Development and evaluation of an information booklet for adult survivors of cancer in childhood. The United Kingdom Children's Cancer Study Group Late Effects Group. *Arch Dis Child*. 1998;78(4):340–344.

32. Langer T, Stohr W, Bielack S, Paulussen M, Treuner J, Beck JD. Late effects surveillance system for sarcoma patients. *Pediatr Blood Cancer*. 2004; 42(4):373–379.

33. Meadows AT, Black B, Nesbit ME, et al. Long-term survival. Clinical care, research, and education. *Cancer.* 1993;71(suppl 10):3213–3215.
34. Neglia JP, Nesbit ME Jr. Care and treatment of long-term survivors of childhood cancer. *Cancer.* 1993;71(suppl 10):3386–3391.
35. Oeffinger KC, Eshelman DA, Tomlinson GE, Buchanan GR. Programs for adult survivors of childhood cancer. *J Clin Oncol.* 1998;16(8):2864–2867.
36. Taylor A, Hawkins M, Griffiths A, et al. Long-term follow-up of survivors of childhood cancer in the UK. *Pediatr Blood Cancer.* 2004;42(2):161–168.
37. Children's Cancer and Leukemia Group. CCLG Web site. www.ukccsg.org. Accessed November 25, 2008.
38. NICE Service guidance for improving outcomes in children and young people with cancer. National Institute for Health and Clinical Excellence Web site. www.nice.org.uk. Accessed November 25, 2008.
39. SIGN Long term follow up of survivors of childhood cancer: a national clinical guideline. Scottish Intercollegiate Guidelines Network Web site. http://www.sign.ac.uk/pdf/sign76.pdf. Updated March 4, 2004. Accessed November 25, 2008.
40. Long-term follow-up guidelines for survivors of childhood, adolescent, and young adult cancers. CureSearch Web site. www.survivorshipguidelines.org. Updated March 2006. Accessed November 25, 2008.
41. Landier W, Bhatia S, Eshelman DA, et al. Development of risk-based guidelines for pediatric cancer survivors: the Children's Oncology Group Long-Term Follow-Up Guidelines from the Children's Oncology Group Late Effects Committee and Nursing Discipline. *J Clin Oncol.* 2004;22(24): 4979–4990.
42. Goldsby RE, Ablin AR. Surviving childhood cancer; now what? Controversies regarding long-term follow-up. *Pediatr Blood Cancer.* 2004;43(3): 211–214.
43. Hollen PJ, Hobbie WL. Establishing comprehensive specialty follow-up clinics for long-term survivors of cancer. Providing systematic physiological and psychosocial support *Support Care Cancer.* 1995;3(1):40–44.
44. Hobbie WL, Hollen PJ. Pediatric nurse practitioners specializing with survivors of childhood cancer. *J Pediatr Health Care.* 1993;7:24–30.
45. Hinkle AS, Proukou C, French CA, et al. A clinic-based, comprehensive care model for studying late effects in long-term survivors of pediatric illnesses. *Pediatrics.* 2004;113(suppl 4):1141–1145.
46. Ginsberg JP, Hobbie WL, Carlson CA, Meadow, AT. Delivering long-term follow-up care to pediatric cancer survivors: transitional care issues. *Pediatr Blood Cancer.* 2006;46(2):169–173.
47. Hobbie WL, Ogle S. Transitional care for young adult survivors of childhood cancer. *Semin Oncol Nurs.* 2001;17(4):268–273.

48. Bhatia S. Late effects among survivors of leukemia during childhood and adolescence. *Blood Cells Mol Dis.* 2003;31(1):84–92.
49. Oeffinger KC, Eshelman DA, Tomlinson GE, Tolle M, Schneider GW. Providing primary care for long-term survivors of childhood acute lymphoblastic leukemia. *J Fam Pract.* 2000;49(12):1133–1146.

PART 4

Medical Issues

19

The Long-Term Cardiac Effects of Cancer Therapy

Lynda E. Rosenfeld, MD

ABSTRACT

Great strides have been made in cancer therapy, resulting in many more long-term survivors. Cardiac complications of such treatment are a relatively infrequent, but important cause of morbidity and mortality in these patients, and some cancer survivors face a higher risk of death from cardiovascular causes than from recurrent cancer. Chemotherapy, most notably anthracyclines and trastuzumab, has been associated with the development of a dilated cardiomyopathy, while radiation treatment may cause effusive and constrictive pericarditis, a restrictive cardiomyopathy, valvular heart disease, sinus node dysfunction, and heart block. Arrhythmias, both atrial and ventricular, may be a primary or secondary consequence of cancer treatment. Research is now focusing on ways to better target cancer therapy, monitor for evidence of early cardiac toxicity, and identify myocardial protectants that do not interfere with the tumoricidal effects of such treatments, all with the hope of producing healthier long-term cancer survivors.

INTRODUCTION

Over the last 30 to 40 years, oncologists have radically altered the prognosis of patients diagnosed with cancer. The number of individuals cured of cancer has dramatically increased, as has the number of patients living with cancer as a chronic disease. In 2004, there were over 10 million cancer survivors in the United States, many living more than 20 years following their diagnosis.[1] This triumph of medical therapy has not come without a price, however, because the powerful agents used to fight cancer often produce collateral damage. Cardiac complications of cancer treatment, although relatively uncommon, have become an important cause of morbidity and mortality in these patients,[2,3] and many cancer survivors have a higher risk of cardiovascular disease than of recurrent cancer.[4]

These complications may result from the systemic effects of treatment such as chemotherapeutic agents or radiation exposure, if the heart is located near the tumor, necessitating its inclusion in radiation ports and, less commonly, in surgical strategies. Importantly, cardiac effects of cancer treatment may be especially prominent in two groups: children, who if cured of their cancer could be expected to live a very long time and have the opportunity to develop such complications,[2] and the elderly, who represent the largest and a rapidly growing population of cancer survivors and may have preexisting cardiovascular disease or other risk factors.[3] It is important to realize that today we must be vigilant to recognize and treat the cardiac effects of both "old" treatments such as the extensive and relatively unsophisticated radiation therapy used to treat lymphoma and breast cancer 20 years ago, and "newer" treatments such as trastuzumab[5] and perhaps other novel drugs such as lapatinib.[6]

This chapter will deal primarily with the long-term cardiac sequelae of cancer treatments, including congestive cardiomyopathy; restrictive cardiomyopathy and effusive or constrictive pericarditis; valvular heart disease; the premature development of coronary artery disease; and arrhythmias such as sinus node dysfunction, atrial fibrillation, and conduction system disease.

CHEMOTHERAPY

A variety of chemotherapeutic agents have been associated with the development of a congestive cardiomyopathy; however, the strongest association has been with anthracyclines and, more recently, trastuzumab and similar agents. Radiation has also been associated with the development of congestive heart failure.[7,8]

Anthracyclines have been used in cancer treatment since the 1960s, when doxorubicin became available, revolutionizing cancer therapy and, in many cases, making long-term survival possible. More than one-half of the pediatric patients enrolled in pediatric oncology group protocols from 1974 to 1990 received anthracyclines, and today it is estimated that 1 in every 570 young adults in the United States is a cancer survivor.[9] Anthracyclines have also been proven very effective in the treatment of a number of hematologic and solid malignancies in adults[7] and remain a mainstay of many treatment protocols.

Anthracyclines show a clear dose–response relationship in treatment efficacy; lower doses are associated with a reduced response rate.[10] However, in the 1970s it also became certain that one of the predominant dose-limiting effects of these drugs was cardiotoxicity.[11–13] Anthracycline cardiotoxicity has been divided into three forms: acute pericarditis-myocarditis, which may be seen immediately after initiation of treatment and can usually be avoided by limiting the initial dose[10,14]; subacute cardiomyopathy, which may occur during or within months of treatment; and delayed cardiotoxicity, which may be seen years after treatment.[10,14] Because congestive heart failure continues to develop in some of these patients over many years or decades of follow-up, long-term observation is indicated.[10]

In a landmark study, Lefrak and colleagues demonstrated that heart failure was much more common in patients who had received a cumulative dose of more than 550 mg/m^2 of adriamycin.[12] While cardiotoxicity was seen in less than 1% of those receiving less than this dose, 30% of those receiving more than 550 mg/m^2 developed heart failure.[12] Equally important was the finding by Alexander and colleagues that serial monitoring of left ventricular function with quantitative radionuclide angiography during a course of anthracycline chemotherapy made possible identification of subtle reductions in left ventricular function and permitted discontinuation of therapy before the development of clinical congestive heart failure.[15] On the basis of their experience with this technique, Schwartz and colleagues were able to formulate guidelines for the discontinuation of anthracycline therapy, including a 10% or more decline in left ventricular function from a normal baseline to 50% or less.[16] This strategy permits administration of the largest possible dose of these agents, with a marked reduction in clinical congestive heart failure. Other measures of left ventricular function such as echocardiography have been used in a similar manner.[10,14] More sensitive indicators of myocardial dysfunction, including dobutamine stress testing, may, in fact, be too sensitive and unnecessarily dose limiting,[10] while more invasive techniques such as endomyocardial biopsy carry obvious risk and may not serve as a reliable indicator of clinical outcome.[14,17]

A number of factors, in addition to drug dose, have been identified as risks for the development of anthracycline cardiotoxicity. These include younger[9] and older[14] age, the dosing schedule,[13] combination therapy with other chemotherapeutic agents[13,18] and mediastinal radiation,[14,18] preexisting cardiac disease,[13,14] and perhaps female sex,[14] trisomy 21, and being African American.[9]

Anthracycline cardiotoxicity is believed to be due to the generation of free radicals and perhaps to the loss of endogenous antioxidants, resulting in increased oxidative stress.[14] Pathologically, this causes a loss of myofibrils and vacuolization of myocytes.[14] Additional mechanisms include interference with mitochondrial function and inhibition of enzymes important in DNA repair and in RNA encoding for sarcoplasmic reticulum Ca^{2+}-adenosine triphosphatase.[9]

Trastuzumab (Herceptin) is a humanized monoclonal antibody that targets HER2 receptors and has proven very effective in the treatment of breast cancers that overexpress this oncoreceptor.[5] Somewhat ironically, like adriamycin, which has a totally different mechanism of action, it also has been associated with the development of a dilated cardiomyopathy.[5,7,19]

Interestingly, initial trials of trastuzumab suggested that it was well tolerated and its major adverse effect was infusion reactions.[19] However, while subsequent studies identified congestive heart failure in 6% to 8.5% of anthracycline naïve patients receiving trastuzumab, an incidence of symptomatic congestive heart failure as high as 28% was seen in those who also received anthracyclines.[5,19] The mechanism of trastuzumab cardiotoxicity is not known, but HER2 may play a role in the maintenance of cardiac contractile function and structure, and may help protect the heart from stress.[19]

Risk factors for trastuzumab cardiotoxicity include, importantly, exposure to anthracyclines as well as preexisting cardiac disease, older age, and chest radiation.[7] It is currently recommended that patients being considered for trastuzumab therapy be assessed for cardiac risk factors and undergo a measurement of left ventricular function. The finding of a reduced ejection fraction should trigger a reassessment of treatment. During treatment with trastuzumab, patients should be monitored closely for signs and symptoms of heart failure and should have their left ventricular ejection fraction periodically reassessed.[5,19] This strategy has been associated with a reduction in the incidence of heart failure.[20]

If a reduction in ejection fraction or signs and symptoms of heart failure are identified, trastuzumab should be discontinued and the patient treated with a standard heart failure regimen including angiotensin-converting enzyme inhibitors, diuretics, and beta-blockers.[5,19,21] Such management has been associated with an improvement in ventricular function in the majority of patients, with a mean time to recovery of 1.5 months[21] (Figure 19.1). Further, most of these patients can then be successfully rechallenged with trastuzumab, with careful monitoring, without a recurrence of heart failure or deterioration of their ejection fraction.[21]

While anthracyclines and trastuzumab have been most prominently linked to the development of a congestive cardiomyopathy, a number of other agents have less frequently been associated with this problem. These agents include high-dose cyclophosphamide (such as that used in bone marrow transplantation), mitomycin and the monoclonal antibodies, alemtuzumab,[20] and bevacizumab.[7] There has also been concern that lapatinib, a small molecule that inhibits the tyrosine kinases of HER2 and epidermal growth factor receptor type 1, may cause left ventricular dysfunction.[6]

RADIATION THERAPY

Radiation is a powerful tool in the treatment of cancer. Its use to treat tumors of the chest and thorax has, however, been associated with damage to virtually all cardiac structures, including:

▷ The myocardium (dilated and restrictive cardiomyopathy)
▷ The pericardium (acute pericarditis and constrictive or effusive pericardial disease, often in association with restrictive cardiomyopathy)

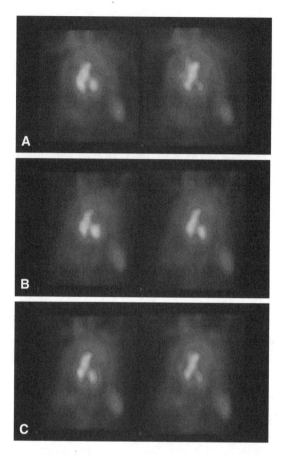

FIGURE 19.1   Images in diastole (left panels) and systole (right panels) from quantitative radionuclide angiocardiograms in a patient (A) before receiving trastuzumab (ejection fraction 62%), (B) after 12 cycles of trastuzumab (ejection fraction 29%), and (C) 2 months after discontinuing trastuzumab and being treated with an angiotensin-converting enzyme inhibitor and beta-blockers (ejection fraction 45%). The patient had previously been treated with 240 mg/m² of doxorubicin.

▷ The valves
▷ The epicardial coronary arteries (premature or accelerated atherosclerotic coronary artery disease)
▷ The specialized conduction system (sinus node dysfunction and conduction system disease)

Radiation damage to the heart is a function of the dose of radiation delivered (generally doses of greater than 30–35 Gy[22]), the delivery technique, the volume of the heart exposed, concomitant cardiotoxic systemic therapy,[22] and other cardiovascular risk factors,[23,24] such as smoking, hyperlipidemia, and hypertension. Hodgkin disease and other lymphomas treated with mantle irradiation, cancers of the breast and lung, as well as esophageal cancer, have most often been associated with cardiac damage. While radiation therapists are using increasingly sophisticated techniques to target tumors, limiting the exposure of normal tissue to the smallest effective doses of radiation, we are now treating the survivors of older, more damaging radiation techniques. In one meta-analysis of patients treated for breast cancer before 1990, radiation reduced the annual mortality from breast cancer by 13% but increased the annual mortality rate from other causes, primarily vascular, by 21%.[25]

Although the slow rate of myocardial cell division makes the heart somewhat radioresistant, diffuse interstitial fibrosis may be seen after relatively low doses of radiation,[26,27] and it, as well as microvascular damage,[28] is well described with longer follow-up. These effects may alter myocardial compliance leading to both systolic and diastolic dysfunction.[29] Echocardiographic studies have demonstrated a reduced left ventricular volume, consistent with a restrictive myopathy[26] in patients who have previously received radiation. Other studies of survivors of radiation therapy have shown a reduction in myocardial mass, which becomes more marked with longer follow-up, a pattern quite opposite that typically seen as patients age. These studies have also shown a greater number of echocardiographically documented wall-motion abnormalities compared with a reference population derived from the Framingham study[30] and myocardial perfusion defects detected by radionuclide techniques.[24] Importantly, these abnormalities became more pronounced as patients were followed for more than 20 years, indicating ongoing risk for progressive myocardial dysfunction with even remote treatment and the need for truly long-term follow-up.

Pericarditis, acute and chronic (both effusive and constrictive), is perhaps the most commonly recognized cardiac manifestation of radiation injury[26,28–30] (Figure 19.2). Fibrin replacement of pericardial adipose tissue and connective tissue deposits in pericardial vascular endothelial cells lead to thickening of pericardial tissue and its adherence to the heart and pleura as well as calcification. Vascular permeability is also affected.[29] Symptoms may be acute, chronic, or intermittent.

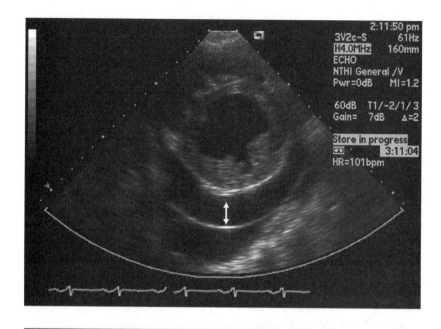

FIGURE 19.2   An echocardiogram from a patient treated with extensive radiation for left-sided breast cancer 2 years earlier. Note the large pericardial effusion (arrow). The effusion was later drained. Cytologic studies were negative for malignancy, and no organisms were identified on Gram stain or by culture.

In one older series of patients treated for Hodgkin disease, almost 30% were noted to have an effusion within 2 years of their cancer therapy.[26] More recent series, utilizing newer radiation techniques, lower doses, and myocardial shielding, have been associated with a much lower incidence of pericarditis.[28] Chronic pericardial disease may present as late as 10 years after treatment, often with symptoms of dyspnea.[31] Patients may require pericardiocentesis, creation of a pericardial window for recurrent effusions, or pericardial stripping for constrictive disease.[21]

Thoracic radiation also has an association with obstructive epicardial coronary artery disease.[7,8,24,28,32–35] In one series of children treated for Hodgkin disease from 1961 to 1991, the risk of fatal myocardial infarction was 41.5 times that of the general population. Clinical events occurred 3 to 22 years after therapy and were limited to patients receiving the highest doses of radiation (> 40 Gy).[34] Other studies have shown evidence of lesser, but still substantial, increases in risk for older patients and those treated for other diseases such as breast cancer (specifically cancer of the left breast[8]), esophageal cancer,[36] and other lymphomas.[8,28,33] Radiation-induced vascular injury may also be clinically silent, manifest as perfusion defects on radionuclide scans,[36] or localized wall-motion abnormalities detected by echocardiography,[30] and may contribute to a global depression of left ventricular function.

Pathologically, radiation-related epicardial coronary artery disease may be due to intimal hyperplasia,[7] leading to long, tapering areas of coronary narrowing[32] or to acceleration of more typical atherosclerotic lesions.[28] Obstructive lesions often are ostial or involve the proximal coronary arteries, and vessels on the anterior surface of the heart may be more vulnerable in those patients treated with anterior radiation ports.[28] Risk appears to be increased by the presence of other standard risk factors for coronary artery disease, such as hypertension,[8,33] hyperlipidemia,[8,37] and smoking.[8] Treatment is by standard techniques, including angioplasty, the placement of stents, and coronary artery bypass grafting. The latter may be made more challenging by radiation-related mediastinal and pericardial fibrosis.[7]

Recent data are somewhat encouraging in suggesting that the refinement of radiation techniques has been associated with a reduction in the incidence of late coronary artery disease in some long-term cancer survivors.[8,32,35]

Less well recognized is the association of thoracic radiation with the development of significant valvular heart disease.[28–30,38] This relation is most notable for left-sided valves and may take the form of stenotic[39] or predominantly regurgitant lesions.[30] Hering and colleagues have described a distinctive radiation-related echocardiographic pattern in which there is calcification of the "aortic mitral curtain"—that is, calcification from the aortic cusps to the adjacent fibrous skeleton to the mitral valve.[39] Of some importance, the prevalence and severity of these valvular lesions, which may be relatively asymptomatic, increase with time since therapy (most notably for the aortic valve).[30] In Heidenreich and colleagues' series of patients treated for Hodgkin disease, older age and female sex were associated with a greater risk of aortic regurgitation.[30] A percentage of these patients will require valve replacement, which may, again, be complicated by radiation-associated mediastinal fibrosis and coronary artery disease.[39,40]

Thoracic radiation may be associated with a number of arrhythmias and conduction disturbances.[28,30] These effects may be indirect, such as the well-known association between pericardial irritation or mitral valve disease and atrial arrhythmias, and the increased risk of life-threatening ventricular arrhythmias associated with depressed left ventricular function. It is now well appreciated that prophylactic placement of a defibrillator in patients with a reduced left ventricular ejection fraction either on the basis of epicardial coronary artery disease[41] or a non-ischemic cardiomyopathy and heart failure, such as might develop after radiation or anthracycline therapy,[42] may be life saving. In patients with cancer, sensitive discussions and a good understanding of long-term prognosis are often required to determine the appropriateness of implanting such devices.

Radiation-related fibrosis of the sinus node, the specialized conduction system, and the myocardium may directly result in electrocardiographic abnormalities such as right bundle branch block,[28] loss of voltage, and other nonspecific abnormalities. It may also produce significant sinus node dysfunction and complete heart block, requiring pacemaker therapy.[43]

Radiation-induced skin changes, the dissection of axillary lymph nodes, the potential need for additional radiation, and the presence of infusion ports may influence decisions about sidedness in placing pacemakers and defibrillators (Figure 19.3).

CARDIAC PROTECTION

Knowledge of the cardiotoxic effects of cancer therapy is a first step in ensuring the heart health of cancer survivors. Recognizing that these patients have a lifelong risk for some of these effects and providing appropriate follow-up and aggressive risk factor modification (e.g., providing smoking cessation counseling and treatment for hypertension, diabetes, and hyperlipidemia) is an important second step. Also important is continued research to identify the most-targeted and least-toxic cancer therapies, delivered in the lowest effective doses that do not significantly compromise their tumoricidal effect.

In addition, recent and continuing studies are evaluating adjuvant therapies and new screening techniques that are designed to minimize

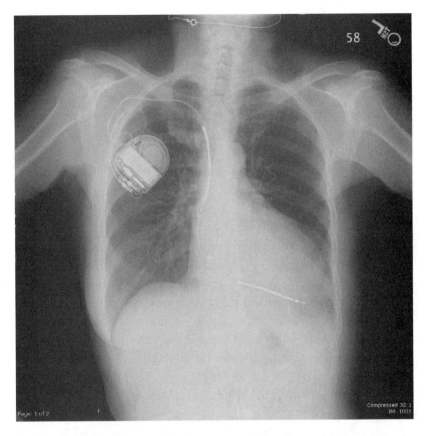

FIGURE 19.3   A chest x-ray from a patient with a chemotherapy-induced cardiomyopathy. A dual-chamber defibrillator was placed via the right cephalic vein. Although defibrillators are usually placed on the left side, this configuration was chosen because the patient previously had a left-sided mastectomy and axillary lymph node dissection as well as radiation to the left side of the chest.

cardiac toxicity while maintaining the effectiveness of cancer therapy. One of the earliest approaches to this problem has been the recognition that monitoring for subclinical declines in ventricular function may be useful in preventing more severe myocardial damage.[9,10,15,16] A tension has always existed between identifying myocardial damage that is clinically significant and limiting life-prolonging cancer treatment. To this end, measures of cardiac dysfunction, such as changes in exercise-induced augmentation of ventricular function, may be too sensitive to be clinically useful.[10] A promising new strategy is the monitoring of troponin levels in association with chemotherapy administration.[44] Persistent elevation of troponin levels has been linked to an increased risk of cardiotoxicity.[44]

Changes in drug delivery strategies[45,46] and drug preparations[9,47] have also been employed. Most notable is liposomal adriamycin, which appears to be associated with reduced cardiac toxicity with no compromise of its antineoplastic efficacy.[7,9,10,47] This preparation is less likely than its parent compound to leave the vascular space at sites where gap junctions are tight; thus its delivery to tumors, where capillaries may be disrupted, is more targeted.[47] Also, its slow release may play a role in preventing cardiotoxicity by reducing peak plasma levels of the drug.[47]

A number of "myocardial protectants" have been administered in conjunction with chemotherapy. Such agents range from products purchased at health food stores to pharmaceuticals that have been studied in controlled trials.[7,9,10,47–50] These substances are primarily antioxidants (probucol, N-acetylcysteine, and others), iron and calcium chelating agents, vitamins (vitamins A, C, and E), and trace elements (selenium and others). Other substances include typical anticongestive drugs such as angiotensin-converting enzyme inhibitors, angiotensin II receptor blockers, and beta-blockers.[51] A body of data supports the use of dexrazoxane as a cardioprotectant in patients receiving adriamycin.[7,10,47] Dexrazoxane acts as an iron chelator, limiting free radical production and presumably oxidative injury.[47] It is currently approved for use in adult patients with metastatic breast cancer who have received 300 mg/m^2 of doxorubicin and would benefit from further treatment.[47] It is not recommended at the start of treatment because of lingering concerns that it might limit the antineoplastic efficacy of the anthracycline.[47]

∾ Case Example 19.1

Julia was a 32-year-old white woman who presented with pericarditis and paroxysmal atrial fibrillation in 1977. Seven years earlier, she had been treated for stage IIB Hodgkin disease with chemotherapy and mantle radiation (4000 R). Her subsequent medical history follows:

1991—More persistent atrial fibrillation. Failure of disopyramide and quinidine to control atrial arrhythmias.

1993—Flecainide initiated. Because of recurrent atrial flutter, an electrophysiology study was performed. Multiple areas of conduction delay were seen in the right atrium, indicating diffuse scarring and disease. Extensive ablations were performed across the tricuspid isthmus and elsewhere in the atrium. Atrial flutter remained inducible at the end of the procedure, and Julia was continued on flecainide.

1995—Breast cancer diagnosed and treated with mastectomy, chemotherapy, and additional radiation.

1996—Repeat attempt at ablation of atrial tachycardia, which was unsuccessful. Permanent pacemaker placement because of sinus arrest. Subsequent atrioventricular (AV) nodal ablation to control the ventricular response to atrial flutter/fibrillation.

1996—Development of congestive heart failure. A diagnosis of constrictive pericarditis was made, and pericardial stripping and right pleurodesis were performed.

1996—Recurrent heart failure with normal left ventricular systolic function. Diagnosis of restrictive cardiomyopathy and severe mitral regurgitation. Mitral valve replacement with a St. Jude mechanical valve. Femoral-femoral bypass required because of adhesions and a "socked in chest."

1999—Right heart failure (volume overload). Amiodarone was begun in an effort to maintain AV synchrony.

1999—Bone metastases from breast cancer, treated locally with radiation.

Julia, unfortunately, exhibited a number of the complications associated with extensive thoracic radiation, including (ultimately) constrictive pericarditis, restrictive cardiomyopathy, atrial arrhythmias, sinus node dysfunction, and mitral valve disease with severe regurgitation, as well as the development of a second malignancy.

∾ Case Example 19.2

Mary Jo is a 63-year-old African American woman with breast cancer. Her medical history follows:

1994—Presented with an invasive carcinoma of the left breast. This was treated with wide excision, axillary dissection, and radiation therapy. She received tamoxifen for 5 years.

2005—Presented with a mass in the left breast.

2006—MRI-guided biopsy revealed invasive carcinoma, which was felt to be a second primary cancer (nuclear grade 3; estrogen/progesterone receptor +; HER2/neu +).

2006—Left mastectomy. Received four courses of doxyrubicin (240 mg/m^2), cytoxan, taxol, and trastuzumab. Left ventricular function was monitored serially and was normal from February to May of 2006.

June, 2006—Admitted with biventricular failure and palpitations, and found to have an atrial tachycardia and a left ventricular ejection fraction of 20% to 25%. A small pericardial effusion was present. Mary Jo was treated with beta-blockers, an angiotensin-converting enzyme inhibitor, and diuretics. Cancer therapy was changed to arimidex.

January, 2007—Admitted with syncope and shortness of breath. Echocardiogram showed a larger pericardial effusion, initially without hemodynamic compromise. Bilateral pleural effusions were present. Monitoring demonstrated both atrial tachycardia and prolonged episodes of nonsustained ventricular tachycardia. The ejection fraction remained significantly reduced at 20% to 25%.

Subsequently, because of concern for hemodynamic compromise, Mary Jo underwent a pericardiocentesis. Because of rapid fluid reaccumulation, a pericardial window was created. All cultures and cytologic studies were negative for infection or malignancy. Amiodarone was begun to control the arrhythmias.

February 2007—Underwent implantation of a defibrillator via the right cephalic vein. With continued diuresis and medical treatment, her condition improved, although her ejection fraction remained significantly depressed.

Mary Jo developed a dilated cardiomyopathy, almost certainly related to her chemotherapy and radiotherapy. She also had pericardial disease, and both atrial and ventricular arrhythmias. Because of her extensive left-sided radiation, a decision was made to place her defibrillator on the right, rather than on the more standard, left side.

CONCLUSION

Over the last 40 years, tremendous strides have been made in cancer therapy, greatly increasing the number of long-term cancer survivors in our population. Unfortunately, these powerful treatments have resulted in a variety of cardiac toxicities in a relatively small, but significant number of patients. We must strive to improve the health and well-being of these individuals using a multipronged approach that includes developing new therapies, myocardial protectants, and new ways of delivering old therapies to minimize cardiac toxicity. This approach should promote continued vigilance of patients who have received cardiotoxic therapies in the past and an awareness of the possibility of cardiac toxicity as a consequence of future treatments. With this approach, we will achieve our goal of producing many more healthy long-term cancer survivors.

REFERENCES

1. Ries LAG, Melbert D, Krapcho M, et al, eds. SEER Cancer Statistics Review, 1975–2004. National Cancer Institute Web site. http://seer.cancer.gov/csr/1975_2004. Published November 2006. Updated November 15, 2008. Accessed November 25, 2008.
2. Oeffinger KC, Mertens AC, Sklar CA, et al. Chronic health conditions in adult survivors of childhood cancer. *N Engl J Med*. 2006;355:1572–1582.
3. Rao AV, Demark-Wahnefried W. The older cancer survivor. *Crit Rev Oncol/Hematol*. 2006;60:131–143.
4. Schultz PN, Beck ML, Stava C, et al. Health profiles of 5836 long-term cancer survivors. *Int J Cancer*. 2003;104:488–495.
5. Cook-Burns N. Retrospective analysis of the safety of herceptin immunotherapy in metastatic breast cancer. *Oncol*. 2001;61:58–66.
6. Geyer CE, Forster J, Lindquist D, et al. Lapatinib plus capecitabine for HER2-positive advanced breast cancer. *N Engl J Med*. 2006;355:2733–2743.
7. Yeh ETH, Tong AT, Lenihan DJ, et al. Cardiovascular complications of cancer therapy: Diagnosis, pathogenesis, and management. *Circulation*. 2004;109:3122–3131.
8. Hooning MJ, Botma A, Aleman BMP, et al. Long-term risk of cardiovascular disease in 10-year survivors of breast cancer. *J Natl Cancer Inst*. 2007;99:365–375.
9. Simbre VC II, Duffy SA, Dadlani GH, et al. Cardiotoxicity of cancer chemotherapy. *Pediatr Drugs*. 2005;7:187–202.

10. Shan K, Lincoff AM, Young JB. Anthracycline-induced cardiotoxicity. *Ann Intern Med.* 1996;125:47–58.
11. Ainger LE, Bushore J, Johnson WW, et al. Daunomycin: a cardiotoxic agent. *J Natl Med Assoc.* 1971;63:261–267.
12. Lefrak EA, Pitha J, Rosenheim S, et al. A clinicopathologic analysis of adriamycin cardiotoxicity. *Cancer.* 1973;32:302–314.
13. Von Hoff DD, Layard MW, Basa P, et al. Risk factors for doxorubicin-induced congestive heart failure. *Ann Intern Med.* 1979;91:710–717.
14. Singal PK, Iliskovic N. Doxorubicin-induced cardiomyopathy. *N Engl J Med.* 1998;339:900–905.
15. Alexander J, Dainiak N, Berger HJ, et al. Serial assessment of doxorubicin cardiotoxicity with quantitative radionuclide angiocardiography. *N Engl J Med.* 1979;300:278–283.
16. Schwartz RG, McKenzie WB, Alexander J, et al. Congestive heart failure and left ventricular dysfunction complicating doxorubicin therapy. *Am J Med.* 1987;82:1109–1118.
17. Isner JM, Ferrans VJ, Cohen SR, et al. Clinical and morphologic cardiac findings after anthracycline chemotherapy. *Am J Cardiol.* 1983;51: 1167–1174.
18. Minow RA, Benjamin RS, Lee ET, et al. Adriamycin cardiomyopathy—risk factors. *Cancer.* 1977;39:1397–1402.
19. Suter TM, Cook-Burns N, Barton C. Cardiotoxicity associated with trastuzumab (herceptin) therapy in the treatment of metastatic breast cancer. *Breast.* 2004;13:173–183.
20. Yeh ETH. Cardiotoxicity induced by chemotherapy and antibody therapy. *Annu Rev Med.* 2006;57:485–498.
21. Ewer MS, Vooletich MT, Durand JB, et al. Reversibility of trastuzumab-related cardiotoxicity: new insights based on clinical course and response to medical treatment. *J Clin Oncol.* 2005;23:7820–7826.
22. Byrd BF III, Mendes LA. Cardiac complications of mediastinal radiotherapy. *J Am Coll Cardiol.* 2003;42:750–751.
23. Recht A. Which breast cancer patients should *really* worry about radiation-induced heart disease—and how much? *J Clin Oncol.* 2006;24: 4059–4061.
24. Prosnitz RG, Marks LB. Radiation—induced heart disease: vigilance is still required. *J Clin Oncol.* 2005;23:7391–7394.
25. Early Breast Cancer Trialists' Collaborative Group. Favourable and unfavourable effects on long-term survival of radiotherapy for early breast cancer: an overview of the randomised trials. *Lancet.* 2000;355:1757–1770.
26. Gottdiener JS, Katin MJ, Borer JS, et al. Late cardiac effects of therapeutic mediastinal irradiation. *N Engl J Med.* 1983;308:569–572.

27. Applefeld MM, Wiernik PH. Cardiac disease after radiation therapy for Hodgkin's disease: analysis of 48 patients. *Am J Cardiol.* 1983;51:1679–1681.

28. Adams MJ, Lipshultz SE, Schwartz C, et al. Radiation-associated cardiovascular disease: manifestations and management. *Semin Radiat Oncol.* 2003;13:346–356.

29. Adams MJ, Hardenbergh PH, Constine LS, et al. Radiation-associated cardiovascular disease. *Crit Rev Oncol Hematol.* 2003;45:55–75.

30. Heidenreich PA, Hancock SL, Lee BK, et al. Asymptomatic cardiac disease following mediastinal radiation. *J Am Coll Cardiol.* 2003;42:743–749.

31. Applefeld MM, Cole JF, Pollock SH, et al. The late appearance of chronic pericardial disease in patients treated by radiotherapy for Hodgkin's disease. *Ann Intern Med.* 1981;94:338–341.

32. Dunsmore LD, LoPonte MA, Dunsmore RA. Radiation-induced coronary artery disease. *J Am Coll Cardiol.* 1986;8:239–244.

33. Moser EC, Noordijk EM, van Leeuwen FE, et al. Long-term risk of cardiovascular disease after treatment for aggressive non-Hodgkin lymphoma. *Blood.* 2006;107:2912–2919.

34. Hancock SL, Donaldson SS, Hoppe RT. Cardiac disease following treatment of Hodgkin's disease in children and adolescents. *J Clin Oncol.* 1993;11:1208–1215.

35. Gaya AM, Ashford RFU. Cardiac complications of radiation therapy. *Clin Oncol.* 2005;17:153–159.

36. Gayed IW, Liu HH, Yusuf SW, et al. The prevalence of myocardial ischemia after concurrent chemoradiation therapy as detected by gated myocardial perfusion imaging in patients with esophageal cancer. *J Nucl Med.* 2006;47:1756–1762.

37. Hull MC, Morris CG, Pepine CJ, et al. Valvular dysfunction and carotid, subclavian, and coronary artery disease in survivors of Hodgkin lymphoma treated with radiation therapy. *JAMA.* 2003;290:2831–2837.

38. Carlson RG, Mayfield WR, Normann S, et al. Radiation-associated valvular disease. *Chest.* 1991;99:538–545.

39. Hering D, Faber L, Horstkotte D. Echocardiographic features of radiation-associated valvular disease. *Am J Cardiol.* 2003;92:226–230.

40. Mittal S, Berko B, Bavaria J, et al. Radiation-induced cardiovascular dysfunction. *Am J Cardiol.* 1996;78:114–115.

41. Moss AJ, Zareba W, Hall WJ, et al. Prophylactic implantation of a defibrillator in patients with myocardial infarction and reduced ejection fraction. *N Engl J Med.* 2002;346:877–883.

42. Bardy GH, Lee KL, Mark DB, et al. Amiodarone or an implantable cardioverter-defibrillator for congestive heart failure. *N Engl J Med.* 2005;352:225–237.

43. Slama MS, Le Guludec D, Sebag C, et al. Complete atrioventricular block following mediastinal irradiation: a report of six cases. *Pacing Electrophysiol.* 1991;14:1112–1118.
44. Cardinale D, Sandri MT, Colombo A, et al. Prognostic value of troponin I in cardiac risk stratification of cancer patients undergoing high-dose chemotherapy. *Circulation.* 2004;109:2749–2754.
45. Torti FM, Bristow MR, Howes AE, et al. Reduced cardiotoxicity of doxorubicin delivered on a weekly schedule. *Ann Intern Med.* 1983;99:745–749.
46. Legha SS, Benjamin RS, Mackay B, et al. Reduction of doxorubicin cardiotoxicity by prolonged continuous intravenous infusion. *Ann Intern Med.* 1982;96:133–139.
47. Wouters KA, Kremer LCM, Miller TL, et al. Protecting against anthracycline-induced myocardial damage: a review of the most promising strategies. *Br J Haematol.* 2005;131:561–578.
48. Granger CB. Prediction and prevention of chemotherapy-induced cardiomyopathy. *Circulation.* 2006;114:2432–2433.
49. Soga M, Kamal FA, Watanabe K, et al. Effects of angiotensin II receptor blocker (candesartan) in daunorubicin-induced cardiomyopathic rats. *Int J Cardiol.* 2006;110:378–385.
50. Siveski-Iliskovic N, Hill M, Chow DA, et al. Probucol protects against adriamycin cardiomyopathy without interfering with its antitumor effect. *Circulation.* 1995;91:10–15.
51. Cardinale D, Colombo A, Sandri MT, et al. Prevention of high-dose chemotherapy-induced cardiotoxicity in high-risk patients by angiotensin-converting enzyme inhibition. *Circulation.* 2006;114:2474–2481.

chapter

20

Pulmonary Problems in Cancer Survivors

Kenneth D. Miller, MD

&

Lynn Tanoue, MD

ABSTRACT

Pulmonary toxicity is very common among people who have been treated for cancer and survived. Many patients will have short-term pulmonary problems during or just after their treatment. Up to 20% of patients who have undergone chemotherapy will have some pulmonary complications in the long term, and up to 50% of patients who have received thoracic radiation also have long-term complications.[1–5] The incidence of pulmonary toxicity with the newer agents, including monoclonal antibodies, small-molecule inhibitors, and other new agents, is still unknown.

INTRODUCTION

In the acute setting, the differential diagnosis is very broad for cancer survivors who present with shortness of breath, cough, fever, or any other pulmonary symptoms and whose chest x-rays or computed tomography (CT) scans reveal abnormalities. Many of these patients have an infection within the first weeks to months after treatment. Nonetheless, there are many other causes of these symptoms, including malignancy itself, both primary and metastatic disease, pulmonary edema, acute lung injury, pulmonary hemorrhage, transfusion reactions, pulmonary emboli, acute drug toxicity, and acute radiation injury.

In contrast, in long-term cancer survivors, lung problems often represent toxicity from chemotherapy as well as radiation, and symptoms can present weeks, months, or years after treatment. Often, the best diagnostic tool is a good medical history, which can give an accurate time frame. A chronic symptom, such as a cough that has been insidiously progressing over months, may represent a consequence of cancer therapy. Patients with pulmonary toxicities are very hard to evaluate. Months and years after the cancer treatment, it is difficult to determine why a person is short of breath and has interstitial lung disease, and if it is related or unrelated to the previous treatment. In addition, the particular chemotherapy agent responsible for the problem is difficult to define, because multiagent regimens are common. Some drugs also serve as radiosensitizers, and when combined with chest radiation, they are more harmful. An insidious onset of symptoms and x-ray findings over weeks to months to years may reflect subtle inflammations as opposed to recurrence of malignancy. Unfortunately, there are no specific diagnostic tests to establish the cause of these problems with certainty. Toxicity associated with chemotherapy or radiation therapy tends to be a diagnosis of exclusion after infection and recurrent malignancy are ruled out. Some patients need a lung biopsy to define the etiology of their symptoms and findings.[6,7]

SHORT-TERM TOXICITY OF CHEMOTHERAPY AND RADIATION THERAPY

Short-term complications related to chemotherapy or radiation are common. Patients can present with cough, dyspnea, or fever and diffuse pulmonary infiltrates. Very acute lung injury is typically due to hypersensitivity reactions, such as those seen in the acute reaction of some patients to treatment with a retinoic acid preparation.[8] Every class of drug can potentially cause pulmonary toxicity, but it is more commonly seen in association with the alkylating agents, antimetabolites, and many of the biological response modifiers. The pathophysiology of lung toxicity with the individual classes of drugs can result in different clinical syndromes that can be distinct or indistinguishable from each other.

Short-Term Pulmonary Toxicity from Chemotherapy (9)

▷ Cytotoxic antibiotics (bleomycin, mitomycin, actinomycin, nitrosoureas)
- Bleomycin
  - 6% to 18% incidence of lung injury, 1% to 10% mortality if toxicity occurs
  - Risks: higher dose, other toxins (O_2, radiotherapy, other chemo), renal dysfunction, older age
▷ Alkylating agents (cyclophosphamide, busulfan, melphalan)
▷ Antimetabolites (methotrexate, Ara-C, fludarabine)
- Methotrexate
  - Up to 7% incidence of lung injury, not dose dependent
  - Syndromes: hypersensitivity, pulmonary fibrosis, pleuritis
- Ara-C: noncardiogenic pulmonary edema
▷ Biological response modifiers and others
- Retinoic acid syndrome
- IL-2—noncardiogenic pulmonary edema
- Gefitinib—pulmonary fibrosis
- Bevacizumab—hemoptysis
- Rituximab—COP
- Taxanes—hypersensitivity reactions

DELAYED AND LONG-TERM PULMONARY TOXICITIES

Most of the long-term toxicity related to chemotherapy involves pulmonary fibrosis, with a chronic impairment related to scarring in the lung. Pulmonary function studies on these patients, including diffusion capacity and lung volumes, and radiographic imaging studies are helpful. Unfortunately, months and years after cancer treatment, pulmonary function tests, x-ray studies, and even a biopsy may be very nonspecific. A biopsy may exclude other causes of lung problems that are treatable other than advanced treatment-related toxicities.

ᐁ Case Example 20.1: Bleomycin-Associated Acute Lung Toxicity

Fred is a 21-year-old man who presented to his primary care physician with shortness of breath. He also had a germ cell tumor and had multiple, "cannonball" metastatic lesions in the lung (Figure 20.1A). He received chemotherapy, and there was a dramatic improvement and response to therapy. Fred then required additional surgery. His preoperative chest x-ray is seen in Figure 20.1B, and his chest x-ray 2 days after surgery, which includes new diffuse infiltrates, is shown in Figure 20.1C. Fred had an acute lung injury related to bleomycin and oxygen cotoxicities. The treatment with bleomycin was completed, but a hypersensitivity to high concentrations of oxygen administered during surgery persisted for many years. Fortunately, Fred's x-ray completely cleared in several weeks.

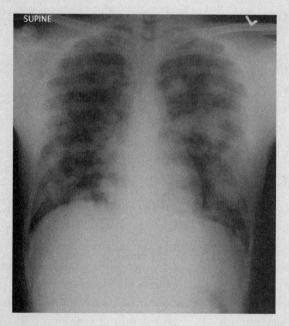

FIGURE 20.1A   Fred's presenting x-ray.

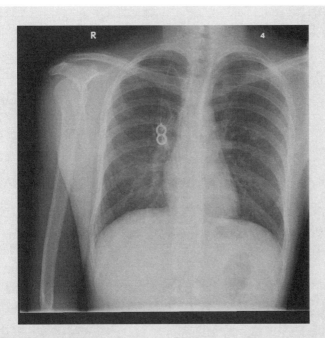

FIGURE 20.1B Fred's preoperative chest x-ray.

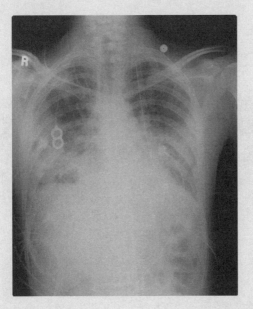

FIGURE 20.1C Fred's chest x-ray 2 days after surgery.

∾ Case Example 20.2: Delayed Bleomycin Lung Toxicity

Giannis, a 21-year-old man who has had a germ cell tumor, was treated with a bleomycin-containing regimen. He was complaining of cough and dyspnea after the first few cycles of treatment, so his therapy was changed to avoid worsening acute bleomycin lung toxicity. Fortunately, later he was cured of his germ cell tumor, and all of the symptoms and radiographic changes completely resolved. Many years later, he has normal pulmonary function and a normal life.

Figure 20.2A shows Giannis's baseline chest x-ray, and Figure 20.2B shows that he has developed diffuse pulmonary infiltrates on bleomycin.

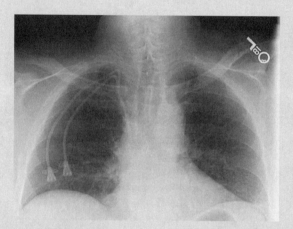

FIGURE 20.2A   Baseline chest x-ray.

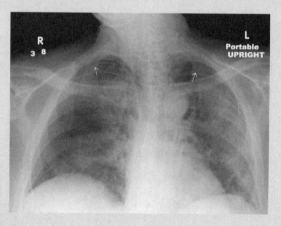

FIGURE 20.2B   Diffuse pulmonary infiltrates.

∽ Case Example 20.3: Lung Toxicity Associated with Nitrosourea Chemotherapy Drugs

Figure 20.3A–C shows the chest x-ray of Norman, a 54-year-old man who had Hodgkin disease at age 25 and was treated with radiation at that time. At age 52, he developed non-Hodgkin lymphoma and was treated with a carmustine-containing regimen and then a bone marrow transplant. In his baseline chest CT scan, there are actually minor fibrotic changes that are hugging the mediastinum related to his prior radiation for treatment of Hodgkin disease, which are classic radiographic changes of radiation injury. The mantle radiation is given right over the mediastinum, and pulmonary fibrosis can be seen years later from radiation pneumonitis, though most patients are unaware of these changes and are clinically asymptomatic. There has been a significant change 18 months after Norman's bone marrow transplant. Six months later, Norman was brought to the intensive care unit with very progressive pulmonary changes and died.

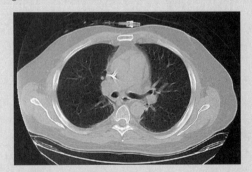

FIGURE 20.3A   Norman's CT scan at the time of diagnosis of Non-Hodgkin Lymphoma.

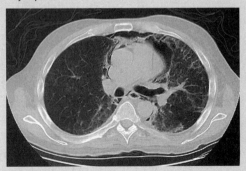

FIGURE 20.3B   Norman's CT scan 18 months later.

(continues)

Case Example 20.3: Lung Toxicity Associated with
Nitrosourea Chemotherapy Drugs (*continued*)

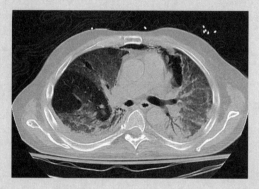

FIGURE 20.3C   Norman's CT scan 24 months later.

RADIATION THERAPY

Radiation therapy can also have short-term pulmonary toxicity, and a large percentage of patients who receive radiation to the chest, either for breast cancer or for any cancer in the thorax, will show evidence of pulmonary inflammation and scarring. Most of these patients do well, and only a minority will eventually have any injury that can be measured by pulmonary function tests or CT scans. Female gender also tends to be a risk factor because women have a smaller thorax and therefore have a deeper penetration of radiation to the lung.[10–12]

Patients with radiation pneumonitis tend to present with low-grade fever, cough, and chest pain. The radiographic hallmark is that the infiltrate on the CT scan or the chest x-ray corresponds to the radiation treatment field. These infiltrates are geographic and do not respect anatomic boundaries. They tend to look like ground glass opacities when viewed early, and they may get more linear and homogenous. They may be associated with a little bit of serositis, pleural effusion, or a small pericardial effusion, though this tends to be a minor component. It is sometimes difficult to determine if there is residual or recurrent tumor in the irradiated area in the lung because of the radiation changes, including scarring and inflammation.

The long-term sequelae of radiation therapy also need to be considered. Radiation fibrosis usually stabilizes and results in whatever damage has been done functionally and radiographically 1 to 2 years after radiation is completed. Radiation fibrosis usually occurs after prior radiation pneumonitis, but a patient does not have to have acute pneumonitis to develop fibrosis later.

Case Example 20.4: Radiation Pneumonitis and Fibrosis

Larry is a 53-year-old man who received combined chemotherapy and radiation for stage IIIA, non-small cell lung cancer. His chest x-ray is shown in Figure 20.4A and B. Chemotherapy was given partly to radiosensitize the tumor and for direct cytotoxicity, and after the radiation was completed, Larry also received additional systemic chemotherapy. Ten months later he was in remission but had clinical radiation pneumonitis with cough and fever. He was subsequently treated with steroids and was feeling well, but there was infiltrate both in the right middle lobe and in the left lower lobe. The beam for radiation was given at all different angles, but as is typical there is one field where it was given most intensively, and in this field some persistent changes were seen. Larry had classical radiation pneumonitis, with pulmonary function test abnormalities. Presently, he is fine and his symptoms have resolved.

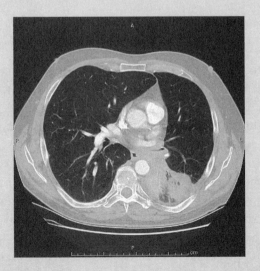

FIGURE 20.4A Larry's CT scan at the time of clinical radiation pneumonitis.

(continues)

Case Example 20.4: Radiation Pneumonitis and Fibrosis
(*continued*)

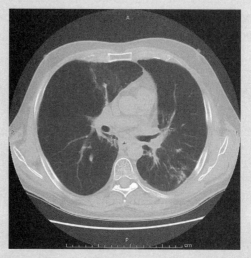

FIGURE 20.4B   Larry's CT scan after resolution of clinical radiation pneumonitis.

LONG-TERM CONSIDERATIONS

A study from Norway of long-term Hodgkin disease survivors found that many had dyspnea with measurable pulmonary function test abnormalities.[13] These patients were not clinically feeling ill, but they were symptomatic from their prior treatment. In this study, the long-term pulmonary toxicity was most strongly related to the combination of bleomycin and anthracycline and not as strongly to treatment with either of them alone.

In a 25-year follow-up, 17 childhood cancer survivors who were treated with carmustine were followed for many years and examined at 10 years and again at 25 years.[14] By the 25-year follow-up, many had died related to pulmonary fibrosis. The chemotherapy saved many of the children's lives, but it put them all at risk for pulmonary fibrosis, which can be a late, chronic, and disabling disease for both chemotherapy and radiation survivors.

Women given thoracic radiation for treatment of Hodgkin disease have an increased risk of developing breast cancer.[15] The risk is related to the dose received as well as younger age at treatment. It is very clear that radiation to the breast is more carcinogenic for the breast at a younger age, whereas radiation to the lung is actually more carcinogenic to the lung when administered at an older age.[16] Hence, childhood cancer survivors need to be screened earlier for the development of breast cancer, and adult cancer survivors who receive radiation therapy to the chest need to be considered at higher risk for lung cancer.

↶ Case Example 20.5: Multiple Effects of High-Dose Radiation

Steven is a 62-year-old man who was diagnosed with Hodgkin disease at age 26 and treated with high-dose radiation (Figure 20.5A–C). He had developed early coronary disease, had small lung volumes on his pulmonary function test, and was complaining of exertional dyspnea. On a recent CT scan, the aorta was completely calcified, and there was a perimediastinal bronchiectatic pattern where the radiation field left a scar in the lung. He has very calcified coronary arteries as well as a cardiomyopathy related to his prior radiation. His CT scans from last year started showing a left upper lobe lesion, which is a new non-small cell lung cancer, and he is actually undergoing treatment for that now.

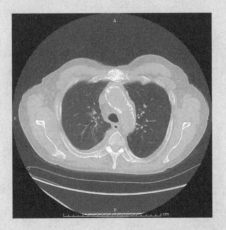

FIGURE 20.5A Stephen's CT scan demonstrating heavy calcification of the aorta.

(continues)

Case Example 20.5: Multiple Effects of High-Dose Radiation (*continued*)

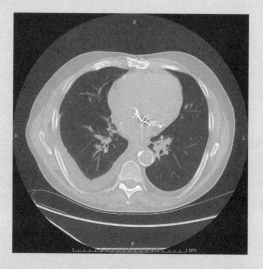

FIGURE 20.5B   Stephen's CT scan demonstrating coronary artery, aortic calcification, and a chronic right pleural effusion.

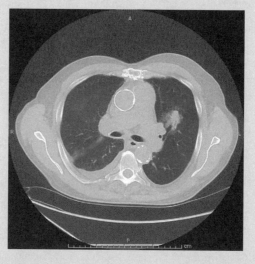

FIGURE 20.5C   Stephen's CT scan demonstrating a left upper lobe lung nodule, which is a non-small cell lung cancer.

CONCLUSION

Pulmonary toxicities and risk of a secondary malignancy are long-term considerations, and clinicians cannot stop being vigilant. Patients who have had a history of cancer and who have fortunately survived are at higher risk for pulmonary disease for the rest of their lives and need to be monitored carefully.

REFERENCES

1. Putterman C, Polliack A. Late cardiovascular and pulmonary complications of therapy in Hodgkin's disease: report of three unusual cases, with a review of relevant literature. *Leuk Lymphoma.* 1992;7(1–2):109–115.
2. Brice P, Tredaniel J, Monsuez JJ, et al. Cardiopulmonary toxicity after three courses of ABVD and mediastinal irradiation in favorable Hodgkin's disease. *Ann Oncol.* 1991;2(suppl 2):73–76.
3. Hohl RJ, Schilsky RL. Nonmalignant complications of therapy for Hodgkin's disease. *Hematol Oncol Clin North Am.* 1989;3(2):331–343.
4. Moreno M, Aristu J, Ramos LI, et al. Predictive factors for radiation-induced pulmonary toxicity after three-dimensional conformal chemoradiation in locally advanced non-small-cell lung cancer. *Clin Transl Oncol.* 2007;9(9):596–602.
5. Sleijfer S. Bleomycin-induced pneumonitis. *Chest.* 2001;120:617–624.
6. O'Sullivan JM, Huddart RA, Norman AR, et al. Predicting the risk of bleomycin lung toxicity in patients with germ-cell tumors. *Ann Oncol.* 2003;14:91–96.
7. Uzel I, Ozguroglu M, Uzel B, et al. Delayed onset bleomycin-induced pneumonitis. *Urology.* 2005;66:195.
8. De Botton S, Dombret H, Sanz M, et al. Incidence, clinical features, and outcome of all trans-retinoic acid syndrome in 413 cases of newly diagnosed acute promyelocytic leukemia. The European APL Group. *Blood.* 1998;92(8):2712–2718.
9. Tanoue L. Pulmonary toxicities in cancer survivors. New Haven, CT: Yale Cancer Center First Annual Symposium on Cancer Survivorship; May 2007.
10. Das SK, Chen S, Deasy JO, Zhou S, Yin FF, Marks LB. Combining multiple models to generate consensus: application to radiation-induced pneumonitis prediction. *Med Phys.* 2008;35(11):5098–5109.
11. Bradley J, Graham MV, Winter K, et al. Toxicity and outcome results of RTOG 9311: a phase I-II dose-escalation study using three-dimensional

conformal radiotherapy in patients with inoperable non-small-cell lung carcinoma. *Int J Radiat Oncol Biol Phys.* 2005;61(2):318–328.

12. Hu X, Bao Y, Chen YY, et al. Efficacy of chemotherapy combined hyper-fractionated accelerated radiotherapy on limited small cell lung cancer. *Ai Zheng.* 2008;27(10):1088–1093.

13. Lund MB, Kongerud J, Nome O, et al. Lung function impairment in long-term survivors of Hodgkin's disease. *Ann Oncol.* 1995;6(5):495–501.

14. Lohani S, O'Driscoll BR, Woodcock AA. Long term (25 year) follow up of 17 childhood brain tumor survivors treated with BCNU. *Chest.* 2004; 126(3):1007.

15. Horwich A, Swerdlow AJ. Second primary breast cancer after Hodgkin's disease. *Br J Cancer.* 2004;90(2):294–298.

16. Swerdlow AJ, Schoemaker MJ, Allerton R, et al. Lung cancer after Hodgkin's disease: a nested case-control study of the relation to treatment. *J Clin Oncol.* 2001;19(6):1610–1618.

chapter

21

Gastrointestinal and Liver Toxicity in Cancer Survivors

Sahar Ghassemi, MD

ABSTRACT

The digestive system comprises various organs, including the liver, esophagus, stomach, small intestine, and colon. Cancer patients commonly have gastrointestinal (GI) issues related to long-term effects of their cancer therapy, such as radiation proctitis, graft versus host disease (GVHD), or esophageal strictures. This chapter provides an introduction to some of the most common types of chronic GI injuries encountered. Attention is placed on chronic causes of toxicity.

INTRODUCTION

The digestive system is critical to an individual's health, and it spans from the esophagus to the anus. Additionally, the cells of the digestive tract are highly mitotic, turning over every 2 to 5 days. Given the large surface area covered by the digestive system and the rapidity of cell turnover, it is easy to understand its sensitivity to the affects of radiation and chemotherapy. This chapter will focus primarily on common GI and hepatic complications seen in the cancer survivor, with focus on issues related to radiation-induced chronic injury, GVHD, and secondary iron overload states. Details on specific drug-induced toxicities are beyond the scope of this review.

NORMAL FUNCTIONS AND ROLE OF THE GASTROINTESTINAL TRACT

The GI tract spans over 20 feet from the esophagus to the anus. Both the innervations and vascular network of the GI tract are extensive. While acute injuries tend to cause immediate denudation of the epithelial surface, chronic insult destroys the integrity of rich vascular supply and innervation. Understanding cancer-related GI complications requires a brief review of the function within each site. Often both gut motility and mucosa integrity are impaired with cancer-related injuries.

The esophagus is approximately 20 inches long and is the main conduit by which food travels from the mouth to the stomach. The stomach, with its bactericidal acidic environment, its production of protein-digesting enzymes, and its unique shape, churns the solid food into a thick chyme that is further processed and digested in the small intestine. The small intestine spans over 15 feet and is the primary site of nutrient absorption. Over 6 to 10 liters of nutrient-rich fluid is absorbed daily within the small intestine. While iron and folate are preferentially absorbed proximally, other nutrients such as vitamin B_{12}, bile salts, and fats or fat-soluble vitamins are absorbed in the distal segment (ileum). Finally, the colon provides 5 feet of absorptive surface where on average a remaining 1 liter of additional fluid is absorbed. All nutrients, medicines, and bacterial products absorbed across the luminal wall are then exclusively shuttled by the portal circulation to the liver where they are sampled, processed, and purified before the blood finally enters the systemic circulation.

Radiation injury to the digestive tract can be categorized into early and late injury. Acute toxicity, however, is not exclusively predicative of late or chronic injury. Acute radiation injury typically occurs within days or a few weeks, and it is reported in the majority of cancer patients. This reaction is because radiation targets cells with rapid DNA turnover. The most radiation-sensitive cells are not only rapidly dividing cancer cells but also intestinal epithelial. Chronic radiation toxicity occurs months to years after exposure. This form of injury targets less mitotically active vascular endothelial and connective tissue cells. Here the injury leads to extensive scarring of the vascular bed, predisposing to mesenteric ischemia, mucosal fibrosis, and motility disturbances.

Risk factors for radiation injury can be divided into 2 categories: patient specific and radiation specific. High doses of radiation over a broad field have a higher risk of inducing complications. Additionally, patients' comorbidities, such as previous abdominal surgeries with adhesions, diabetes, hypertension, chemotherapy, or preexisting inflammatory diseases, impact the likelihood of toxicity. In patients with extensive pelvic adhesions, the bowel is fixed and cannot move away from the irradiated field. Patients with vascular damage, either from chronic high blood pressure, diabetes, or inflammatory vasculitis, have inherent compromise to intestinal blood flow.

ESOPHAGEAL RADIATION INJURY

Acute injury to the esophagus occurs within 2 weeks of initiating radiation therapy. Symptoms include difficulty swallowing (dysphagia) or substernal burning. In malnourished or immune-suppressed patients, it is important to evaluate for coexisting thrush resulting from a superimposed fungal infection. In acute radiation injury, symptoms abate within 2 to 3 days of holding radiation therapy but can persist for over a week. Viscous lidocaine may provide temporary relief of pain symptoms. Additionally, patients are recommended to eat small frequent meals, avoiding foods that can produce acid reflux such as alcohol and coffee. Though proton pump inhibitors have not been studied in patients receiving radiation therapy, they may reduce the risk of ulcer formation or symptoms of reflux. Chronic changes typically form months to years after radiation therapy and manifest as fibrotic strictures of the esophagus or motility disorders. Given that the main role of the esophagus is to pass food to the stomach, symptoms of difficulty swallowing are common and will require endoscopic evaluation with possible dilation. With careful endoscopic dilation, most patients can resume a near-normal diet.

STOMACH

Radiation-induced injury to the stomach is rare. It is unclear if this resistance to injury is related to inherent protective elements of the stomach or if it is simply because there are fewer cancers that require radiation exposure to the stomach. Acute injury manifests as ulcers, and chronic injury includes scarring and decreased motility (gastroparesis). Treatment is primarily focused on symptoms. Though injury is primarily secondary to ischemia to the mucosa, proton pump inhibitors are still given.

SMALL INTESTINE

Perhaps the most devastating site of radiation injury is the small intestine. The small intestine spans 20 feet of tissue and resides within the field of the stomach, pancreas, rectum, and gynecological system. The mobility of the small intestine within the abdomen serves as a protective factor; however, in patients with preexisting scars, the small intestine is trapped within the irradiated field.

Acute injury manifests in the form of abdominal pain, diarrhea, nausea, and vomiting. Often patients are on concomitant chemotherapeutic medicines with confounding side effects. Any patient with fever and elevated white blood cell count needs critical consideration for infectious causes such as clostridium difficile colitis (predominant colonic infection that results in diarrhea). Symptoms typically remit within 2 to 5 weeks of the cessation of radiation therapy.

Chronic symptoms in radiation enteritis result from chronic mesenteric ischemia, tissue scarring, loss of mucosal surface area, and alterations in motility. Risk factors for chronic ischemic injury include female gender, older age, prior abdominal surgeries, diabetes, and high blood pressure. Given that it is the site of 90% of nutrient absorption, loss of critical function in the small intestine can lead to diarrhea, obstructive symptoms, malnutrition, alterations in motility, and bacterial overgrowth. It is important to note that patients can lose function of their small intestine either because large segments are surgically removed to treat obstructive symptoms, or because they suffer functional loss in which the vascular obliteration of the vessels and ischemia have compromised that intestinal segment.

The site of radiation injury can predict the type of nutrition disturbance; specifically, if patients have their ileum irradiated, they may present with vitamin B_{12} deficiency or fat malabsorption. Small bowel obstructions not alleviated with conservative medical management of bowel rest may require surgical lysis of adhesions and segmental bowel removal. All patients suspected of radiation enteritis should undergo radiographic evaluation (e.g., small bowel series or CT scan) to evaluate for stricture, fistulas, and related concerns. Additionally, if feasible, a lactose breath test should be done to evaluate for treatable bacterial overgrowth in this patient population.

COLONIC INJURY

Radiation proctitis is a common complication particularly encountered in patients treated for prostate cancer and in patients with radiation therapy to their bladder, testes, cervix, rectum, or uterus. Symptoms again can manifest months to years after therapy, with patients presenting to their physician with nonspecific complaints of fatigue secondary to anemia or with symptoms of fecal urgency and blood mixed with stool. Additional symptoms include urgency or tenesmus, diarrhea, or difficulty evacuating stool (stricture). A sigmoidoscopy will reveal superficial and friable capillary beds that bleed with minimal contact. Both endoscopic therapy and medical therapy are available to control the chronic bleeding from the site, although there have been no large controlled trials to suggest the optimal course of therapy.

LIVER

Radiation-induced liver injury typically manifests within a few weeks to 4 months after completion of radiation therapy. Clinically, patients present with ascites, hepatomegaly, and elevation alkaline phosphatase out of proportion to elevation in liver transaminases. Radiation fields covering greater than 25% of the liver surface often place the patient at increased risk of liver injury. Concomitant use of chemotherapeutic agents such as chlorambucil, platinum-based drugs, and busulfan increase the risk of liver damage.

GRAFT VERSUS HOST DISEASE

A common complication of patients receiving allogeneic hematopoietic cell transplants GVHD. Both acute and chronic forms of GVHD can occur in the liver and digestive tract. The absence of skin findings does not rule out hepatic or intestinal manifestations. Though the precise mechanism of pathogenesis is not known, our current understanding of this disease is that the donor-grafted cells recognize the patient's host cells as foreign, thus resulting in inflammation. This disease is principally T-cell mediated, and therapy involves the addition of an immunosuppressant agent, predisposing the patient to infection.

The liver is the second most common organ involved in acute GVHD (first is skin). Clinically, patients present with symptoms of jaundice, and lab work reveals elevations of alkaline phosphatase as well as conjugated bilirubin. Often concomitant skin rash makes the diagnosis of GVHD most plausible; however, it is important to note other common confounding conditions with this patient population, including acute viral hepatitis, drug-induced toxicity, and hepatic veno-occlusive disease (VOD). Often patients require a liver biopsy (either transcutaneously or transjugular in patients with coagulopathy) to determine the etiology for hepatic cholestasis.

Acute GVHD can occur along the entire length of the GI tract. Upper tract involvement presents with symptoms of nausea, vomiting, food intolerance, and dyspepsia, while lower tract symptoms are predominately diarrhea and cramping abdominal pain. The severity of luminal disease is graded by the extent of diarrhea, nausea, and/or the development of ileus. Diarrhea must be quantitated, especially when severe and intravenous fluid replacement becomes paramount. Severity of the diarrhea can exceed 10 liters a day and can transition from watery stools to bloody stools. Again, confounding diagnosis of infections such as cytomegalovirus, clostridium difficile, and drug toxicity should be considered in the differential. Endoscopy with biopsies can often clarify the diagnosis and should be pursued promptly. Chronic colonic GVHD is rare in the absence of acute GVHD and is commonly associated with complaints of diarrhea, abdominal cramping, and nausea. It must be stressed that during the first year and a half after transplant, the predominant reason for GI symptoms remains acute GVHD and infection. Beyond 1.5 years after transplant, the likelihood of acute GVHD falls significantly, and other issues such as chronic GI dysmotility and medication effects are more common causes of symptoms.

SECONDARY IRON OVERLOAD

Iron deposition in the liver is a common complication in survivors of hematologic malignancies. Mechanisms include ineffective erythropoiesis and frequent red cell transfusions. Patients often require a significant number of blood transfusions. Each unit of transfused blood introduces 250 mg of elemental iron into the body. Since our bodies cannot readily excrete excessive iron, it becomes deposited first into resident macrophages, and when these are overloaded into organs such as the liver and heart, end organ dysfunction from free radical-induced oxidative damage results. Elevated ferritin in a patient without active malignancy or inflammation is a possible indicator of elevated hepatic iron levels. Concurrent liver disease such as hepatitis C virus may accelerate fibrosis to the liver. Long-term survivors suspected of iron overload should have liver biopsy with quantitative iron measurements. Therapy with phlebotomy (if patient is not anemic) or chelation should be considered in these patients.

VENO-OCCLUSIVE DISEASE

Veno-occlusive disease (VOD) is a devastating complication that can be caused by chemotherapeutic agents and radiation therapy. Endothelial injury induced by high-dose chemotherapy results in thrombosis of the small central hepatic venules. Patients typically present with abdominal pain, ascites, an enlarged liver, and jaundice. Clinical course varies from mild self-limited disease to multi-organ dysfunction and death. Thrombolytics are successful in a minority of patients. Oral ursodiol is often provided as an adjunct to lower free-radical injury from excessive bile acid cholestasis. Treatment largely remains supportive, given that there are currently no effective therapies for VOD.

> ↶ Case Example 21.1
>
> John is a 70-year-old man with a history of prostate cancer requiring radiation therapy. He presents 12 months after his cancer therapy to the emergency room with months of generalized fatigue and over 6 months

(continues)

Case Example 21.1 (*continued*)

of episodic blood and mucus from his rectum. On his admission, his hematocrit is 22 with an MCV of 67. Iron studies support significant iron deficiency anemia with a ferritin of 7, iron saturation of 7%, and iron level of 13. The patient has a colonoscopy, which is notable for significant cluttering of friable superficial vessels in his rectum.

The primary question in this case is "What is the cause of these vascular changes, and could it still be related to John's cancer therapy after 12 months?"

John's case highlights a very common diagnosis of radiation-induced proctitis. It is important to note that symptoms may not manifest for months to years after radiation exposure. As noted, radiation can cause chronic ischemia to the vascular endothelium, leading to formation of superficial friable vessels (telangiectasias). These vessels are prone to bleed and rupture upon contact from luminal stool contents. Local endoscopic ablation therapy with argon plasma beam therapy using high-frequency energy can obliterate small vessels, thus minimizing the risk of bleeding over multiple sessions. Additionally, there may be marginal benefit to local sucralfate enemas (2 gm bid).

John received local endoscopic therapy and was able to avoid chronic blood transfusions.

∿ Case Example 21.2

Delia is a 50-year-old survivor of ovarian cancer. She complains of bouts of significant abdominal bloating and discomfort. She suspects the cause is irritable bowel syndrome, noting, "I have the same symptoms as those ladies on the commercials." She recently underwent a colonoscopy, which was "unremarkable." On her lab work today, you note her blood count is 30 with an MCV of 120. She has been feeling somewhat tired but attributes this to "the winter."

The primary question in this case is "What are some possible causes of Delia's abdominal symptoms, and is there a connection between her bowel symptoms and her anemia?"

Delia's history of radiation therapy along with evidence of macrocytic anemia suggests the possibility of small bowel involvement. Lab work shows she is vitamin B_{12} deficient. Other causes of macrocytic anemia such as thyroid function and folate levels remain normal.

Either direct injury to a sufficient length of distal small bowel (ileum) or delayed motility resulting in chronic bacterial overgrowth can give rise to vitamin B_{12} deficiency. Although there is over 10 to 15 feet of small intestine, with significant reserve, only the distal ileum is responsible for vitamin B_{12} absorption. In the context of chronic radiation injury, the vascular flow to this area could be compromised, resulting in the essentially nonfunctional fibrotic tissue. Additionally, many cancer survivors who have undergone chemotherapy and radiation therapy may have alterations in the motility of their gut. Either slowed motility or radiation-induced fibrosis can predispose a person to luminal content stasis. This condition favors the overpopulation of local enteric bacteria. Thus, bacterial overgrowth can occur in this patient population.

In Delia's case, a small bowel series was done, which was unremarkable for strictures but markedly slowed in transit time. Delia had a lactose breath test that suggested bacterial overgrowth. She underwent a trial of antibiotic therapy for bacterial overgrowth and had marked improvement of her symptoms.

RECOMMENDED READING

Coia L, Myerson R, Tepper J. *Int J Radiat Oncol Biol Phys.* 1995;31(5): 1213–1236.

Ross W, Couriel D. Colonic graft verses host disease. *Curr Opin Gastroenterol.* 2004;21:64–69.

22

Neurologic Sequelae of Cancer Therapy

Joachim Baehring, MD

&

Guido Wollmann, MD

ABSTRACT

Cancer therapy affects central and peripheral portions of the nervous system. Surgical intervention for retrieval of diagnostic material or tumor resection can damage neural structures. Ionizing radiation gives rise to radiation necrosis, a calcific vasculopathy in the brain, and peripheral neuropathies. A variety of chemotherapeutic agents are toxic to peripheral nerves or the brain when a threshold dose is exceeded. This chapter describes the most common adverse effects of cancer therapy, provides diagnostic criteria, and discusses treatment options.

SURGERY

Central nervous system (CNS) complications of surgical interventions include wound infections and neurologic disability. The risk of wound healing problems and infection is increased after implantation of chemotherapy-impregnated wafers and brachytherapy. In rare instances, placement of an Ommaya reservoir for intrathecal chemotherapy administration is complicated by hemorrhage or infection. Morbidity of neurosurgical procedures largely depends on tumor type and location. Infiltrative growth in functionally important areas increases the surgical risk, and procedures are often limited to stereotactic biopsy. When compressive growth—as frequently encountered in brain metastases—results in a focal neurologic deficit, complete resection restores function. A peculiar syndrome comprised of seizures, hemiparesis, or aphasia is frequently observed after operations within the supplementary motor area (SMA). The severity of the SMA syndrome is dependent upon the extent of resection. While frequently dramatic upon awakening from anesthesia, it is fully reversible within days to weeks.[1] Transient mutism is a complication of cerebellar tumor resection in children.[2,3] Modern imaging techniques such as functional magnetic resonance imaging, diffusion-tensor imaging with fiber tractography, and intraoperative stimulation with the patient awake have decreased neurosurgical morbidity.

Peripheral nervous system structures are at risk for surgical injury when compressive or infiltrative tumor masses or lymph node metastases are removed. Laryngeal nerve palsy after thyroid surgery leads to vocal cord paralysis. Neck dissection can compromise the cervical plexus or accessory nerve. Phrenic nerve injury results in diaphragmatic weakness. Axillary lymphadenectomy may lead to lymphedema, brachial plexus injury, and complex regional pain syndrome type I. For early-stage breast cancer patients, a less invasive approach (sentinel lymph node biopsy) is preferred, because it has been shown to reduce this risk.[4]

RADIATION THERAPY

Adverse reactions to ionizing radiation are dependent upon dose, volume, treatment duration, and fraction size. They are best classified by their time of onset in relationship to exposure. When they arise during or shortly after completion of therapy, they are generally reversible (early acute and early delayed adverse reactions). Late effects occurring months to years after radiation tend to be irreversible.

Adverse Reactions Affecting the Central Nervous System

Constitutional complaints such as fatigue or loss of appetite and anosmia characterize *early* effects of radiation therapy. The somnolence syndrome is characterized by excessive drowsiness, an inability to concentrate, lethargy, mental slowness, and fatigue.[5] Vasogenic cerebral edema leads to signs and symptoms of increased intracranial pressure and worsening of focal neurologic deficits. Its occurrence is directly correlated to single fraction dose and size of the exposed field. Not uncommonly, this reaction is accompanied by imaging changes suggestive of tumor growth (contrast enhancement and enlargement of tumor mass). Corticosteroids or osmotic diuretics are useful in the acute stage and most commonly required after stereotactic radiosurgery to targets at the upper size limit of the technique. Surgical procedures within the radiation field shortly after irradiation are avoided, because wound healing problems might occur. Patients frequently complain of diminished hearing after radiotherapy involving middle and inner ear. A sterile otitis media resolves spontaneously, whereas high-frequency hearing loss as a result of inner ear exposure is permanent. After radiation of the cervical spinal cord, less than 5% of patients may complain of tingling dysesthesias radiating down the spine and into the limbs upon neck flexion (Lhermitte sign).[6]

In the modern era, there has been a notable reduction in the *long-term* neurologic complications of ionizing radiation, which typically occur within 6 to 18 months of exposure. Increasingly, emphasis is placed on use of radiation doses and fractionation schedules below levels that would produce irreversible gray and white matter damage; the lower levels thus prevent cognitive decline or neuroendocrine difficulties. Previous combinations of drugs and radiation were associated with damaged white matter, cognitive changes or neuroendocrine difficulties.[7-9] These changes reflect a calcific angiopathy predominantly affecting small vessels.

Endocrine deficiencies arise from irradiation of the hypothalamus and pituitary region.[10] Not surprisingly, this late complication is most commonly encountered after irradiation of midline tumors such as germ cell neoplasms or central neurocytoma. Radiation necrosis is a serious complication of radiation protocols that apply 55 Gy and higher. It is true incidence is difficult to ascertain, because few cases are biopsied and coexistence with tumor progression is frequent.[11] It is directly related to total dose and fraction size. Not surprisingly, the highest incidence of radiation necrosis is seen after brachytherapy, a technique now largely abandoned and used only for selected patients with cystic primary tumors or metastases.

An increased risk for developing radionecrosis is also encountered after stereotactic radiosurgery, particularly if lesions are larger than 10 cm³.¹² Radiographic distinction from relapsed tumor is difficult even when metabolic and perfusion imaging studies are used. Corticosteroids, nonsteroidal anti-inflammatory agents, anticoagulation with warfarin, and hyperbaric oxygen therapy have been used with limited success. Frequently, the process is self-limited, but some patients require surgical debulking. The recent report of clinical and radiographic responses after bevacizumab use is encouraging but requires prospective evaluation.¹³

Myelopathies of varying degrees have been described as a late complication of radiation therapy. When the optic apparatus (e.g., nerve, chiasm) is included in the radiation field, painless vision loss can occur. Accelerated atherosclerosis arises in large vessels exposed to ionizing radiation (e.g., the internal carotid artery after radiation for head and neck cancer). Patients benefit from anti-platelet therapy, carotid endarterectomy, or stent placement.

A 7-fold excess of all cancers and a 22-fold increase in the risk of CNS tumors have been observed in leukemia patients, especially those who received whole brain radiation therapy when younger than 5 years of age.¹⁴ High grade gliomas (median latency 9 years) and meningiomas (median latency 19 years) occur with equal frequency. The risk is dose dependent,¹⁵ but meningiomas have been observed even after low-dose irradiation for tinea capitis.

Adverse Results Affecting the Peripheral Nervous System

Brachial or lumbosacral plexopathies are encountered when total radiation doses exceed 60 Gy. The brachial plexus is typically included in the radiation field in breast cancer, lung cancer, Hodgkin disease (mantle field), and non-Hodgkin lymphoma. Early acute brachial plexopathy can mimic Parsonage-Turner syndrome, with pain followed by weakness.¹⁶ The late form tends to be irreversible and has to be distinguished from tumor relapse. Electrophysiologic evaluation may be helpful in the differential diagnosis. Myokymia is present in at least 50% of patients with radiation plexopathy but absent with neoplastic infiltration.¹⁷,¹⁸ Lumbosacral plexopathies are typically bilateral, because radiation fields for advanced prostate or rectal cancer include both sides. Exposure of peripheral nerves to radiation increases the risk of malignant peripheral nerve sheath tumor. These rare malignancies occur years to decades after irradiation.¹⁹ Herpes zoster frequently affects corresponding dermatomes after irradiation of segmental nerve or plexus, or infiltration thereof by cancer (e.g., perianal zoster in metastatic prostate cancer).

CHEMOTHERAPY

Adverse Reactions Affecting the Central Nervous System

Chemotherapy is often associated with neurotoxicity affecting both the central and peripheral nervous system. In the following, chemotherapy-associated neurological syndromes and disturbances are presented followed by a discussion of individual drugs.

CLINICAL SYNDROMES

Drug toxicities affecting the CNS occur in the setting of various types of chemotherapy. Because treatment usually involves polychemotherapy or even various therapeutic modalities, the effect of any single agent is difficult to ascertain. Thus, for some of the neurologic syndromes listed in this section, only circumstantial evidence exists for a pathogenetic link between drug and reaction. The clinical manifestations of chemotherapy-related neurotoxicity are a complex function of dose, mode of administration (e.g., intravenous, intra-arterial, or intrathecal), exposure time, and the genetic background of the affected individual.

Encephalopathic symptoms linked to chemotherapy treatment can present in an acute, delayed, or chronic fashion. In the early days of intracarotid chemotherapy using drugs like nitrosureas, cisplatin, or etoposide, patients were reported to be at high risk for acute encephalopathic toxicity and visual symptoms, including loss of vision, orbital myositis, and retinal vasculitis. Newer studies, however, report lower incidences of severe toxicities, which may indicate improved drug selection, dose adaptation, angiographic technique (ie, catheter tip placement distal to origin of ophthalmic artery), and protocol design.

Delayed acute leukoencephalopathy with stroke-like presentation (DLEPS) is an uncommon complication after administration of various chemotherapeutic agents, including methotrexate (MTX), 5-fluorouracil (5-FU), carmofur, and capecitabine. Symptoms may fluctuate over a few days and spread to involve both hemispheres; these symptoms generally resolve without clinical residual findings. Almost all patients with DLEPS after MTX are children or adolescents with acute leukemia or lymphoblastic lymphoma, whereas DLEPS after 5-FU, carmofur, or capecitabine has been described in adults. Patients develop seizures, severe headache, or transient focal neurologic symptoms (e.g., sensory disturbance, aphasia, weakness). Diffusion-weighted MRI shows areas of restricted proton diffusion in the deep white matter of the cerebral hemispheres.[20]

Spinal fluid circulation abnormalities are rare manifestations of chemotherapeutic toxicity and often cannot be separated from direct disease effects. "Normal pressure" hydrocephalus is characterized by the triad of cognitive decline, gait apraxia, and cortical bladder dysfunction. Pseudotumor cerebri in recipients of retinoic acid presents with headache and transient obscured vision.

Various immunosuppressive or chemotherapeutic drugs have been associated with *reversible posterior leukoencephalopathy syndrome*.[21] It presents with headache, cortical blindness, altered mental status, and seizures. Its pathogenesis remains uncertain, but a disorder of autoregulation of cerebral perfusion predominantly affecting the posterior circulation is suspected.

Chemotherapy-induced thrombocytopenia can give rise to *cerebral or subdural hemorrhage*. These events are typically acute and present with headache, progressive somnolence, and focal neurologic findings. *Meningitis* results from chemical irritation by intrathecally administered drugs (especially liposomal cytarabine). Clinical presentation with nausea, neck stiffness, photophobia, and vomiting is indistinguishable from infectious etiologies. *Psychiatric symptoms* including anxiety, sleep disorders, and depression complicate the use of glucocorticoids and a variety of antiepileptic drugs (e.g., levetiracetam). *Myelopathies* have been described after both intravenous and intrathecal chemotherapy administration (MTX, cytarabine). Patients complain of leg weakness, sensory loss below the level of cord involvement, and neurogenic bladder dysfunction.

SPECIFIC DRUG REACTIONS

Methotrexate. Methotrexate neurotoxicity is dependent upon mode of administration, cumulative dose, and association with other neurotoxins, especially ionizing radiation. In addition, it has been proposed that polymorphisms in the enzyme 5,10-methylenetetrahydrofolate reductase may lead to increased susceptibility to MTX neurotoxicity.[22,23]

Intrathecal methotrexate. This drug may cause chemical meningitis within hours of injection. High-dose intravenous administration can cause a transient syndrome characterized by encephalopathy, headache, nausea, and seizures. DLEPS occurs within days of intravenous administration of intermediate to high doses or intrathecal provision. Complete recovery is the rule. Reexposure to MTX is possible without recurrence of the neurologic syndrome, but depending on severity of neurotoxicity, the dose is frequently reduced or leukovorin rescue is intensified.[24] A chronic leukoencephalopathy with MRI evidence of demyelination as seen on T2 or FLAIR images is seen in recipients of intrathecal MTX administered after whole brain radiation therapy (WBXRT) or recipients of high-dose systemic MTX after cranial irradiation. Patients suffer from progressive cognitive decline. Underlying these changes is a calcific microangiopathy afflicting white matter.[25]

Cytarabine. Cytarabine induces cerebellar and spinal cord toxicity.[26] The gait instability and incoordination, within weeks of therapy, is more pronounced in recipients of high-dose drug, elderly patients, and those with impaired renal function. Therapy should be ceased.

L-asparaginase. This drug has been linked to thrombotic and hemorrhagic cerebrovascular complications in 1% to 2% of patients. Patients are at risk for arterial as well as venous thrombosis within days of treatment initiation until a few days after its completion.[27] These complications are likely due to depletion of plasma proteins involved in coagulation and fibrinolysis. Fresh frozen plasma is provided as an emergency treatment but also as prophylaxis in patients who suffered a complication during a previous cycle.

Ifosfamide. Global cerebral dysfunction manifesting as confusion, delirium, or frank psychosis characterizes ifosfamide neurotoxicity. Retrospective series have identified elevated serum creatinine and low albumin as possible predisposing factors. The syndrome is completely reversible. Methylene blue (50 mg in a 2% aqueous solution given up to six times daily) administered by slow intravenous injection is available for treatment and prophylaxis of this complication. Re-exposure may not result in recurrence of symptoms.[28]

5-fluorouracil. Central neurotoxicity has been reported in prolonged 5-FU infusions as used in protocols for colorectal cancer. While DLEPS is reversible upon cessation of therapy, multifocal inflammatory leukoencephalopathy causes severe and irreversible neurologic disability.[29] Both conditions may be different stages of the same pathological process. As one would anticipate, risk of central neurotoxicity is increased in patients with dihydropyrimidine dehydrogenase deficiency.

Bevacizumab. Out of concern for intratumoral hemorrhage, experience with bevacizumab and other antiangiogenic agents has been limited in patients with cerebral metastases and primary brain tumors. Results of early studies in primary cerebral neoplasms do not seem to suggest an increased risk of hemorrhage.[30]

Central neurologic syndromes in recipients of immunomodulatory therapy (interferon alpha, interleukin-2) are poorly characterized. These syndromes tend to be reversible upon cessation of drug exposure, and an immune-mediated pathomechanism is suspected.

OPPORTUNISTIC INFECTIONS

The spectrum of opportunistic nervous system infections (e.g., meningitis, encephalitis with or without abscess formation) in cancer patients reflects the cellular or serologic immune deficit inherent in the disease itself and its treatment. Patients with leukemia and lymphoma represent 25% of all patients with cancer with CNS infections. Overall, bacterial meningitis is the most common clinical syndrome.

Disruption of physiologic barriers such as neurosurgical procedure, placement of central lines, or implantation of venous or ventricular access devices (e.g., Ommaya reservoir) are ports of entry for *Staphylococcus aureus* or *Streptococcus pneumoniae*. Dysfunction of neutrophil granulocytes predisposes to bacterial infections derived from the skin, GI tract, or respiratory tract, or to fungal disorders (e.g., aspergillus, candida). Patients with impairment of the serologic immune response are at risk for infection by encapsulated bacteria (*Hemophilus influenzae*, *Streptococcus pneumoniae*). Impaired T-cell–mediated immunity as encountered in recipients of allogeneic stem cell transplantations (ASCTs), Hodgkin disease, or the chronic leukemias predispose to infections with or reactivation of *Mycobacterium tuberculosis*, *Toxoplasma gondii*, *Nocardia*, JC virus, herpes simplex virus,

Epstein-Barr virus (EBV), varicella-zoster virus, human herpesvirus 6, cytomegalovirus, *Cryptococcus neoformans*, and intracellular pathogens such as *Listeria monocytogenes*.

Routine screening and prophylactic administration of acyclovir and gancyclovir for high-risk patients have essentially eliminated cytomegalovirus encephalitis.[31]

Progressive multifocal leukoencephalopathy, a fatal white matter disorder caused by reactivation of JC virus infection, afflicts patients with chronic leukemias. Rare cases are reported after use of rituximab.[32]

COMPLICATIONS OF BONE MARROW AND STEM CELL TRANSPLANTATION

Reversible posterior leukoencephalopathy syndrome complicates chronic immunosuppression with cyclosporine or tacrolimus. Blood pressure, symptomatic seizure management, and modification of immunosuppressive therapy usually lead to complete recovery. Cerebral involvement by graft versus host disease is rare, and a pathogenetic link between graft and CNS disease is difficult to establish. A few cases of primary CNS angiitis have been described in recipients of allogeneic bone marrow or peripheral blood stem cell transplants.[33] Posttransplant lymphoproliferative disorder (PTLD) complicates ASCT and reflects EBV reactivation or recent infection in the majority of cases. Isolated CNS manifestations are rare. If identified at an early stage of transformation, the process can be reversed by administration of corticosteroids, reduction of the dose of immunosuppression, or provision of radiation therapy. Whether antiviral therapy is of additional benefit is unproven. For later stage systemic disease or disease unresponsive to these manipulations, treatment with rituximab may be successful,[34] although its poor penetration into the CNS makes it unlikely to be useful in primary CNS PTLD.

Adverse Reactions Affecting the Peripheral Nervous System

CLINICAL SYNDROMES

Peripheral neuropathy is one of the most common neurologic complications of chemotherapy. Type and severity depend upon the chemotherapeutic agent, the individual as well as the cumulative dose. Known risk factors are preexisting peripheral neuropathies (e.g., Charcot-

Marie-Tooth disease, diabetes mellitus). Typically, patients present with symmetric fiber-length–dependent sensory neuropathies. Less common are asymmetric manifestations or mononeuropathy. Involvement of large nerve fibers or the dorsal root ganglion results in proprioceptive deficits. When small nerve fibers are affected, pain and temperature sensation are reduced; patients complain of uncomfortable dysesthesias (burning, tingling) and allodynia; autonomic nerve damage manifests as orthostatic hypotension, abdominal pain, nausea as a result of gastroparesis, sexual dysfunction, urinary retention, and decreased sweating. At least partial recovery is possible, but the neuropathy may continue to deteriorate for weeks or months after discontinuation of the neurotoxic agent.

Myopathies in cancer patients are characterized by proximal muscle weakness and preservation of tendon stretch reflexes.

SPECIFIC DRUG REACTIONS

Vincristine. Administration of vincristine produces a dose-related axonal disorder predominantly of sensory nerves in the face or extremities giving rise to tingling or burning paresthesias or jaw pain. Autonomic involvement leads to gastrointestinal dysmotility and abdominal cramping in one-third of patients. When treatment is continued, distal weakness (e.g., foot drop, weak grip) ensues.[35,36] Nearly complete improvement is noted with cessation of the medication at an early stage of neuropathy. However, rare cases of severe vincristine neurotoxicity with quadriplegia and incomplete recovery have been reported. The provision of gabapentin or amitriptyline suppresses painful paresthesias. Vincristine is believed to cause neuropathy by disrupting axonal transport because it binds to tubulin and prevents microtubule formation.

Platinum compounds. Cisplatin gives rise to a sensory neuropathy predominantly affecting large fibers when cumulative doses exceed 300 to 400 mg/m^2. Patients have poor proprioception, and a Lhermitte's sign may be present. Improvement may be slow and incomplete with significant functional disability in severe cases.[37] In addition, cisplatin causes sensorineural hearing loss.

Two forms of peripheral neurotoxicity are encountered in recipients of oxaliplatin.[38] An acute neuropathy may begin during the infusion or within hours of completion and affects most patients. A characteristic feature is its aggravation by cold exposure. This complication is usually self-limited and may be prevented by calcium and magnesium solutions, antiepileptic drugs, glutathion, and alpha-lipoic acid.[39] Chronic oxaliplatin neuropathy arises after cumulative doses over 540 mg/m^2 and mimics the one seen in cisplatin recipients.

Taxanes. Both paclitaxel and to a lesser degree docetaxel cause a fiber-length neuropathy dependent upon both individual and cumulative dose. In patients treated with 250 to 350 mg/m^2 per cycle, neuropathy may develop as early as after the first or second cycle and sometimes within 24 hours of the first infusion. Neurotoxicity is less likely with 24-hour infusions compared to bolus injection.[40] Most patients improve after discontinuation of the drug. Reports of benefit from prophylactic administration of glutamine are available, but confirmation by prospective randomized evaluation is pending.[41,42]

Bortezomib. Bortezomib causes a predominantly sensory axonal peripheral neuropathy in one-third of patients. Not uncommonly, onset of symptoms is acute rather than gradual. Dose reduction or discontinuation leads to resolution to baseline or improvement in the majority of patients. Preexisting neuropathy or diabetes mellitus are predisposing factors.[43]

Thalidomide. Thalidomide therapy gives rise to a predominantly sensory axonal, fiber-length–dependent polyneuropathy. Up to two-thirds of patients are affected. Within the first few months of therapy, patients complain of tingling paresthesias, numbness, and neuropathic pain in hands and feet. Decreased vibratory sensation may be present, but neither proprioception nor vegetative function are affected. Motor involvement has been described and may predominantly affect proximal muscles. Electrophysiologic studies demonstrate decreased amplitudes of sensory and motor action potentials. Neurotoxicity is likely cumulative, and a critical threshold dose may exist (20 g).[44]

Other drugs. Suramin gives rise to a mild, reversible, and dose-dependent distal axonal sensorimotor polyneuropathy. Less common is a subacute demyelinating polyradiculoneuropathy resembling Guillain-Barré syndrome (GBS) evolving over 2 to 9 weeks. *Etoposide* provided at high doses causes a predominantly sensory-distal axonal polyneuropathy. Occasionally, severe autonomic involvement is seen. *Procarbazine* gives rise to a fiber-length–dependent peripheral neuropathy and myalgias in 10% to 20% of cases. A severe sensorimotor polyneuropathy resembling GBS is a rare complication of high-dose *cytarabine* therapy. *Fludarabine* affects the peripheral nervous system and CNS only at high doses. Chronic use of *glucocorticoids* gives rise to myopathy. In addition to the obvious alterations in physiognomy (e.g., Cushingoid appearance), patients complain of proximal muscle weakness. Psychiatric side effects ranging from anxiety and insomnia to severe depressive episodes are seen in more than 10% of patients.

COMPLICATIONS OF BONE MARROW AND STEM CELL TRANSPLANTATION

Various peripheral neurologic syndromes have been described in recipients of ASCTs. Differential diagnosis always includes graft versus host disease, neurotoxicity of the myeloablative conditioning regimen, or immunosuppressive therapy. Acute or chronic inflammatory neuropathies develop in 1% to 10% of patients. Much less common are inflammatory muscle disorders (e.g., polymyositis, dermatomyositis, fasciitis) and myasthenic syndromes. Myositides have been described 7 to 24 months after ASCT. These complications occasionally improve with corticosteroid treatment, sometimes in combination with other immunosuppressive drugs. Myasthenia gravis represents a late complication of stem cell transplantation (manifestation after 3 years) and almost always is associated with chronic graft versus host disease. Standard therapies (e.g., acetylcholine esterase inhibitors, immunosuppression) are applied.[45]

∽ Case Example 22.1: Bortezomib Polyneuropathy

Oscar, a 58-year-old man with a history of multiple myeloma, started experiencing intermittent excruciating, throbbing pain in his legs. Days without any discomfort were followed by prolonged episodes of relentless pain radiating from his buttocks into his feet. The pain was not aggravated by position, physical activity, or Valsalva maneuver. During the pain-free intervals, his feet felt "spongy," and his balance was off. There were no sensory symptoms in his hands, the center of his face, or his trunk. Symptoms of autonomic or motor dysfunction were completely absent.

Oscar's plasma cell disorder had been diagnosed 21 months before the onset of his pain syndrome. Treatment had included vincristine and thalidomide. Bortezomib had been initiated for worsening monoclonal gammopathy after an autologous stem cell transplant. In retrospect, he admitted that he had had slight numbness in his feet ever since treatment with vincristine. Neurologic examination revealed normal strength, muscle bulk, and tone in his upper extremities. There was mildly diminished muscle bulk in his feet. Iliopsoas, anterior tibialis, gastrocnemius, and extensor hallucis longus muscle strength was diminished (4+/5). Achilles tendon reflexes were absent, and patellar reflexes diminished symmetrically. A fiber-length–dependent loss of sensation to thermal, tactile, and vibratory stimuli was found in his legs. Romberg sign was negative. Magnetic resonance imaging of the spine only demonstrated known compression fractures causing mild spinal canal stenosis in the lumbar area. Lambda free light chain level was 22.6 mg/dL compared to 58.4 mg/dL when taken 3 months before. Serum thyrotropin, vitamin B_{12}, and rapid plasma reagin tests were normal.

With the clinical diagnosis of a multifactorial peripheral neuropathy (exposure to bortezomib, vincristine, and thalidomide) with predominant involvement of small fibers, symptomatic therapy with gabapentin was initiated, which provided him with good relief from his pain. A few months after completing bortezomib, Oscar was tapered off gabapentin, which was followed by recurrence of neuropathic pain in his feet and hands. Gabapentin was resumed but was no longer effective. He had nearly complete resolution of pain upon initiation of amitriptyline therapy.

↝ Case Example 22.2: Delayed Methotrexate-Related Leukoencephalopathy

Gina, a 17-year-old girl, was treated for pre-B-cell acute lymphoblastic leukemia with a high-risk chemotherapy protocol including prednisone, L-asparaginase, vincristine, daunorubicin, 6-mercaptopurine, cyclophosphamide, and intrathecal MTX. Seven days after receiving vincristine (2 mg intravenously), L-asparaginase, and intrathecal MTX (12 mg)—now 4 months after her initial leukemia diagnosis—she suffered the acute onset of right hemiparesis and hemianesthesia. Diffusion-weighted MRI (DWI) showed a well-demarcated area of moderately high signal intensity in the white matter of the left frontal and parietal lobes. An extensive neuroimaging workup for cerebrovascular accident was unrevealing.

(continues)

Case Example 22.2: Delayed Methotrexate-Related Leukoencephalopathy (*continued*)

Gina recovered completely within the next 24 hours. Four days after the initial neurologic presentation, she acutely developed weakness and hemibody numbness on the opposite side. DWI after this second presentation showed signal abnormalities in the white matter of both frontoparietal regions. Four-vessel cerebral angiography showed no vascular abnormalities. Gina again recovered. She was continued on the same chemotherapy protocol. Three months later, she suffered another episode of delayed leukoencephalopathy, 12 days after intrathecal MTX administration. After complete recovery, she completed her chemotherapy regimen without further neurologic events.

REFERENCES

1. Zentner J, Hufnagel A, Pechstein U, Wolf HK, Schramm J. Functional results after resective procedures involving the supplementary motor area. *J Neurosurg*. 1996;85(4):542–549.
2. Rekate HL, Grubb RL, Aram DM, Hahn JF, Ratcheson RA. Muteness of cerebellar origin. *Arch Neurol*. 1985;42(7):697–698.
3. Ammirati M, Mirzai S, Samii M. Transient mutism following removal of a cerebellar tumor. A case report and review of the literature. *Childs Nerv Syst*. 1989;5(1):12–14.
4. Langer I, Guller U, Berclaz G, et al. Morbidity of sentinel lymph node biopsy (SLN) alone versus SLN and completion axillary lymph node dissection after breast cancer surgery: a prospective Swiss multicenter study on 659 patients. *Ann Surg*. 2007;245(3):452–461.
5. Faithfull S, Brada M. Somnolence syndrome in adults following cranial irradiation for primary brain tumours. *Clin Oncol (R Coll Radiol)*. 1998; 10(4):250–254.
6. Fein DA, Marcus RB Jr, Parsons JT, Mendenhall WM, Million RR. Lhermitte's sign: incidence and treatment variables influencing risk after irradiation of the cervical spinal cord. *Int J Radiat Oncol Biol Phys*. 1993; 27(5):1029–1033.
7. Butler RW, Hill JM, Steinherz PG, Meyers PA, Finlay JL. Neuropsychologic effects of cranial irradiation, intrathecal methotrexate, and systemic methotrexate in childhood cancer. *J Clin Oncol*. 1994;12(12):2621–2629.
8. Mulhern RK, Fairclough D, Ochs J. A prospective comparison of neuropsychologic performance of children surviving leukemia who received 18-Gy, 24-Gy, or no cranial irradiation. *J Clin Oncol*. 1991;9(8):1348–1356.

9. Duffner PK. Long-term effects of radiation therapy on cognitive and endocrine function in children with leukemia and brain tumors. *Neurologist*. 2004;10(6):293–310.

10. Arlt W, Hove U, Muller B, et al. Frequent and frequently overlooked: treatment-induced endocrine dysfunction in adult long-term survivors of primary brain tumors. *Neurology*. 1997;49(2):498–506.

11. Giglio P, Gilbert MR. Cerebral radiation necrosis. *Neurologist*. 2003;9(4): 180–188.

12. Korytko T, Radivoyevitch T, Colussi V, et al. 12 Gy gamma knife radiosurgical volume is a predictor for radiation necrosis in non-AVM intracranial tumors. *Int J Radiat Oncol Biol Phys*. 2006;64(2):419–424.

13. Gonzalez J, Kumar AJ, Conrad CA, Levin VA. Effect of bevacizumab on radiation necrosis of the brain. *Int J Radiat Oncol Biol Phys*. 2007;67(2): 323–326.

14. Neglia JP, Meadows AT, Robison LL, et al. Second neoplasms after acute lymphoblastic leukemia in childhood. *N Engl J Med*. 1991;325(19): 1330–1336.

15. Walter AW, Hancock ML, Pui CH, et al. Secondary brain tumors in children treated for acute lymphoblastic leukemia at St Jude Children's Research Hospital. *J Clin Oncol*. 1998;16(12):3761–3767.

16. Malow BA, Dawson DM. Neuralgic amyotrophy in association with radiation therapy for Hodgkin's disease. *Neurology*. 1991;41(3):440–441.

17. Harper CM Jr, Thomas JE, Cascino TL, Litchy WJ. Distinction between neoplastic and radiation-induced brachial plexopathy, with emphasis on the role of EMG. *Neurology*. 1989;39(4):502–506.

18. Kori SH. Diagnosis and management of brachial plexus lesions in cancer patients. *Oncology (Williston Park)*. 1995;9(8):756–760.

19. Foley KM, Woodruff JM, Ellis FT, Posner JB. Radiation-induced malignant and atypical peripheral nerve sheath tumors. *Ann Neurol*. 1980;7(4): 311–318.

20. Haykin ME, Gorman M, van Hoff J, Fulbright RK, Baehring JM. Diffusion-weighted MRI correlates of subacute methotrexate-related neurotoxicity. *J Neurooncol*. 2006;76(2):153–157.

21. Hinchey J, Chaves C, Appignani B, et al. A reversible posterior leukoencephalopathy syndrome. *N Engl J Med*. 1996; 334(8):494–500.

22. Strunk T, Gottschalk S, Goepel W, Bucsky P, Schultz C. Subacute leukencephalopathy after low-dose intrathecal methotrexate in an adolescent heterozygous for the MTHFR C677T polymorphism. *Med Pediatr Oncol*. 2003;40(1):48–50.

23. Ulrich CM, Yasui Y, Storb R, et al. Pharmacogenetics of methotrexate: toxicity among marrow transplantation patients varies with the methyl-

enetetrahydrofolate reductase C677T polymorphism. *Blood.* 2001;98(1): 231–234.

24. Mahoney DH Jr, Shuster JJ, Nitschke R, et al. Acute neurotoxicity in children with B-precursor acute lymphoid leukemia: an association with intermediate-dose intravenous methotrexate and intrathecal triple therapy—a Pediatric Oncology Group study. *J Clin Oncol.* 1998;16(5): 1712–1722.

25. Lovblad K, Kelkar P, Ozdoba C, Ramelli G, Remonda L, Schroth G. Pure methotrexate encephalopathy presenting with seizures: CT and MRI features. *Pediatr Radiol.* 1998;28(2):86–91.

26. Damon LE, Mass R, Linker CA. The association between high-dose cytarabine neurotoxicity and renal insufficiency. *J Clin Oncol.* 1989;7(10): 1563–1568.

27. Feinberg WM, Swenson MR. Cerebrovascular complications of L-asparaginase therapy. *Neurology.* 1988;38(1):127–133.

28. Pelgrims J, De Vos F, Van den BJ, Schrijvers D, Prove A, Vermorken JB. Methylene blue in the treatment and prevention of ifosfamide-induced encephalopathy: report of 12 cases and a review of the literature. *Br J Cancer.* 2000;82(2):291–294.

29. Hook CC, Kimmel DW, Kvols LK, J et al. Multifocal inflammatory leukoencephalopathy with 5-fluorouracil and levamisole. *Ann Neurol.* 1992;31(3):262–267.

30. Vredenburgh JJ, Desjardins A, Herndon JE, et al. Phase II trial of bevacizumab and irinotecan in recurrent malignant glioma. *Clin Cancer Res.* 2007;13(4):1253–1259.

31. Maschke M, Dietrich U, Prumbaum M, et al. Opportunistic CNS infection after bone marrow transplantation. *Bone Marrow Transplant.* 1999; 23(11):1167–1176.

32. Freim Wahl SG, Folvik MR, Torp SH. Progressive multifocal leukoencephalopathy in a lymphoma patient with complete remission after treatment with cytostatics and rituximab: case report and review of the literature. *Clin Neuropathol.* 2007;26(2):68–73.

33. Ma M, Barnes G, Pulliam J, Jezek D, Baumann RJ, Berger JR. CNS angiitis in graft vs host disease. *Neurology.* 2002;59(12):1994–1997.

34. Milpied N, Vasseur B, Parquet N, et al. Humanized anti-CD20 monoclonal antibody (rituximab) in post transplant B-lymphoproliferative disorder: a retrospective analysis on 32 patients. *Ann Oncol.* 2000; 11(suppl 1):113–116.

35. Macdonald DR. Neurologic complications of chemotherapy. *Neurol Clin.* 1991;9(4):955–967.

36. Hildebrand J, Kenis Y, Mubashir BA, Bart JB. Vincristine neurotoxicity. *N Engl J Med.* 1972;287(10):517.

37. Roelofs RI, Hrushesky W, Rogin J, Rosenberg L. Peripheral sensory neuropathy and cisplatin chemotherapy. *Neurology*. 1984;34(7):934–938.

38. Cersosimo RJ. Oxaliplatin-associated neuropathy: a review. *Ann Pharmacother*. 2005;39(1):128–135.

39. Gamelin L, Boisdron-Celle M, Delva R, et al. Prevention of oxaliplatin-related neurotoxicity by calcium and magnesium infusions: a retrospective study of 161 patients receiving oxaliplatin combined with 5-fluorouracil and leucovorin for advanced colorectal cancer. *Clin Cancer Res*. 2004; 10(12, pt 1):4055–4061.

40. Postma TJ, Vermorken JB, Liefting AJ, Pinedo HM, Heimans JJ. Paclitaxel-induced neuropathy. *Ann Oncol*. 1995;6(5):489–494.

41. Stubblefield MD, Vahdat LT, Balmaceda CM, Troxel AB, Hesdorffer CS, Gooch CL. Glutamine as a neuroprotective agent in high-dose paclitaxel-induced peripheral neuropathy: a clinical and electrophysiologic study. *Clin Oncol (R Coll Radiol)*. 2005;17(4):271–276.

42. Vahdat L, Papadopoulos K, Lange D, et al. Reduction of paclitaxel-induced peripheral neuropathy with glutamine. *Clin Cancer Res*. 2001; 7(5):1192–1197.

43. Richardson PG, Briemberg H, Jagannath S, et al. Frequency, characteristics, and reversibility of peripheral neuropathy during treatment of advanced multiple myeloma with bortezomib. *J Clin Oncol*. 2006;24(19): 3113–3120.

44. Plasmati R, Pastorelli F, Cavo M, et al. Neuropathy in multiple myeloma treated with thalidomide: a prospective study. *Neurology*. 2007;69(6): 573–581.

45. Padovan CS, Sostak P, Reich P, Kolb HJ, Muller-Felber W, Straube A. [Neuromuscular complications after allogeneic bone marrow transplantation]. *Nervenarzt*. 2003;74(2):159–166.

23

Kidney Concerns for Cancer Survivors

Rex L. Mahnensmith, MD

ABSTRACT

Kidney injury is a frequent complication of cancer and its treatments. Kidney injury may be acute and reversible, or it may be chronic and irreversible. Acute kidney injury, defined as a sudden decrease in glomerular filtration rate (GFR) leading to an acute rise in blood urea nitrogen and serum creatinine levels, appears to be the more common and is a major source of morbidity and mortality. Unfortunately, acute kidney injury may result in a context wherein cancer chemotherapy must be reduced or limited because of impaired clearance or associated infection, and this may subsequently render the chemotherapy less effective.

~ Case Example 23.1

Nina is a 57-year-old woman. She developed breast carcinoma, had local resection, and underwent hormonal therapy with anastrozole. She was well, receiving 4 mg of zolendronate intravenously every month. Computed technology intravenous (IV) scans every 3 months with IV radiocontrast exhibited no tumor masses. Serum creatinine was stable at 0.8 to 0.9 mg/dL with measured creatinine clearance 89 mL/min through 2006. Then, in January 2007, serum creatinine jumped to 1.9 mg/dL. Evaluation revealed that Nina received IV radiocontrast and IV zolendronate the same

(continues)

> **Case Example 23.1** (*continued*)
>
> week. A concurrent urinalysis revealed 0 to 2 tubular cells per high power field, a rare granular case, and trace proteinuria. A spot urine protein to creatinine ratio was slightly elevated at 289 mg total protein/g creatinine. Creatinine clearance is now 33 mL/min. Her serum creatinine remains 1.7 mg/dL, and urine now has cleared of tubular cells and casts. Her urine protein to creatinine ratio remains slightly elevated at 207 mg/g creatinine.

RECOGNITION AND DIAGNOSIS OF KIDNEY INJURY

Acute and chronic kidney injury are recognized with blood and urine testing. A 25% increase in the patient's serum creatinine concentration is accepted as the most sensitive indicator of acute kidney injury. Some clinicians prefer to see a 50% increase in a patient's serum creatinine concentration over baseline before declaring that acute kidney injury is evolving. International consensus now exists that a 25% increase in serum creatinine indicates an "at risk" status, and a 50% increase indicates actual "injury." This definition is highly specific but if rigidly applied will miss a significant proportion of patients experiencing true and clinically significant kidney injury. Figure 23.1 illustrates the reason: a person with serum creatinine in the lower ranges, such as 0.8 to 1.2 mg/dL, can experience sufficient kidney injury to cause a decline in GFR by 30% to 50%, and the serum creatinine will not rise by 50%. In fact, a person may lose 50% of GFR and exhibit only a 0.2 to 0.4 mg/dL increase in serum creatinine concentration. Hence, even 0.2 to 0.3 mg/dL increases in serum creatinine may indicate a clinically significant decline in GFR. Measuring creatinine clearance is far more precise, sensitive, and specific in diagnosing a patient's declining kidney function.

Recommendation: Measure the patient's serum creatinine at routine visits and frequently during chemotherapy or radiation therapy. A baseline creatinine clearance is essential prior to chemotherapy or radiation therapy. If a patient's serum creatinine increases by more than 0.2 mg/dL, then repeat the creatinine clearance and measure the serum creatinine more frequently. Repeat creatinine clearance measurements if serum creatinine increases by more than 0.5 mg/dL.

Secondly, proteinuria, red blood cells, white blood cells, tubular cell casts, or granular casts in routine urinalyses can indicate kidney injury.

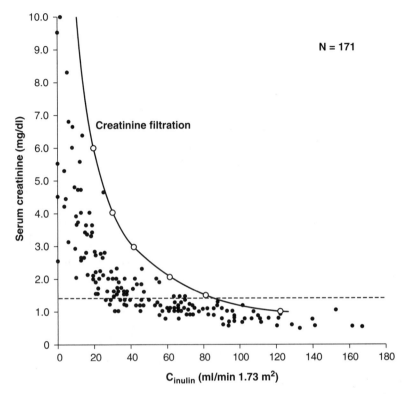

FIGURE 23.1 Relationship between glomerular filtration rate, measured as inulin clearance, and serum creatinine concentration.

Each requires interpretation, because any of these abnormalities can reveal kidney injury. However, determining site or etiology of injury requires further evaluation. Proteinuria most commonly indicates glomerular or tubular injury. Proteinuria can be quantified by a 24-hour measurement or a spot urine protein to creatinine ratio. Proteinuria arising from renal tubular injury typically ranges 300 to 800 mg per 24 hours, or protein to creatinine ratio less than 800 mg/g. Proteinuria arising from glomerular injury can reach 20,000 mg per 24 hours, or a protein to creatinine ratio exceeding 10,000 mg/g. Red blood cells may arise from a bladder injury or tumor presence. Further testing is required because of this nonspecificity. White blood cells in a urine specimen most commonly indicate infection, either lower tract or upper urinary tract. However, an allergic interstitial injury or radiation injury will also cause white cells to appear in the urine. Granular casts indicate tubular injury, typically acute. Etiology may be ischemic, or toxic, such as from a drug-induced tubular injury, or inflammatory, such as in the context of allergic tubular-interstitial inflammation.

Recommendation: Assess urinalysis at initial evaluation and throughout therapy. Include spot urine protein to creatinine ratio, because this brings more precision to the evaluation. Whenever serum creatinine increases by more than 0.2 mg/dL, include a fresh urinalysis in the evaluation. If a component abnormality is discovered, perform deeper evaluation to determine causation.

Diagnosing the cause of a patient's kidney injury requires comprehensive evaluation with a nephrologist. Etiologic diagnosis is possible through history, physical exam, medication timing, urinalysis, comprehensive blood test profiles, and diagnostic imaging in virtually all cases. On occasion, a kidney biopsy will be necessary to establish certainty. Table 23.1 lists the more common causes of kidney injury in cancer patients. These are discussed in more detail in the following section.

CAUSES OF KIDNEY INJURY IN CANCER PATIENTS

Chemotherapy Agents

Most chemotherapeutic agents are not kidney toxic. However, some medications have a strong risk, and these must be used with extra caution and surveillance. These include the platinum compounds, gemcitabine and mitomycin C, ifosfamide and cyclophosphamide, nitrosoureas, methotrexate, and IV bisphosphonates (Table 23.1).

Platinum compounds injure tubular cells. Injury is typically mild. Hydration with saline can mute toxicity. Cisplatin is the more toxic in this family and can produce a non-oliguric acute or chronic injury that typically includes renal magnesium wasting. Carboplatin is less kidney toxic at doses 400 to 600 mg/m^2. When doses exceed 1200 mg/m^2, as in patients being prepared for bone marrow transplant, kidney toxicity is more common. Oxaliplatin is the least kidney toxic of this family. Tubular injury may manifest simply with reduced GFR. Tubular cells and granular casts indicate more severe injury.

Methotrexate kidney toxicity emerges with doses exceeding 1 mg/m^2. A metabolite of methotrexate, 7-OH-methotrexate, can precipitate in tubular urine and obstruct nephrons. Injury will be manifest

TABLE 23.1 Causes of Kidney Injury in Cancer Patients

1. Chemotherapy
   a. Mitomycin C
   b. Ifosfamide
   c. Platinum compounds
   d. Gemcitabine
   e. Nitrosoureas
2. Bisphosphonates
   a. Pamidronate
   b. Zolendronate
3. Antimicrobial Medications
   a. Aminoglycosides
   b. Amphotericin B
   c. Anti-viral agents
4. Tumor Lysis
   a. Uric acid release
   b. Xanthine release
   c. Phosphate release
5. Radiocontrast
6. Sepsis
7. Paraprotein precipitation

by falling GFR, crystalluria, hematuria, tubular cells, tubular protein-uria, and/or granular casts.

Mitomycin C may induce acute, sub-acute, or chronic kidney in-jury. Mitomycin C has a propensity to incite a thrombotic microan-giopathy and hemolytic uremic syndrome. The kidney is injured from microthrombi in pre-glomerular arterioles and glomerular capillaries. This will manifest with falling GFR, falling platelets and hematocrit, and rising lactate dehydrogenase. Urinalysis will reveal mild proteinuria, granular casts, and possibly red blood cells. Such injury with mitomycin C appears to be dose related. Gemcitabine may also induce microan-giopathy and hemolytic uremic syndrome. Injury with gemcitabine may be less severe.

Ifosfamide and cyclophosphamide rarely cause kidney injury. Of the two, ifosfamide has the greater potential for tubular injury, causing a proximal tubular injury that can result in reduced GFR, glucosuria, acidosis, phosphate wasting, and potassium wasting. Low-grade proteinuria will be present.

Pamidronate and zolendronate are now recognized as causing kidney injury. Pamidronate is associated with glomerular injury manifest by proteinuria with or without reduced GFR. Zolendronate is associated with tubular injury manifest by reduced GFR, low-grade proteinuria, and granular casts.

Recommendation: Be informed of the potential for kidney injury with any chemotherapy agent. Adjust dosages according to hepatic or renal clearances. Ensure adequate hydration before and after administration. Assess serum creatinine and urinalyses before and after. Chart accumulative dosages. Be aware of concurrent nonchemotherapy kidney injury risks.

Radiocontrast Agents

The risk of kidney injury with IV radiocontrast agents is associated with dose, state of hydration, level of GFR, osmolality of the agent, and concurrence of other potential kidney injurious agents. Patients with reduced GFR or proteinuria of any type have high risk of radiocontrast injury. Radiocontrast injury can be muted with deliberate saline or sodium bicarbonate IV administration before and after the administration of the radiocontrast intravenously. Oral hydration is not sufficient. Avoid furosemide or other diuretic agents, because these may amplify risk of contrast nephropathy. Concurrent treatment with N-acetylcysteine can also mitigate risk of kidney injury.

Recommendation: Follow a radiocontrast injury prevention protocol that includes IV saline or sodium bicarbonate, cessation of diuretics, and oral N-acetylcysteine with each radiocontrast study in cancer patients who have proteinuria and/or serum creatinine greater than 1.2 mg/dL.

Anti-Microbial Agents

Risk of infection in patients receiving cancer chemotherapy is high, particularly as neutropenia evolves. Sepsis itself can induce kidney injury through two mechanisms: ischemia from reduced blood pressure and liberated cytokines. Cancer patients do acquire wide-ranging virulent infections owing to an immunocompromised state, and many of the anti-microbials are directly renal tubular toxic. High-risk agents include amphotericin B, foscarnet, aminoglycosides, and varied antiviral agents. Mechanisms of injury include direct cellular toxicity and intra-tubular precipitation. Risk is associated with dose, frequency, level of GFR, state of hydration, and whether other kidney injury risks coexist.

Recommendation: Be informed of the potential for kidney injury with any anti-microbial agent. Adjust dosages according to hepatic or renal clearances. Ensure adequate hydration before and after administration. Assess serum creatinine and urinalyses routinely and regularly during anti-microbial therapy. Be aware of concurrent kidney injury risks and aim to mitigate these as well.

Tumor Lysis-Associated Kidney Injury

A tumor lysis syndrome may emerge following rapid tumor cell death from radiation or chemotherapy. On occasion, rapidly growing tumors produce a self-tumor lysis. Dying cells release uric acid, xanthine, and phosphate, and high concentrations precipitate either in the renal tubular lumens or renal interstitium. Acute kidney injury results from either uric acid and/or xanthine precipitation, calcium-phosphate precipitation, or both. Combined precipitations are common. Hyperkalemia often accompanies tumor lysis syndrome owing to its high release from dying cells and acute kidney injury. Hypocalcemia may evolve as it is precipitated with phosphate. Intentional prevention should be routine. High tumor burden, dehydration, tumor sensitivity to the therapy, and level of GFR are the principal variables. Allopurinol is preventative, although its action does allow xanthine to accumulate, which is less soluble than uric acid in the nephron. Intentional IV hydration with sodium bicarbonate also dilutes uric acid in the tubules and increases its solubility. However, calcium phosphate precipitation may be promoted by alkalinization, and tetany or hypotension may evolve from abrupt declines in plasma-ionized calcium from IV alkali therapy. Thus, saline hydration is preferred now. Rasburicase reduces uric acid more effectively and safely than allopurinol and is preferred in high-risk settings.

Recommendation: Be aware of your patient's particular risk for tumor lysis syndrome. Provide deliberate IV saline hydration, and measure serum creatinine, phosphate, potassium, calcium, and uric acid daily during the period of high risk. Avoid alkali. Provide rasburicase in high-risk settings.

CLINICAL COURSE OF KIDNEY INJURY

Acute kidney injury may resolve completely, partially, or not at all. Chronic kidney disease may then emerge as a new chronic problem for the patient. Chronic kidney disease is now staged according to level of GFR (Table 23.2). New problems emerge when GFR settles below 60 mL/min. It is important to remember that a patient's serum creatinine may still range less than 2 mg/dL with GFR in the 25 to 40 mL/min range. Significant clinical problems derive from this level of kidney impairment, including reduced erythropoietin production, chronic anemia, reduced calcitriol production, associated secondary hyperparathyroidism, progressive immune impairments, hyperphosphatemia, accelerated vascular disease, secondary hypertension, progressive left ventricular hypertrophy, dyslipidemia, progressive osteodystrophy, and progressive nutritional declines. These problems require active surveillance, discovery, and management.

TABLE 23.2　∿　Stages of Chronic Kidney Disease

Stage	Glomerular Filtration Rate
1	> 90 + parenchymal damage
2	60–90 mL/min
3	30–60 mL/min
4	15–30 mL/min
5	< 15 mL/min

FURTHER READING

Berns JS, Ford PA. Renal toxicities of antineoplastic drugs and bone marrow transplantation. *Semin Nephrol.* 1997;17:54–66.

de Jonge MJ, Verweij J. Renal toxicities of chemotherapy. *Semin Oncol.* 2006;33:68–73.

Kintzel PE. Anticancer drug-induced kidney disorders. *Drug Safety.* 2001; 24:19–38.

Lameire NH, Flombaum CD, Moreau D, Ronco C. Acute renal failure in cancer patients. *Ann Med.* 2005;37:13–25.

Levey AS, Coresh J, Balk E, et al. National Kidney Foundation practice guidelines for chronic kidney disease: evaluation, classification, and stratification. *Ann Intern Med.* 2003;139:137–147.

Perazella MA. Drug-induced nephropathy: an update. *Expert Opin Drug Safety.* 2005;4:689–706.

Ocular Manifestations of Cancer

Rajeev K. Seth, MD

&

Ron Afshari Adelman, MD, MPH, FACS

ABSTRACT

Ocular manifestations of non-ocular, systemic cancer are either (1) directly related to the cancer itself (e.g., metastasis or infiltration), (2) indirectly related to systemic effects of the cancer (e.g., anemia, thrombocytopenia), or (3) secondary to treatment of the cancer. This chapter touches on metastatic cancers to the eye and elaborates on various ocular manifestations of cancer therapy. Primary ocular and orbital malignancies are beyond the scope of this chapter and are not covered here.

INTRODUCTION

Some have described the eye as a window into the whole body, while others have stated that it is a window into the soul. The eye is a unique organ that contains or is supported by many tissue elements of other systems (including the bony orbit, eyelid skin, collagen in the cornea and sclera, extraocular muscles and muscles of the eyelid, mucosal membranes of the conjunctiva, nervous tissue of the retina and optic nerve, and vascular tissue). For this reason, many disease processes (including cancer) that affect different tissue components can have ocular manifestations.

The eye is the only part of the body, other than the skin and hair, that allows an observer to directly visualize each of its components. Furthermore, by examination of the fundus, the examiner can directly see vascular and nervous tissue, because the retina is considered part of the central nervous system (CNS).

The eye must remain in a state of complete balance, where each component is crucial to the preservation of sight. For example, damage to the eyelid compromises the integrity of the ocular surface and leads to corneal and conjunctival damage, which can lead to vision loss. Our senses allow us to perceive and interact with our surrounding environment. Damage to any of our senses, including sight, can not only lead to physical handicaps, but also emotional distress and depression.

It is for these reasons that the eye is truly a window into the whole body as well as the soul, and it is important to recognize secondary ocular manifestations of cancer and its treatment.

METASTATIC CANCER TO THE EYE

The most common intraocular tumor of the eye or orbit in adults is metastatic cancer. A recent study showed that the most common primary cancers that metastasize to the eye are breast (47%), then lung (21%), gastrointestinal tract (4%), kidney (2%), skin (2%), and prostate (2%).[1] Overall, the incidence is equal among men and women, but in men, the most common primary site of malignancy is the lung, while in women it is the breast.

The most common route of metastasis to the eye is via hematogenous spread, so it makes sense that the most vascularized site of the eye, the choroid, is the most frequent site of metastasis. Rarely, other parts of the eye can also serve as secondary sites of spread. However, the choroid is affected 10 to 20 times more frequently than either the iris or ciliary body.[1,2]

Metastatic disease to the choroid is seen as discrete, elevated subretinal/choroidal masses, usually cream or light yellow in color. Diagnosis of metastatic cancer to the eye is through careful examination of the eye, with the aid of ultrasound examination to differentiate it from primary ocular amelanotic melanomas. Patients may present with decreased vision, because occasionally metastatic disease to the choroid can affect the overlying retina; but most times the patient is asymptomatic. Occasionally, a choroidal lesion seen on routine eye examination can be the first sign of a systemic malignancy.

LEUKEMIA AND LYMPHOMA

Leukemia and lymphoma can also have a variety of ocular manifestations. Ocular manifestations are either from direct infiltration or involvement of the eye, or they are indirectly from effects such as secondary anemia, thrombocytopenia, and leukocytosis[3-7](these effects are detailed in this chapter). Ocular manifestations are seen more commonly in acute leukemias than in chronic forms. In lymphomas, ocular involvement is most commonly seen with large B-cell, non-Hodgkin lymphomas. Clinically, the retina and vitreous are the most frequently involved sites, but histologically, the choroid is most commonly involved.[3-7]

Studies have shown that 30% to 40% of patients with leukemia have ocular manifestations,[3-7] and the overall 5-year survival rate in children is 21% with ocular manifestations, compared to 45% without ocular manifestations.[5]

Metastasis to the orbit can present as proptosis. Leukemia or lymphoma can occasionally present as a pink, fleshy-appearing conjunctival mass often referred to as a salmon patch.

As in metastatic carcinomas, leukemia or lymphoma can present with choroidal involvement. However, unlike the discrete masses of metastatic carcinomas, choroidal leukemic or lymphomatous involvement is a more flat and possibly diffuse thickening. Occasionally, patients with lymphoma first present with bilateral vitritis (inflammatory cells within the vitreous cavity), unresponsive to anti-inflammatory therapy. Biopsy of the vitreous with cytology and flow cytometry will reveal atypical, lymphomatous cells. Elderly patients with vitritis unresponsive to treatment should be suspected of having ocular lymphoma and referred for vitreous biopsy.[8] CNS workup with neuroimaging and lumbar puncture should also be performed.[8]

As noted, the retina is a common clinical site of involvement in leukemia and lymphoma. Retinal manifestations include direct retinal infiltration, retinal hemorrhages, retinal venous dilation and tortuosity, perivascular infiltrates, nerve fiber layer infarcts (cotton-wool spots), retinal detachment, or vascular occlusion (secondary to hyperviscosity states).[9] The optic nerve can also have direct infiltration, presenting as decreased vision with optic nerve swelling, edema, and peripapillary hemorrhages. One may also see papilledema related to increased intracranial pressure with CNS involvement. Optic nerve involvement necessitates CNS imaging and lumbar puncture to assess for CNS involvement or increased intracranial pressure. (See Figure 24.1.)

Treatment of leukemic or lymphomatous involvement of the eye includes systemic treatment for the disease process. Local radiation therapy and intrathecal chemotherapy is sometimes included as part of the regimen for intraocular lymphoma associated with CNS involvement.[10]

OCULAR MANIFESTATIONS FROM SYSTEMIC EFFECTS OF CANCER

Many malignancies and their treatment result in systemic effects, such as anemia, thrombocytopenia, leukopenia, leukocytosis, immunosuppression, or increased intracranial pressure with some CNS malignancies. These secondary effects can also have various ocular manifestations.

Anemia and thrombocytopenia can manifest as retinal hemorrhages or nerve fiber layer infarcts (cotton-wool spots). Extreme leukocytosis can lead to a hyperviscosity state, predisposing a patient to central retinal vein or artery occlusions. Patients may also present with amaurosis fugax symptoms (intermittent, short-duration loss/blackening of vision)

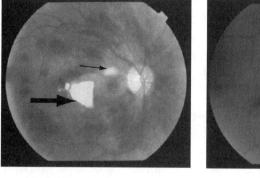
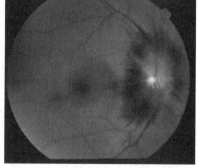

A   B

FIGURE 24.1   (A) Retinal hemorrhages and large retinal infiltration in a patient with acute myelocytic leukemia. Cotton-wool spot is also present (small arrow). (B) Optic nerve involvement with optic nerve edema and peripapillary hemorrhages in a patient with acute myelocytic leukemia.

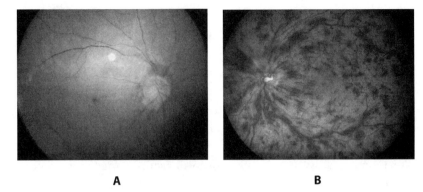

A   **B**

FIGURE 24.2 (A) Central retinal artery occlusion with ischemic white retina, narrowed retinal arteries, and "cherry-red spot." (B) Central retinal vein occlusion with diffuse retinal hemorrhages.

with transient ischemic attacks associated with hyperviscosity states. (See Figure 24.2.)

OPPORTUNISTIC INFECTIONS

Many cancer patients are immunocompromised either directly from their malignancy or indirectly from chemotherapy or radiation. Immunocompromised states place the patient at risk for opportunistic infections, which are a source of morbidity and mortality in cancer patients.

Bacterial Endophthalmitis

Immunocompromised patients are susceptible to endogenous bacterial infections of the eye. The route is by hematogenous spread to the choroid, retina, and/or vitreous. The most common bacteria causing endogenous endophthalmitis are *Streptococcus* species and *Staphylococcus aureus*.[11,12] Patients present with decreased vision and floaters. The lesions appear as early flat lesions involving the retina and choroid, which later enlarge and may spread into the vitreous.[11,12] Treatment is with systemic as well as intravitreal injections of antibiotics.

Fungal Endophthalmitis

Even more common than bacterial infections are endogenous fungal infections of the eye in an immunocompromised patient. The most common cause of fungal endophthalmitis is *Candida* species.[9] Risk factors for endogenous fungal endophthalmitis include indwelling catheters, immunosuppression, chronic antibiotic use, abdominal surgery, hyperalimentation, and diabetes mellitus.[9] Cancer patients have many of these risk factors. Patients again present with decreased vision and floaters. Fungal endophthalmitis presents as single or multiple yellow-white choroidal lesions or subretinal infiltrates that can progress and grow into an elevated lesion that projects into the vitreous cavity. Treatment consists of systemic antifungal agents, namely intravenous amphotericin B or azoles. If there is no response to systemic treatment, intravitreal injections of amphotericin B can be done as well.[9]

Opportunistic Viral Infections

Immunosuppressed patients are also at risk for reactivation of viral disease, most commonly herpes simplex (HSV), herpes zoster (HZV), or cytomegalovirus (CMV). HSV and HZV may affect any part of the eye and can cause a vesicular eyelid rash, conjunctivitis, a painful keratitis (inflammation of the cornea), iritis (inflammation within the anterior part of the eye), or a retinitis causing significant retinal destruction and visual compromise. Treatment depends on site of involvement, but includes systemic antivirals, topical antivirals, or topical steroids.

Unlike HSV or HZV, which can affect any part of the eye, CMV usually affects the retina. The hallmark of CMV retinitis is a slowly progressive infection of the retina with areas of hemorrhage, exudates, necrosis, and vasculitis. Patients present with significant visual loss and floaters, and retinal detachment is a common occurrence. Treatment is with systemic ganciclovir or foscarnet, with intravitreal injection of ganciclovir or ganciclovir implant done for a small number of cases.

OCULAR MANIFESTATIONS OF CHEMOTHERAPY

A wide variety of chemotherapeutic agents affect the eyes. Table 24.1 highlights the more common ocular side effects.[13]

Table 24.2 outlines the various methods reported to decrease the ocular side effects of chemotherapy.[13]

TABLE 24.1 Common Ocular Side Effects of Chemotherapy

Site	Side Effect	Agent	Likelihood[a]
Orbit	Periorbital edema	5FU Methotrexate	Somewhat common
	Eye pain	5FU	Somewhat common
	AV shunts	Carmustine	Somewhat common
Lacrimal drainage	Epiphora	5FU	Common
Conjunctiva	Keratoconjunctivitis sicca	Cyclophosphamide Busulfan	Somewhat common
	Conjunctivitis	5FU Deoxycoformycin	Somewhat common
Cornea	Keratitis	Cytosine arabinoside 5FU Deoxycoformycin	Common Somewhat common
	Corneal opacities	Cytosine arabinoside	Somewhat common
Retina	Macular pigment changes	Cisplatin	Somewhat common
	Crystalline Retinopathy	Tamoxifen	
	Retinal hemorrhages	Carmustine	Somewhat common
	Arterial narrowings	Carmustine	Somewhat common

(continues)

TABLE 24.1 ᐭ Common Ocular Side Effects of Chemotherapy (*continued*)

Site	Side Effect	Agent	Likelihood[a]
Optic nerve	Papilledema	Carmustine	Somewhat common
Cranial nerves 3, 4, 5, and 6	Cranial nerve palsies	Plant alkaloids	Somewhat common
	Ptosis	Plant alkaloids	Somewhat common
Central nervous system	Focal demyelination in optic nerves	Carmustine	Somewhat common
Vision	Blurred vision	Busulfan 5FU	Somewhat common
	Photophobia	5FU	Somewhat common

[a] Common = 50–100%; somewhat common = 20–49% probability

Source: Adapted with modifications from Schmid KE, Kornek GV, Scheithauer W, Binder S. Update on ocular complications of systemic cancer chemotherapy. *Surv Ophthalmol.* 2006;51(1):19–40.

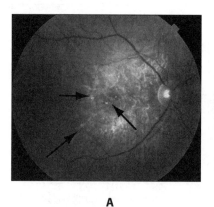
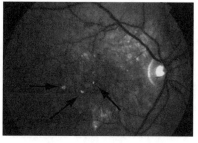

A   B

FIGURE 24.3 (A) Fundus photograph of retina showing tamoxifen crystals (arrows). (B) Red-free fundus photograph of same eye highlighting the tamoxifen crystals (arrows).

TABLE 24.2 Agents and Treatment Suggestions

Agent	Treatment Suggestions
Cisplatin	Infusion catheter should be advanced beyond the ophthalmic artery if intracarotid administration is inevitable
Carmustine/BCNU	Infusion catheter should be advanced beyond the ophthalmic artery if intracarotid administration is inevitable
Cytosine arabinoside	• Glucocorticoid eyedrops applied prior to therapy • Eye washing with normal saline and instillation of 0.1% sodium bethamethazone phosphate eyedrops applied prior to therapy
5FU	• Ocular ice packs for 30 minutes, starting 5 minutes prior to therapy • Methylcellulose eyedrops • Dexamethasone eyedrops
Methotrexate	Artificial Tears
Docetaxel	Early temporary silicone intubation in symptomatic patients receiving weekly docetaxel

Source: Adapted with modifications from Schmid KE, Kornek GV, Scheithauer W, Binder S. Update on ocular complications of systemic cancer chemotherapy. *Surv Ophthalmol.* 2006;51(1):19–40.

Corticosteroids

Corticosteroids are often used in the treatment of malignancies and can have serious ocular side effects, namely glaucoma and cataract.

Glaucoma is a disease in which there is gradual damage to the optic nerve, most commonly from an increase in the intraocular pressure

(IOP). All forms of steroids, including systemic, topical (cutaneous or ocular), or inhaled, are known to possibly cause an elevation of IOP. Those already with a history of glaucoma (unrelated to steroid use) are at an increased risk of developing a steroid-induced rise in IOP.

If the rise in IOP is only moderate, the patient may be asymptomatic until the glaucoma has progressed significantly. This is because glaucoma first damages the part of the optic nerve responsible for peripheral vision, and the central vision is unaffected until the late stages of the disease (Figure 24.4). However, if there is a significant IOP elevation, the patient may have symptoms of throbbing eye pain and cloudy vision (from corneal edema caused by significant IOP rise). Treatment for steroid-induced glaucoma includes IOP-lowering medications and glaucoma surgery.

Cataract is clouding of the lens, a part of the eye that is responsible for focusing light rays onto the retina. Steroids cause a type of cataract known as posterior subcapsular cataract, in which there is a clouding of the posterior surface of the lens. In addition to blurry or cloudy vision, patients typically have more glare symptoms, particularly at night. If visually significant, patients can undergo cataract extraction with synthetic lens implantation.

OCULAR MANIFESTATIONS OF RADIATION THERAPY

Radiation therapy is commonly used in the treatment of cancer. Although radiation is typically applied to a particular area, damage to nearby areas can occur. Ocular manifestations usually occur with radiation therapy to the head and neck, the CNS, or the eye itself.

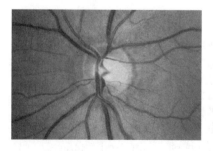 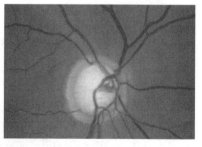

A   **B**

FIGURE 24.4   (A) Normal optic nerve; (B) Optic nerve after glaucomatous damage.

Table 24.3 summarizes the ocular effects of radiation therapy by anatomic site and the amount of radiation typically necessary to produce such damage.[14,15]

The lens is the most sensitive part of the eye to radiation; therefore, cataracts are common in these patients. Acutely, the most common ocular surface complication from radiation is dry eye and corneal epitheliopathy with pain, burning, foreign body sensation, and dryness.

TABLE 24.3 Ocular Effects of Radiation Therapy

Tissue	Effect	Total Dose (Gy)
Conjunctiva	Conjunctivitis	55–75
	Telangiectasia	30
Cornea	Keratitis, edema, epithelial defect	30–50
	Ulcer, scarring, perforation	> 60
Lens	Cataract	16
Retina	Retinopathy	> 46.5
Optic nerve	Neuropathy	> 55
Lacrimal system	Atrophy	50–60
	Stenosis	65–75
Eyelid	Lash loss	40–60
	Erythema	30–40
	Telangiectasia	> 55
Orbit	Implant extrusion	Not specified

Source: Adapted from Bardenstein D, Char DH. Ocular toxicity. In: Madhu J, Flam MS, eds. *Chemoradiation: An Integrated Approach to Cancer Treatment*, Philadelphia: Lea & Febiger, 1993, pp. 591–598 and Barabino S, Raghavan A, Loeffler J, Dana R. Radiotherapy-induced ocular surface disease. *Cornea.* 2005;24(8):909–914.

(Please see the following section on graft versus host disease (GVHD) for a complete discussion on dry eye and its treatment.) Late complications of radiation injury to the ocular surface include poor tear production secondary to lacrimal gland dysfunction, poor wound healing, decreased corneal sensation, and corneal epitheliopathy or ulceration.[14]

Perhaps the most significant and irreversible loss of vision secondary to damage from radiation occurs when the retina or optic nerve is involved. Radiation retinopathy may present as a vascular disease of the retina that can mimic diabetic retinopathy. It is characterized by cotton-wool spots, retinal hemorrhages, microaneurysms, telangiectasias, retinal ischemia, and macular edema.[16,17] Optic neuropathy is characterized by optic disc edema and later by optic atrophy, which is clinically seen as a pale optic nerve.

OCULAR MANIFESTATIONS OF BONE MARROW TRANSPLANTATION

Graft-Versus-Host Disease (GVHD)

Graft-versus-host disease is a major cause of morbidity following allogenic bone marrow transplantation, which is most commonly used to treat hematopoietic malignancies. Graft versus host disease can either be acute or chronic (occurring more than 3 months after transplantation). Ocular manifestations of GVHD are common in both the acute and chronic form, occurring in 60% to 90% of all cases, although ocular complications are most common and most devastating with chronic GVHD.[18–20]

Keratoconjunctivitis sicca: The most frequent complication of GVHD is keratoconjunctivitis sicca, or dry eye, occurring in 40% to 76% of patients with GVHD. It may be the presenting symptom of GVHD.[18–20] Furthermore, most patients who develop dry eye with GVHD will continue to have dry eye even after remission of their GVHD.[18]

In general, dry eye symptoms result from either decreased tear production, excessive evaporation of tears, or poor quality of tears. All forms of dry eye also have an inflammatory component. The dry eye associated with GVHD is from decreased tear production as a result of lacrimal gland dysfunction.[18] Symptoms of dry eye include irritation, burning, dryness, grittiness, or foreign body sensation. Symptoms usually are worse toward the end of the day, in dry climates, or in the winter when humidity levels are lowered by indoor heating systems.

Signs include conjunctival injection, decreased tear meniscus, irregular corneal surface, and punctuate staining of the cornea and conjunctiva seen with the use of fluorescein stain (Figure 24.5). In severe forms of GVHD, profound corneal epitheliopathy can lead to recurrent or persistent corneal erosions/abrasions and corneal ulceration[18,20] with significant permanent vision loss.

Patients may also develop a filamentary keratopathy, in which filaments, composed of damaged and denuded epithelial cells with mucus, become attached to the cornea. This condition may be quite painful, because these filaments are firmly attached to the well-innervated cornea.

In addition to treatment of GVHD itself with immunomodulatory agents, treatment of dry eye includes a stepladder approach as outlined below:[21–23]

1. Artificial tears
2. Lubricating ointments
3. Moist environment (humidifier, moisture shields)
4. Punctal plugs, in which the puncta (entrance of the drainage system for tears) are occluded either reversibly with plugs or irreversibly by cautery or surgery
5. Autologous serum tears
6. Tarsorrhaphy in severe cases

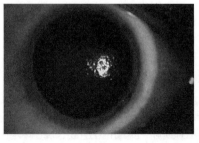 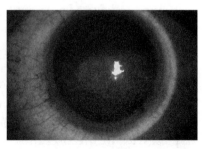

A   B

FIGURE 24.5 (A) Patient with dry eyes with irregular corneal epithelium. (B) Same eye with fluorescein dye instilled, showing diffuse, punctuate, green staining of the corneal epithelium.

7. Avoidance, if possible, of systemic medications that exacerbate dry eyes (e.g., diuretics, antihistamines, anticholinergic agents, and psychotropic drugs)

8. For filamentary keratopathy, treatment includes controlling dry eye with the preceding methods, manual debridement of filaments from the cornea, and acetylcysteine as a mucolytic agent

Conjunctivitis: GVHD is also associated with a noninfectious, immune-mediated chronic conjunctivitis resulting from a T-lympho-cyte–mediated attack on the conjunctiva itself.[18] Up to 12% of GVHD patients develop this conjunctivitis.[24] Findings include conjunctival injection, chemosis, serosanguinous discharge with membrane formation, scarring, and damage to the corneal surface leading to vision loss.[18] Treatment for this complication includes systemic control of GVHD with immunomodulatory agents.

OCULAR PARANEOPLASTIC DISORDERS

Although rare, clinicians should be aware of two paraneoplastic disorders affecting the eye: cancer-associated retinopathy (CAR) and melanoma-associated retinopathy (MAR). Occasionally, these disorders can be the first presentation of previously undiagnosed cancer.

These paraneoplastic disorders are secondary to antibodies produced by the patient's immune system against tumor antigens.[2] However, there is a cross-reactivity of these tumor antigens with innate proteins of the patient. In the case of ocular paraneoplastic disorders, the tumor expresses antigens that cross-react with retinal rod and cone proteins.[2]

Cancer-associated retinopathy is most commonly seen with small cell carcinoma of the lung. Other malignancies associated with CAR include gynecologic, breast, and endocrine malignancies.[2] Cancer-associated retinopathy is associated with antirecoverin antibodies. Recoverin is a 23-kDa protein of photoreceptors (rod and cones) that is involved in the visual transduction pathway of the retina, and its gene is located on chromosome 17.[2] It is hypothesized that various cancers atypically express recoverin or a protein very similar to recoverin, thereby inducing the production of antibodies that cross-react with this photoreceptor protein, causing visual compromise.

Symptoms of CAR include progressive, bilateral peripheral or central visual loss over months, nyctalopia (night-blindness), or photopsias (shimmering lights). Examination can be normal in the early stages but shows retinal arterial narrowing and retinal pigment alterations late in the disease course.[2] Treatment is difficult but includes immunomodulatory agents and periocular steroid injections.[2]

Melanoma-associated retinopathy is similar to CAR in that there is cross-reactivity of a tumor-expressed antigen with a photoreceptor protein.[2] Most patients with MAR have a previously diagnosed melanoma. Symptoms, clinical appearance, and treatment are similar to CAR.

MISCELLANEOUS OCULAR MANIFESTATIONS OF SYSTEMIC MALIGNANCY

Gardner Syndrome

Familial adenomatous polyposis is an autosomal dominant condition characterized by numerous polyps of the intestine with potential malignant transformation. Gardner syndrome is characterized by familial adenomatous polyposis, soft tissue tumors, and skeletal hamartomas.[2,25,26] Ocular manifestations of Gardner syndrome include heavily pigmented, multifocal, round/ovoid, small, and often bilateral retinal lesions.[2,25,26] They histologically represent congenital hypertrophy of the retinal pigment epithelium. Patients are asymptomatic with normal vision, because these lesions are usually in the periphery and do not affect central vision. Presence of multiple such lesions triggers a referral for gastrointestinal evaluation and colonoscopy.[2,25,26]

von Hippel-Lindau Disease

von Hippel-Lindau disease is an autosomal-dominant inherited condition characterized by vascular cerebellar hemangioblastomas and retinal capillary hemangiomas. This disease is associated with renal cell carcinoma, pheochromocytoma, and cysts of the kidney, pancreas, liver, and genitourinary tract. A retinal hemangioma appears as a round orange/reddish retinal vascular tumor that is fed by a dilated artery and drained by a large vein. Leakage from this vascular tumor can cause retinal exudation or serous detachment of the retina, leading to decreased vision.

SUMMARY

Ocular manifestations of non-ocular, systemic cancer are either (1) directly related to the cancer itself (e.g., metastasis or infiltration),

(2) indirectly related to systemic effects of the cancer (e.g., anemia, thrombocytopenia), or (3) secondary to treatment of the cancer.

Metastatic disease is the most common tumor of the eye in adults, with the most common primary cancers being breast and lung. Leukemia and lymphomas can also cause various ocular manifestations, primarily affecting the retina, vitreous, and choroid. Opportunistic infections, particularly endogenous fungal infections, can cause significant morbidity in immunocompromised cancer patients.

Various chemotherapeutic agents have different ocular manifestations, and systemic corticosteroids can cause glaucoma or cataract. Radiation therapy can cause significant visual compromise by causing a cataract, a retinal vascular disease similar to diabetic retinopathy, or an optic neuropathy. Bone marrow transplantation is associated with GVHD, which can have adverse effects on the ocular surface, primarily dry eye syndrome.

REFERENCES

1. Shields CL, Shields JA, Gross NE, Schwartz GP, Lally SE. Survey of 520 eyes with uveal metastases. *Ophthalmology*. 1997;104:1265–1276.
2. Solomon SD, Smith JH, O'Brien J. Ocular manifestations of systemic malignancies. *Curr Opin Ophthalmol*. 1999;10:447–451.
3. Schachat AP, Markowitz JA, Guyer DR, Burke PJ, Karp JE, Graham ML. Ophthalmic manifestations of leukemia. *Arch Ophthalmol*. 1989;107(5): 697–700.
4. Reddy SC, Jackson N, Menon BS. Ocular involvement in leukemia—a study of 288 cases. *Ophthalmologica*. 2003;217:441–445.
5. Ohkoshi K, Tsiaras WG. Prognostic importance of ophthalmic manifestations in childhood leukaemia. *Br J Ophthalmol*. 1992;76(11):651–655.
6. Leonardy NJ, Rupani M, Dent G, Klintworth GK. Analysis of 135 autopsy eyes for ocular involvement in leukemia. *Am J Ophthalmol*. 1990;109(4): 436–444.
7. Sharma T, Grewal J, Gupta S, Murray P. Ophthalmic manifestations of acute leukemias: the ophthalmologist's role. *Eye*. 2004;18:663–672.
8. Gill MK, Jampol LM. Variations in presentation of primary intraocular lymphoma: case reports and a review. *Surv Ophthalmol*. 2001;45:463–471.
9. Regillo C, Chang TS, Johnson MW, et al. Retina and vitreous. In: Liesegang TJ, Skuta GL, Cantor LB, eds. *Basic and Clinical Science Course,*

American Academy of Ophthalmology. American Academy of Ophthalmology; 2005:sect 12.

10. Valluri S, Moorthy RS, Khan A, Rao NA. Combination treatment of intraocular lymphoma. *Retina.* 1995;15:125–129.

11. Binder MI, Chua J, Kaiser PK, Procop GW, Isada CM. Endogenous endophthalmitis: an 18-year review of culture-positive cases at a tertiary care center. *Medicine (Baltimore).* 2003;82:97–105.

12. Okada AA, Johnson RP, Liles WC, D'Amico DJ, Baker AS. Endogenous bacterial endophthalmitis: report of a ten-year retrospective study. *Ophthalmology.* 1994;101:832–838.

13. Schmid KE, Kornek GV, Scheithauer W, Binder S. Update on ocular complications of systemic cancer chemotherapy. *Surv Ophthalmol.* 2006; 51(1):19–40.

14. Barabino S, Raghavan A, Loeffler J, Dana R. Radiotherapy-induced ocular surface disease. *Cornea.* 2005;24(8):909–914.

15. Bardenstein D, Char DH. Ocular toxicity. In: Madhu J, Flam MS, eds. *Chemoradiation: An Integrated Approach to Cancer Treatment.* Philadelphia: Lea & Febiger; 1993:591–598.

16. Brown GC, Shields JA, Sanborn G, et al. Radiation retinopathy. *Ophthalmology.* 1982;89:1494–1501.

17. Mukai D, Guyer DR, Gragoudas ES. Radiation retinopathy. In: Albert DM, Jakobiec FA, eds. *Principles and Practice of Ophthalmology.* 2nd ed. Philadelphia: Saunders; 2000:2232–2235.

18. Anderson NG, Regillo C. Ocular manifestations of graft versus host disease. *Curr Opin Ophthalmol.* 2004;15:503–507.

19. Bray LC, Carey PJ, Proctor SJ, Evans RG, Hamilton PJ. Ocular complications of bone marrow transplantation. *Br J Ophthalmol.* 1991;75:611–614.

20. Franklin RM, Kenyon KR, Tutschka PJ, Saral R, Green WR, Santos GW. Ocular manifestations of graft-vs-host disease. *Ophthalmology.* 1983; 90:4–13.

21. Stutphin JE, Chodosh J, Dana MR, et al. Cornea and external disease. In: Liesegang TJ, Skuta GL, Cantor LB, eds. *Basic and Clinical Science Course, American Academy of Ophthalmology.* American Academy of Ophthalmology; 2005:sect 8.

22. Pflugfelder SC, Solomon A, Stern ME. The diagnosis and management of dry eye: a twenty-five-year review. *Cornea.* 2000;19(5):644–649.

23. Preferred Practice Pattern Committee, Cornea Panel. Dry Eye Syndrome. San Francisco: American Academy of Ophthalmology; 1998.

24. Jabs DA, Wingard J, Green WR, Farmer ER, Vogelsang G, Saral R. The eye in bone marrow transplantation. III. Conjunctival graft-vs-host disease. *Arch Ophthalmol.* 1989;107(9):1343–1348.

25. Amin AR, Jakobiec FA, Dreyer EB. Ocular syndromes associated with systemic malignancy. *Int Ophthalmol Clin.* 1997;37:281–302.
26. Iwama T, Mishima Y, Okamoto N, et al. Association of congenital hypertrophy of the retinal pigment epithelium with familial adenomatous polyposis. *Br J Surg.* 1990;77:273–276.

Otologic Consequences of Cancer Therapy

Elias Michaelides, MD

ABSTRACT

As a component of the skull base, the temporal bone is integral to both its structure and function. Multiple cranial nerves and large vessels pass through the temporal bone from the intracranial cavity into the neck. In addition, the temporal bone houses the organs of hearing and balance. Treatment of cancer can lead to dysfunction and/or disease of any of these systems.

Problems associated with cancer therapy can be broadly categorized into sensory disorders and structural disease. Tinnitus, hearing loss, imbalance, and vertigo are sensory disorders caused by malfunction of the inner ear organs, the cochlea, and the vestibule. Eustachian tube dysfunction and osteoradionecrosis are processes related to structural changes that can occur with treatment.

QUALITY-OF-LIFE CONSIDERATIONS

Both the hearing and the balance consequences of cancer therapy must be considered when selecting therapies. Patients should be informed of the potential risks to the inner ear and the impact on their quality of life.

Hearing Loss

Helen Keller said that blindness cuts you off from things, but deafness cuts you off from people. Of the senses, hearing is most important for communication. Although most clinicians understand the basic pathophysiology of chemotherapeutic agent and radiation damage to the inner ear and subsequent hearing loss, many of them may not have full understanding of what the quality-of-life consequences of a significant hearing loss can be to their patients. For example, patients may have more difficulty communicating with their clinicians and families members, which makes clinical interactions and decisions more difficult. In addition, patients with significant hearing loss may become socially isolated if they are unable to hear conversations easily. Patients suffering from hearing loss will avoid situations in which many people are speaking or in which there is significant background noise. Hearing clearly in social situations, such as at a restaurant or in church, may become impossible, and patients eventually give up participating in these events to avoid the frustration. Also, having a significant loss in hearing can decrease situational safety. Being unable to hear smoke alarms in the home or traffic sounds while driving or crossing the street are some basic examples.

Tinnitus

Tinnitus (ringing or roaring sounds) often accompanies the hearing loss associated with cancer therapy. Tinnitus may be mild and infrequently noticed. However, it can become a pervasive distraction leading to sleep disturbances and severe depression.

Balance Problems

Damage to the vestibular system can also significantly impact patients' quality of life. When cancer treatments cause vestibular weakness, patients may end up with chronic nausea and imbalance, which can exacerbate the nausea induced by radiation or chemotherapeutic agents. With significant imbalance, patients may restrict their activities because they feel unsafe walking outdoors on uneven ground or without support. Also, driving can become more difficult due to altered sense of acceleration. Patients with imbalance and vertigo are also at higher risk for injury from falls.

CONSEQUENCES OF RADIATION THERAPY

Radiation therapy may have otologic consequences when the irradiated field includes the temporal bone, brain, or nasopharynx. Sensory complications such as hearing loss and vestibular loss are typical inner ear manifestations. Physical complications can also occur and are manifested in disease of the temporal bone, eustachian tube dysfunction, and secondary oncogenesis.

Hearing Loss

Hearing loss may occur if the irradiated field includes the cochlea or cochlear nerve. It typically manifests as a slowly progressive sensorineural hearing loss. This hearing loss is irreversible and will usually cause losses in both pure tones and speech recognition. There are several mechanisms through which the hearing can be damaged. Vascular damage to the microvasculature in the cochlea may cause intracochlear cell death. Direct radiation effects to the hair cells within the cochlea may also occur. Radiation neuropathy of the cochlear nerve may also contribute to slowly progressive hearing loss. Conductive hearing loss, which is often reversible, may also occur, secondary to middle ear mucositis, ossicular sclerosis, and serous otitis media with effusion.

Vestibular Disease

Similar to the mechanisms of hearing loss, the hair cells of the vestibular system can be damaged by radiation, leading to overall hypofunction of the vestibular system. This may manifest in chronic imbalance, oscillopsia, and increased risk of falling. When the semicircular canals are within the irradiated field, approximately 20% of patients will develop temporary true vertigo, whereas 45% of patients have demonstrated reduced vestibular function.[1] Patients may demonstrate long-term imbalance when permanent damage has occurred to the vestibular hair cells.

Temporal Bone Disease

Radiation to the parotid gland, brain, and nasopharynx can lead to changes in the surrounding bony structures. The primary effect on the temporal bone from radiation therapy is damage to the microvasculature. This damage can lead to osteoradionecrosis, ear canal stenosis, and tympanic membrane perforation. Radionecrosis is caused by an avascular necrosis and sequestration of bone, especially in the ear canal. Onset may occur many years after treatment and make the patient vulnerable to infections. This condition may lead to chronic drainage and pain, and is difficult to treat. For small areas, local debridement may be adequate, but surgical treatment may be necessary for larger areas of necrosis or if local or intracranial complications occur.

Eustachian Tube Dysfunction

When the nasopharynx or the temporal bone is within an irradiated field, the eustachian tube may often be affected. In normal patients, the eustachian tube allows for equalization of middle ear pressure and drainage of mucosal secretions. During radiation therapy, an initial phase of edema can cause blockage of the eustachian tube. This blockage usually will lead to a secretory middle ear effusion. In contrast to otitis media from infectious disease, tympanostomy tubes are not always the most appropriate treatment, because mucosal inflammation can lead to chronic drainage and infection. Subsequently, scar tissue can form in the nasophyarnx, causing a permanent obstruction. In patients who develop middle ear effusions and conductive hearing loss from eustachian tube dysfunction in radiation therapy, amplification with hearing aids is often a better solution.

CONSEQUENCES OF CHEMOTHERAPY

Ototoxicity secondary to chemotherapeutic agents is a common occurrence. The primary classes of medications that may cause ototoxicity are platinum compounds and vinca alkaloids. In addition, practitioners need to be aware that concurrent treatment of infectious processes with aminoglycoside antibiotics during treatment courses can also lead to significant ototoxicity.

Platinum Compounds

Of ototoxic chemotherapeutic agents, cisplatin is the most commonly used and also the most ototoxic. Other platinum compounds have slightly different toxicity profiles, but discussion of cisplatin will encompass the general topic.[2] Up to 60% of patients treated with cisplatin may develop some level of hearing loss. Fortunately, cisplatin has little vestibular toxicity.

The hearing loss noted in platinum compound ototoxicy is generally characterized as bilateral, symmetric, and high frequency. Progression of the hearing loss to lower frequencies occurs with cumulative dose. Hearing loss is permanent but usually stabilizes following cessation of therapy. Cisplatin ototoxicity is typically found to be based on cumulative dose and not on peak concentrations. Cumulative dosage above 400 mg will frequently lead to noticeable hearing loss.[3]

Although the pathophysiology of ototoxicity is multifactorial, it is thought that damage to the outer hair cells of the cochlea is the primary disturbance, with spiral ganglion and stria vascularis damage contributing less. Outer hair cell damage interferes with frequency tuning, which in turn leads to poor auditory discrimination, especially in noise. It is also proposed that neurotoxicity of the cochlear nerve may contribute to the hearing loss.[4]

Although hearing loss is the most easily recognized otologic consequence of cisplatin treatment, the majority of patients who undergo platinum compound therapy develop some level of tinnitus. Tinnitus can be extremely disabling and distracting, which can lead to depression and sleep disturbances. The pitch of the tinnitus is often associated with the level of hearing loss.

Vinca Alkaloids

All vinca alkaloids (vincristine, vinblastine, and vinorelbine) have been associated with ototoxicity and hearing loss, especially when they are given at higher doses. However, it is difficult to fully assess their ototoxicity, because these medications are often given in combination with platinum therapy. Neurotoxicity of the spiral ganglion or auditory nerve as well as direct cochlear damage may contribute to the hearing loss seen with vinca alkaloids.

MANAGEMENT

Being aware of the different otologic consequences of cancer therapy can be beneficial both in selecting appropriate treatment protocols and in detecting problems early to ensure rapid treatment. It is important to note that if there are similar treatment protocols that have different side effect profiles, these risks should be explained to patients. For example, a professional musician or singer may opt for a treatment protocol that decreases the exposure to ototoxic medications.

If appropriate alternatives are not available, treatments that may cause otologic consequences should be monitored carefully. An institutional ototoxicity monitoring protocol is important to identify hearing loss early so that patients may be treated before their quality of life is significantly impacted. Monitoring protocols should include an audiogram before treatment and then routine follow-ups. The testing performed should include a high frequency pure tone audiogram, along with otoacoustic emission testing. After identification, early use of hearing aids or FM listening devices for amplification is important to restore normal functional levels and communication. Also of note, the patient should be counseled to be vigilant about hearing protection during subsequent noise exposure, because they may no longer have any painful reflexes to loud noise. The cochlea, however, is still at risk for noise-induced trauma. It is also thought that ototoxic agents may predispose patients to noise trauma.

Identification of balance disorders is more difficult. Patients' complaints of dizziness may be mistakenly attributed to other causes. Complaints of spinning vertigo and imbalance should be addressed through vestibular testing, including electronystamography testing. Management of balance disorders includes pharmacologic vestibular suppression, vestibular exercises, and the use of stabilization devices. Vestibular rehabilitation with vestibular-ocular and vestibular-spinal exercises to readapt the cerebellum to new vestibular inputs can be very beneficial. For patients whose normal function of stabilization is not restored by these exercises, devices such as canes and walkers may be necessary to prevent falls. If a patient develops significant vertigo during treatment, vestibular suppressants such as meclizine and diazepam may be considered.

∾ Case Example 25.1

Jacquelyn, a 15-year-old, was treated with four rounds of cisplatin-based chemotherapy for a germ cell tumor. She was entered into an ototoxicity monitoring program. Initial audiogram obtained at the beginning of therapy was normal. Repeat audiograms performed as her treatment progressed showed a progressive, high-frequency sensorineural hearing loss, which then stabilized at the end of treatment. She had noted difficulty with conversations and talking on the telephone. Hearing teachers at school was also difficult. Amplification was recommended, and Jacquelyn was fitted with bilateral hearing aids with good results.

∾ Case Example 25.2

Madhu is an 80-year-old with a history of a high-grade mucoepidermoid tumor of the parotid gland. It was initially treated with resection and 50 Gy external beam radiation therapy. Recurrence was treated with re-resection, intraoperative brachytherapy, and 45 Gy external beam radiation therapy. Madhu presented for hearing loss and otorrhea. Audiogram showed a moderately severe mixed hearing loss, consistent with both cochlear and middle ear hearing loss. Physical exam demonstrated purulent otorrhea coming from exposed bone in the external ear canal. A serous effusion was also noted behind an intact tympanic membrane. Treatment for osteonecrosis of the temporal bone was initiated with gentle local debridement and ototopical antibiotic drops. After several weeks, the otorrhea completely resolved, but the serous effusion persisted, indicating eustachian tube obstruction. Madhu was fitted with appropriate amplification and returned for routine cleaning of the external ear canal.

REFERENCES

1. Gabriele P, Orecchia R, Magnano M, et al. Vestibular apparatus disorders after external radiation therapy for head and neck cancers. *Radiother Oncol.* 1992;25:25–30.
2. Gratton MA, Smyth BJ. Ototoxicity of platinum compounds. In: Roland PS, Rutka JA, eds. *Ototoxicity.* Hamilton, Ontario: BC Decker Inc; 2004: 60–75.
3. Honore HB, Bentzen SM, Møller K, et al. Sensori-neural hearing loss after radiotherapy for nasopharyngeal carcinoma: individualized risk estimation. *Radiother Oncol.* 2002;65:9–16.
4. Walsh T, Clark A, Parhad L, et al. Neurotoxic effects of cisplatin therapy. *Arch Neurol.* 1982;39:719–720.

FURTHER READING

Leonetti JP, Orgirano T, Anderson D, et al. Intracranial complications of temporal bone osteoradionecrosis. *Am J Otol.* 1997;18:223–229.

Ondrey FG, Greig JR, Herscher L. Radiation dose to otologic structures during head and neck cancer radiation therapy. *Laryngoscope.* 2000;110: 217–221.

Scott AR, Prepageran N, Rutka JA. Iron-chelating and other chemotherapeutic agents: the vinca alkaloids. In: Roland PS, Rutka JA, eds. *Ototoxicity.* Hamilton, Ontario: BC Decker Inc; 2004:76–81.

26

Endocrine Consequences of Cancer Treatment

Elizabeth H. Holt, MD, PhD

ABSTRACT

The endocrine system consists of a diverse group of glandular tissues with target tissues located throughout the body. The endocrine glands produce hormones broadly responsible for metabolism, growth, reproduction, and maintenance of homeostasis. The adverse effects of cancer therapy on the endocrine system usually lead to a loss of hormonal function. The loss of function may be due to damage to a gland by the tumor if the tumor infiltrates or metastasizes to the gland. Surgery to remove a tumor may lead to damage to an adjacent or involved endocrine gland. Radiation treatment may lead to loss of hormonal production if a gland is in the radiation field. Steroids and some types of chemotherapy may also adversely affect endocrine function. The skeleton is subject to metabolic control by the endocrine system, and as a result cancer treatments can affect skeletal health through a variety of mechanisms.

ADRENAL GLANDS

The adrenal glands consist of an inner medulla and an outer cortex. The cortex produces steroid hormones, including glucocorticoids (e.g., cortisol), mineralocorticoids (e.g., aldosterone), and androgens. Production of glucocorticoids by the adrenal cortex is under control of the hypothalamus and pituitary gland in a classical endocrine feedback loop. The hypothalamus releases corticotrophin-releasing hormone, which in turn activates release of adrenocorticotropic hormone (ACTH) from the pituitary gland, and this in turn stimulates release of cortisol from the adrenal glands.

The most common adverse effect of cancer treatment on the adrenal glands is suppression of glucocorticoid production by treatment with exogenous glucocorticoids (e.g., prednisone, dexamethasone) over a prolonged period. Treatment times longer than 2 weeks are likely to cause suppression of adrenal function. This suppression occurs via negative feedback of the synthetic glucocorticoid onto control of the adrenal gland by the hypothalamus and pituitary gland. Over time, the adrenal gland may atrophy due to lack of stimulation by ACTH. Oral and intravenous steroids are not the only cause of adrenal suppression. Steroids delivered in inhaled form, oral rinses, and skin creams may enter the circulation and have all been associated with adrenal suppression. Topical application of steroids to large areas of inflamed tissue is of special concern because of the increased blood supply and lack of protective barrier, both of which increase systemic absorption of the steroids.[1,2]

Testing for adrenal insufficiency may be performed in medically stable outpatients with a fasting serum cortisol drawn between 7:30 and 8:00 AM. A level at or above 20 mcg/dL is considered normal, while a level of 3 mcg/dL or below is a likely indicator of adrenal insufficiency. Cosyntropin (synthetic ACTH) stimulation testing may be needed when morning levels cannot be performed or do not yield definitive results.[1] Many exogenous glucocorticoids will interfere with the cortisol assay, so it is recommended that these stimulated measurements be done while the patient is taking either dexamethasone or a low dose of hydrocortisone. Hydrocortisone should be held on the morning of testing until after the blood has been drawn.

Prolonged treatment with glucocorticoids should be followed by a gradual taper in dosage to allow the patient's own control of adrenal function to "wake up." These tapers may take weeks or even months to complete, depending on the length of time and dosage of glucocorticoid treatment the patient received. During the taper, patients should be advised to watch for symptoms of fatigue and nausea, which may indicate the taper needs to be done more gradually.[2]

The possibility of continued adrenal insufficiency should be borne in mind for patients who are no longer taking glucocorticoids. In acute illness, the response of healthy adrenal glands is to produce very high levels of glucocorticoids, which are needed to fight disease and facilitate healing. Patients who have recovered adrenal function sufficient for day-to-day life may still be unable to mount an adequate response when faced with an acute illness that may strain the body's ability to produce high levels of glucocorticoids. Symptoms that should raise concern for adrenal insufficiency include hypotension, fever, abdominal discomfort, and vomiting. When these symptoms develop, it may be necessary to test for adrenal insufficiency and then treat empirically with "stress-dose" steroids while serum cortisol levels are pending.[1-3] (See Table 26.1.)

TABLE 26.1 Adrenal Dysfunction

- Both primary and secondary adrenal insufficiency following cancer therapy are rare, but if present may become an endocrine emergency.
- Secondary adrenal insufficiency may follow very high doses of total brain radiation (> 4000 cGy), but mainly only when the radiation is directed at the hypothalamus or pituitary for treatment of residual pituitary macroadenomas following surgery.
- Up to 10 years may elapse before the development of adrenal insufficiency.
- Most chemotherapy itself does not cause primary adrenal insufficiency, with the exception of mitotane, which is used for the treatment of adrenal carcinoma.
- Glucocorticoids, when used as chemotherapeutic agents, frequently cause a "secondary" adrenal insufficiency and induce adrenal gland atrophy.
- Patients treated with glucocorticoids as cancer therapy can remain adrenally insufficient up to a year after cessation of the steroids.
- Even patients who do not require daily replacement of glucocorticoids may require stress-doses with major illnesses or surgeries.

GONADAL FUNCTION

Loss of gonadal (testicular and ovarian) function is usually an unintentional effect of cancer treatment and is caused by surgery, chemotherapy, or radiation. Hypogonadism can result from insults to the gonads, or indirectly if there is injury to the pituitary gland or hypothalamus. For tumors whose growth depends on gonadal hormones (e.g., prostate, breast), a hypogonadal state may be the intent of therapy. Effects of treatment on gonadal function may be transient or permanent.

Surgery or radiation treatment to the brain may result in injury to the pituitary gland, compromising production of the gonadotropin hormones, the hormones needed to control fertility and sex hormone (estrogen and testosterone) production. These effects may not be seen immediately after radiation is completed; it may take several years before they become evident.[3,4]

Chemotherapy and radiation may cause direct damage to testicles or ovaries, impairing both fertility and production of sex steroids. Cyclophosphamide and other alkylating agents are well-described causes of testicular and ovarian failure,[5,6] but many other agents have also been implicated. Men who are of reproductive age at the time of treatment can save healthy sperm by cryopreservation before they begin chemotherapy. Cryopreservation of unfertilized eggs is a method for preserving fertility of female patients but is not widely available. Cryopreservation of fertilized eggs (embryos) has also been offered to female patients who are expected to lose fertility. Unfortunately, this is a time-consuming process requiring hormone treatments, and it is not always practical given the urgency of treating the malignancy. A comprehensive review of the literature on fertility preservation in pediatric and adolescent cancer patients was recently published.[7]

Sex hormones can be restored with synthetic testosterone preparations in teenage boys and men, and with birth control pills or other forms of hormone therapy in teenage girls and women. If hypothalamic or pituitary damage is the cause of gonadal failure, women who desire fertility can be treated with injections of gonadotropin hormones to restore fertility.[8] There is little published literature regarding the use of these treatments in male cancer survivors, although they are widely used in men with central hypogonadism due to other conditions. Hormone treatments may not be appropriate for all patients because some cancers grow more rapidly in the presence of sex steroids. (See Table 26.2.)

PITUITARY GLAND

The pituitary gland controls a variety of hormonal and metabolic functions, either through direct effects of its hormones or indirectly by modulating the activity of target glands. Pituitary function may be lost due to destruction of the pituitary gland by a tumor, by surgery, or by

TABLE 26.2 Gonadal Dysfunction

- Radiation can cause central hypogonadism by loss of gonadotropin-releasing hormone (GnRH), luteinizing hormone (LH), or follicle-stimulating hormone (FSH).
- Laboratory testing shows low or inappropriately-normal levels of LH and FSH with low estradiol or testosterone.
- Chemotherapy most often causes primary hypogonadism, which would appear as high LH and FSH with low estradiol or testosterone.
- Clinically, female patients present with primary or secondary amenorrhea, both males and females have infertility, or males may present with symptoms of low testosterone.
- Primary ovarian failure (POF) causes both a low estrogen/ postmenopausal state and infertility.
- High doses of pelvic radiation and the alkylating agents (ie, cyclophosphamide, ifosfamide, and procarbazine) given in chemotherapy are particularly prone to cause POF.
- The ovaries are more tolerant to high dose chemotherapy than germ cells in males, where sperm production (in the seminiferous tubules) is more sensitive to radiation and alkylating chemotherapeutic agents.
- Leydig cells can tolerate higher doses of chemotherapy, so these men may have normal testosterone production but be infertile with azoospermia.
- Although chemotherapy effects on azoospermia occasionally reverse over time, this is not the case with radiation-induced azoospermia.

radiation therapy. Craniopharyngioma is an example of a childhood central nervous system malignancy that is associated with hypopituitarism due to mass effect on the pituitary or as a complication of surgery and radiation. Surgery may immediately impair pituitary function, while the loss of pituitary function due to radiation therapy may take several years to manifest.[9] Primary cancers of the pituitary gland are rare, but metastases to the pituitary gland may cause hypopituitarism. Breast and lung cancer are the most common cancers to metastasize to the pituitary.[10] Effects of cancer therapies on the adrenal glands and the gonads have been described in the preceding sections. In addition to these effects, loss of thyroid hormone, growth hormone (GH), and vasopressin (VP) are seen.

Pituitary Control of Thyroid

Control of the thyroid gland starts with the hypothalamus, where thyrotropin-releasing hormone (TRH) is produced. This hormone then stimulates the pituitary to produce thyroid-stimulating hormone (TSH), which acts on the thyroid gland to cause thyroid hormone release. Loss of thyroid function will result from absence of production of TRH by the hypothalamus and/or lack of TSH release by the pituitary, which in turn impairs release of thyroid hormone from the thyroid gland. Affected individuals will experience the familiar symptoms of hypothyroidism, including fatigue, cold intolerance, constipation, and so on. It is important to note that patients with pituitary hypofunction will not experience a rise in TSH when they are hypothyroid, because the pituitary is not working normally. Serum TSH measurement may be normal or even slightly low and will be misleading if simultaneous thyroid hormone levels are not obtained. The typical pattern of laboratory studies in patients with central hypothyroidism is a normal or low TSH and low thyroid hormone indices.[10] In patients taking thyroid hormone supplementation, the TSH will not be a reliable indicator of whether the dose is appropriate, so thyroid hormone levels should be followed.

Pituitary Control of Growth Hormone

Growth hormone is produced by the pituitary gland in response to growth hormone releasing hormone from the hypothalamus. Growth hormone directs linear growth in children. In adults it continues to be important as a regulator of metabolism and in maintenance of bone and lean body mass. Growth hormone deficiency may result if there is damage to the pituitary or hypothalamus. Children may be identified as GH deficient if they fail to grow along the predicted trajectory for their age.[11] Adults will have nonspecific symptoms such as fatigue or mild weight gain. Often, GH deficiency is suspected in oncology patients because of the location of a tumor or because of known deficiencies of other pituitary hormones. Screening for GH deficiency may be done with a serum IGF-I level. Confirmatory testing is usually done by an endocrinologist and typically consists of interventions (e.g., exercise, amino acid infusion) expected to raise GH above a certain level. Recombinant GH injections are given to deficient patients.[11] GH supplementation is prescribed with caution in patients with a history of malignancy because of the theoretical concern that GH could cause residual tumor to recur more quickly.[12]

Pituitary Control of Vasopressin

Vasopressin, or anti-diuretic hormone, is synthesized in the hypothalamus and released by the posterior pituitary. Vasopressin acts on the kidney to increase water resorption by the kidney. Stimuli for VP release include hypovolemia and hyperosmolarity. Normal release of vasopressin may be interrupted by damage to the hypothalamus or pituitary by a tumor or surgery, causing diabetes insipidus (DI). Symptoms of DI include polyuria and polydipsia. Patients with DI who are unable to compensate for the large water losses will become dehydrated and hypernatremic. Physical examination will reveal signs of dehydration. Laboratory results may reveal hypernatremia and an inappropriately dilute urine specimen. Treatment of inpatients with synthetic VP injection, or of outpatients with desmopressin acetate tablets or nasal spray, will readily reverse this condition.[13] It should be noted that patients who have untreated DI and compensate with increased fluid intake at home can become rapidly dehydrated in the hospital if they do not receive adequate fluid. Thus vigilance is necessary for any patients who may be at risk for this condition. (See Table 26.3.)

TABLE 26.3   ᑐ   Pituitary Dysfunction

Acute

- Central diabetes insipidus (DI) and syndrome of inappropriate excretion of antidiuretic hormone (SIADH) can both be acute disorders after brain tumor surgery affecting the pituitary stalk.
- The patient may experience the "triple phase" response by first developing DI in the days that follow surgery, followed a week or two later by SIADH, and finally may normalize or develop chronic central DI.

Chronic

- Radiation therapy to the brain can cause permanent pituitary failure.
- Radiation directed in the area of the pituitary gland is particularly causative.
  - *Reports have noted that patients who received external beam radiation of a pituitary adenoma have up to a 50% chance of developing new ACTH, TSH, or gonadotropin deficiency during the subsequent years.*
  - *The newer gamma or proton beam source of radiation or linear accelerator (so called "stereotactic") for treatment of pituitary adenomas also cause high rates of hypopituitarism in following 10 years.*

THYROID GLAND

The thyroid gland produces thyroid hormone, which regulates growth in children and is important for metabolism by nearly all tissues in the body. Loss of thyroid function due to damage to the hypothalamus or pituitary gland is considered earlier in the chapter. The thyroid may also be affected by radiation treatments to the neck or mantle areas. Radiation treatments may lead to permanent hypothyroidism, sometimes developing several years after treatment.[10] This side effect can easily be corrected with thyroid hormone supplements.

A more concerning consequence of thyroid irradiation is an increased risk for thyroid neoplasia, both benign and malignant.[14] Patients who have had radiation to the neck area should undergo periodic ultrasound of the thyroid to look for nodules. If appropriate, a fine needle aspiration biopsy can be performed under ultrasound guidance to rule out malignancy. Fortunately, thyroid malignancies that arise in

TABLE 26.4 Thyroid Dysfunction

- Both central or secondary thyroid dysfunction and primary thyroid abnormalities can occur with cancer therapy.
- Thyrotropin-releasing hormone from the hypothalamus stimulates thyroid-stimulating hormone from the anterior pituitary, which directly stimulates the thyroid to increase thyroid hormone production and release.
- Hyperthyroidism following cancer therapy is rare, but can be seen acutely with high doses of radiation.
- Hypothyroidism is the most common clinical abnormality of the thyroid.

the setting of prior radiation therapy are not more aggressive than sporadic thyroid cancers. However, like all cancers, early detection leads to the best chance for cure. (See Table 26.4.)

OSTEOPOROSIS

Low bone mass and osteoporosis develop for a variety of reasons after cancer treatment. Chemotherapy may have direct toxic effects on the living cells in bone and can impair bone mineralization. Cancer treatments can also adversely affect growth hormone and gonadal hormone production, thus indirectly interfering with bone health. Chemotherapy is often accompanied by glucocorticoid treatment. Glucocorticoids cause bone loss by inhibiting function of the bone-forming osteoblasts. They also inhibit absorption of calcium from the gut, thus depriving bone of this important nutrient.[15]

Considerable data are available on the effects of chronic glucocorticoid treatment on bone health. For example, at daily doses as low as 7.5 mg over several weeks, prednisone treatment can result in bone loss and increased fracture risk.[16] In children, long-term use of glucocorticoids can also impair linear growth of the skeleton.[17] Many chemotherapy regimens include pulses of high-dose glucocorticoids such as dexamethasone or methylprednisolone. There are few clinical trial data regarding the effects of these brief, but high doses of glucocorticoids on bone.

In children, chronic illness and the effects of chemotherapy and high-dose glucocorticoids may directly impair growth of the skeleton, and peak adult bone mass may not be attained as a result. This under-development is a setback in later adult life when the effects of declining sex hormones in both men and women result in bone loss. Individuals who have never reached peak bone mass will begin their age-related bone loss from a lower point, meaning they may develop osteoporosis at an earlier age than expected.

As described earlier, many treatments for cancer may result in hy-pogonadism. Loss of gonadal hormones results in bone loss. Supple-mentation with estrogen in teenage girls and women of premenopausal age should be considered if there are no contraindications. In teenage boys and men, testosterone supplements similarly may be appropriate.

Treatment for breast cancer may include use of aromatase inhibitors that block the production of estrogen from other steroid hormones. These agents are effective in reducing estrogen levels and thus prevent-ing recurrence of the cancer. Unfortunately, the lack of estrogen has ad-verse effects on bone health. Similar consequences occur in men whose treatments for prostate cancer include therapies aimed at reducing testosterone levels.

Patients considered at risk for low bone mass due to cancer treat-ments should be screened for osteoporosis with bone densitometry. Supplementation with calcium and vitamin D according to age-appropriate guidelines is recommended, because most individuals do not receive adequate amounts of these nutrients in their diets. Treatment with anti-resorptive therapy should be considered for those whose bone density or prior fracture history indicates that they are at risk for future fractures. Modifiable risk factors for bone loss, such as lack of exercise, smoking, and excessive alcohol intake should be discouraged.[15,16]

SUMMARY

The endocrine system is a complex system of glands and hormones that regulates many aspects of growth, metabolism, and reproduction. Cancers and their therapies impact the endocrine system on multiple levels. Clinicians should be aware of consequences for the endocrine function of cancer patients so they may counsel patients appropriately and make efforts to minimize treatment complications. Many of the adverse effects of cancer treatment on the endocrine system present years later, when the cancer may no longer be foremost in the mind of the patient or the healthcare team. It is important to remember these late-developing complications, because they may adversely impact the health and quality of life of a patient who has survived the cancer itself.

REFERENCES

1. Oelkers W. Adrenal insufficiency. *N Engl J Med.* 1996;335:1206–1212.
2. Hopkins RL, Leinung MC. Exogenous Cushing's syndrome and gluco-corticoid withdrawal. *Endocrinol Metab Clin North Am.* 2005;34:371–384.
3. Van Aken MO, Lamberts SWJ. Diagnosis and treatment of hypopitu-itarism: an update. *Pituitary.* 2005;8:183–191.
4. Littley MD, Shalet SM, Beardwell CG, et al. Hypopituitarism following external radiotherapy for pituitary tumours in adults. *Q J Med.* 1989;70: 145–160.
5. Watson AR, Rance CP, Bain J. Long term effects of cyclophosphamide on testicular function. *Br Med J.* 1985;291:1457–1460.
6. Koyama H, Wada T, Nishizawa Y, et al. Cyclophosphamide-induced ovarian failure and its therapeutic significance in patients with breast can-cer. *Cancer.* 1977;39:1403–1409.
7. Fallat ME, Hutter J. Preservation of fertility in pediatric and adolescent patients with cancer. *Pediatrics.* 2008;121:e1461–e1469.
8. Jones AL. Fertility and pregnancy after breast cancer. *Breast.* 2006;15: S41–S46.
9. Bhandare N, Kennedy L, Malyapa RS, et al. Primary and central hy-pothyroidism after radiotherapy for head-and-neck tumors. *Int J Radiat Oncol Biol Phys.* 2007;68:1131–1139.
10. Sioutos P, Yen V, Arbit E. Pituitary gland metastases. *Ann Surg Oncol.* 1996;3:93–99.
11. Bakker B, Oostdijk W, Geskus RB, et al. Growth hormone (GH) secretion and response to GH therapy after total body irradiation and haematopoi-etic stem cell transplantation during childhood. *Clin Endocrinol.* 2007;67: 589–597.
12. Darendeliler F, Karagiannis G, Wilton P, et al. Recurrence of brain tu-mors in patients treated with growth hormone: analysis of KIGS (Pfizer International Growth Database). *Acta Pediatr.* 2006;95:1284–1290.
13. Matarazzo P, Genitori L, Lala R, et al. Endocrine function and water me-tabolism in children and adolescents with surgically treated intra/ parasellar tumors. *J Pediat Endocrinol Metab.* 2004;17:1487–1495.

14. Metayer C, Lynch CF, Clarke EA, et al. Second cancers among long-term survivors of Hodgkin's disease diagnosed in childhood and adolescence. *J Clin Oncol.* 2000;18:2435–2443.

15. Wasilewski-Masker K, Kaste SC, Hudson MM, et al. Bone mineral density deficits in survivors of childhood cancer: long-term follow-up guidelines and review of the literature. *Pediatrics.* 2008;121:e705–e713.

16. Devogelaer JP, Goemaere S, Boonen S, et al. Evidence-based guidelines for the prevention and treatment of glucocorticoid-induced osteoporosis: a consensus document of the Belgian Bone Club. *Osteoporos Int.* 2006;17: 8–19.

17. Pantelakis SN, Sinaniotis CA, Sbirakis S, et al. Night and day growth hormone levels during treatment with corticosteroids and corticotrophin. *Arch Dis Child.* 1972;47:605–608.

27

Rheumatic Problems in Cancer Survivors

Antoine G. Sreih, MD

&

Elias Obedid, MD, MPH

ABSTRACT

Rheumatic diseases may develop in cancer survivors. They can occur following chemotherapy or later in the remission phase. The most common rheumatologic manifestations are post-chemotherapy rheumatism, drug- or radiation-induced connective tissue and musculoskeletal diseases, and metabolic bone diseases. These conditions are generally self-limited and treatable.

INTRODUCTION

More patients with cancer are surviving their disease due to early diagnosis and advances in adjuvant therapy. Healthcare providers are faced with a growing population of cancer survivors with a new constellation of physical and mental illnesses resulting from the malignancy itself or its treatment. Various rheumatic conditions can occur in the remission period following cancer treatment and can be a major cause of morbidity. The most common disorders are post-chemotherapy rheumatism, drug- or radiation-induced musculoskeletal diseases, and metabolic bone abnormalities (Table 27.1). It is important to recognize these diseases to ensure appropriate therapy. In this chapter, we will discuss the different rheumatic manifestations in cancer survivors, their proposed pathogenesis, and appropriate therapy.

TABLE 27.1 ❧ Summary of Musculoskeletal Diseases Associated with Cancer Therapy

Post-chemotherapy rheumatism	5-fluorouracil Cyclophosphamide Methotrexate Tamoxifen
Gout	Cytotoxic drugs causing tumor lysis syndrome Cyclosporine
Raynaud's phenomenon	5-fluorouracil Bleomycin Cysplatin Vinblastine Vincristine
Hand and foot syndrome	5-fluorouracil Capecitabine
Systemic sclerosis	Bleomycin Radiation therapy Taxanes
Myalgias, arthralgias, and fibromyalgia-like symptoms	Paclitaxel Tamoxifen
Autoimmune diseases (Rheumatoid arthritis, Lupus, Vasculitis, Thyroid disease, etc . . .)	Interferon-α and -γ
Osteonecrosis	Bisphosphonates Bone marrow transplantation Glucocorticoids Radiation therapy
Osteopenia and Osteoporosis	5-fluorouracil Anti-androgens Aromatase inhibitors (Anastrazole and Letrozole) Cyclophosphamide Doxorubicin Methotrexate

> ### ᔍ Case Example 27.1
>
> Roberta, a 43-year-old female, underwent mastectomy for stage 1 breast cancer. She then received 6 cycles of cyclophosphamide-based combination chemotherapy. Eight weeks following the final dose, she developed joint swelling, pain, and morning stiffness. Rheumatologic evaluation showed mild edema in the periarticular soft tissues but no other positive findings. Rheumatoid factor, anti-nuclear antibody, erythrocyte sedimentation rate, C-reactive protein, creatinine kinase, aldolase, total complement levels, and radioactive joint scan were all negative. Naproxen (500 mg, taken twice daily) was ineffective in relieving her pain. The symptoms resolved 6 months later without any additional treatment.

POST-CHEMOTHERAPY RHEUMATISM

Post-chemotherapy rheumatism has been most frequently described in patients treated for breast cancer but has also been reported in other malignancies, including ovarian cancer and non-Hodgkin lymphoma.[1-3] This syndrome is usually a migratory, non-inflammatory, self-limited arthropathy. It typically develops a few weeks to several months after the completion of chemotherapy and often includes arthralgias, myalgias, morning stiffness, and periarticular swelling without true arthritis. All joints may be affected; however, the syndrome predominantly involves the knees, ankles, and the small joints of the hands.[1] The presentation can mimic other inflammatory arthritides and is often mistaken for rheumatoid arthritis (RA) based on its symptoms. But, unlike RA, most patients have little or no evidence of synovial thickening on examination and have no radiographic or serologic evidence to suggest RA.

The pathogenesis of this disorder remains unclear. Siegel[4] has suggested that this syndrome may be a symptom of chemotherapy-induced menopause; however, cases of pre-menopausal rheumatism and arthritis affecting male patients have been described in the literature.[3,5] Another proposed mechanism is the administration of corticosteroids either as an antiemetic or as part of the chemotherapy protocol, resulting in a corticosteroid withdrawal syndrome. Although this theory could explain the development of symptoms shortly after chemotherapy, it would be an unlikely cause of the later onset of symptoms; nor could it explain the cases in which steroids were not administered.[6] This disorder is usually self-limited, lasting less than a year, and is best treated conservatively. Nonsteroidal anti-inflammatory drugs are generally ineffective. Codeine-containing analgesics may relieve the pain. Rarely, a short course of steroids is required to control the symptoms. Evaluation should be performed to exclude recurrent carcinoma or other inflammatory conditions.

The medications that have been most linked to this phenomenon include cyclophosphamide, 5-fluorouracil, methotrexate, and tamoxifen.[3,7] Interestingly, many of these medications have also been used to treat rheumatic diseases. For instance, methotrexate is a well-established therapy for many inflammatory arthritides including RA and systemic lupus erythematosus. In addition, cyclophosphamide is frequently administered to patients with lupus nephritis, cerebritis, or systemic vasculitis. To this date, it remains unclear why these chemotherapeutic agents may treat or result in arthropathy, but it is a phenomenon not completely foreign to oncology whereby chemotherapy can either treat or cause cancer.

The incidence of these syndromes remains unknown and can be determined only by large prospective studies. The difficulty stems from the fact that both fibromyalgia and polyarthritis, like many cancers, are fairly common in the general population of adult patients. It would seem likely that perimenopausal women are at the greatest risk of developing these symptoms after adjuvant therapy, as are patients with preexisting rheumatic syndromes or a family history of a rheumatic disease.

An awareness of these potential complications of systemic adjuvant therapy on the part of their healthcare providers would spare many cancer patients unnecessary repeated workups. Because the management of an inflammatory arthritis differs from the management of post-chemotherapy rheumatism, the establishment of a firm rheumatologic diagnosis is of utmost importance. Healthcare providers should consider referring these patients to a rheumatologist.

DRUG- AND RADIATION-INDUCED MUSCULOSKELETAL DISORDERS AND CONNECTIVE TISSUE DISEASES

Cancer survivor patients may develop musculoskeletal disorders in the remission phase. These features may be the result of direct chemotherapy or radiation toxicity.

Acute and chronic gouty arthritis may occur in the setting of tumor lysis syndrome following the administration of cytotoxic drugs for malignancy. They are often caused by the massive release of nucleic acids from killed tumor cells, particularly lymphomas and related lymphoproliferative diseases. In addition, the use of cyclosporine following bone marrow transplantation also increases the risk of gout (Figure 27.1). Treatment consists of controlling the acute attacks with antiinflammatory drugs, colchicine or prednisone depending on the individual patient's comorbidities. Hypouricemic agents (e.g., allopurinol) may be indicated to prevent recurrent attacks.

Raynaud's phenomenon may occur after treatment with bleomycin, vinblastin, vincristine, and cisplatin.[8] In addition, digital ischemia and necrosis have been associated with 5-fluorouracil.[9] Symptoms can be unilateral or bilateral. Pathogenesis is thought to be due to alterations in the small blood vessels and sympathetic tone by the chemotherapeutic agents leading to vasospasm. Smoking cessation and avoidance of cold exposure may alleviate the symptoms of Raynaud's phenomenon. Occasionally, vasodilators, such as calcium channel blockers or angiotensin receptor inhibitors may be required to control symptoms.

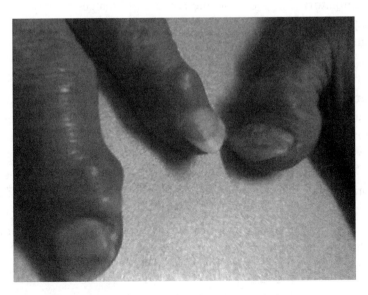

FIGURE 27.1 Cyclosporine-induced tophaceous gout.

The hand-foot syndrome is characterized by burning and painful swelling in the hands and feet. This syndrome is seen with use of 5-fluorouracil or its derivative capecitabine. Management requires dose interruption or reduction.[10]

Systemic sclerosis characterized by skin thickening, Raynaud's phenomenon, and pulmonary fibrosis has been reported with bleomycin, radiation therapy, and rarely with taxanes.[11,12] In fact, a murine model of bleomycin-induced scleroderma is a well-established experimental model.[13] The toxic effects of bleomycin are thought to be due to induction of free radicals leading to chromosome breaks. These breaks may occur in response to oxidative stress and may preferentially lead to the formation and release of unique autoantigens.[14,15] Cutaneous toxicity usually occurs at total doses of between 200 and 300 U, and pulmonary fibrosis at doses greater than 400 U. The most effective way to prevent cutaneous as well as pulmonary fibrosis is to lower the total cumulative dose of bleomycin and to avoid the concurrent use of radiation therapy.[16] Others recommend using continuous infusions, which may induce less pulmonary toxicity than bolus injections.[17]

Dose-related myalgias and arthralgias are a particular problem and may develop within 72 hours of paclitaxel treatment.[18] These symptoms are much less common with weekly regimens compared to every-3-weeks regimens.[19] The pathophysiology is unclear. Nonsteroidal anti-inflammatory drugs or codeine-containing analgesics may lead to symptomatic improvement. In severe cases, a short course (5–7 days) of glucocorticoids may be warranted. Prophylactic gabapentin, given at 300 mg three times daily for 1 or 2 days prior to each dose and continued for 5 days afterward, has been reported to decrease the frequency of myalgias and arthralgias with both taxanes.[20] Paclitaxel-induced arthralgia or myalgia may be worsened by granulocyte colony-stimulating factor,[21] which was also noted once to be the cause of synovitis and fever.[22]

Tamoxifen has been associated with new fibromyalgia-like syndromes, exacerbations of preexisting arthritis, and symmetrical inflammatory polyarthropathy.[3,7] It has been suggested that tamoxifen may exacerbate or induce arthritis through its anti-estrogenic effect, similar to the RA flares seen in the postpartum period when estrogen levels are falling rapidly.[23]

Various rheumatic manifestations also have been seen in association with the use of immunomodulatory agents such as interferon-α and -γ. Such features include the development of myalgia, arthralgia, autoantibody formation, and features suggestive of systemic lupus erythematosus, vasculitis, and autoimmune thyroid disease.[24,25] In one study, more than two-thirds of the patients with chronic myelogenous leukemia treated with interferon were found to have antinuclear antibodies. Of these, half of the studied group reported symptoms related to rheumatic diseases, although few fulfilled the classification criteria for systemic lupus erythematosus. Interferon-α induced the development of a seropositive symmetric polyarthritis similar to RA in a patient being treated for melanoma.[26] The data indicate that interferon treatment may trigger the development of autoimmunity and should not be used in patients with clinical and laboratory features characteristic of autoimmune diseases.

Scoliosis and kyphosis have occurred in patients, specifically children, who have received radiation to the spine, abdomen, or chest, especially when combined with surgery. Similar cases can result from the direct invasion of the tumor to the spine and subsequent surgical removal. Treatment consists of bracing, physical therapy, and surgery in some cases.

BONE DISORDERS

Osteonecrosis and Osteoradionecrosis

Osteonecrosis, also known as avascular necrosis or osteochondritis dessicans, is a pathological condition that affects bone vasculature leading to the death of bone and marrow cells. It is a progressive disease that usually results in joint destruction in 3 to 5 years. Multiple causes have been implicated in this condition. The majority of cases, however, have been associated with high doses of glucocorticoids. Many patients have bilateral involvement at the time of diagnosis. Osteonecrosis most commonly involves the hips, knees, and shoulders. A high index of suspicion is necessary in patients with risk factors to prevent deterioration and loss of joint mobility. Osteonecrosis has been associated with other therapeutic modalities used in cancer including bisphophonates and hematopoeitic cell transplantation (HCT). Patients treated with bisphophonates for multiple myeloma or metastatic breast and prostate cancer were found to be at an increased risk of developing osteoecrosis of the jaw.[27] The presentation can range from mild nonprogressive disease to severe necrosis necessitating reconstructive surgery. Due to the tremendous difficulty of treating jaw osteonecrosis, the focus should be on prevention. When intravenous or high-dose oral bisphosphonates are considered, complete dental assessment and treatment before initiation of therapy are warranted.

When used for patients with myelo- or lymphoproliferative diseases, HCT has also been associated with osteonecrosis. Graft versus host disease, chronic myelogenous leukemia, and female gender have all been identified as steroid-independent risk factors for severe hip osteonecrosis after allogeneic stem cell transplant.[28,29]

Radiation can also cause osteonecrosis. In patients treated for head and neck cancer, osteoradionecrosis has been reported in the jaw.[30]

Osteoporosis

Osteopenia and osteoporosis are not uncommon in cancer survivors. They may occur as a side effect of chemotherapy, steroids, radiation therapy, or from a hypogonadal state. Hypogonadism seen in cancer survivors is often induced by the treatment of hormone-dependent tumors such as breast and prostate cancer, or as a result of chemotherapy for nonhormone-dependent tumors, such as lymphomas. In premenopausal women with breast cancer, hypogonadism develops in at least 63% of patients who receive adjuvant chemotherapy with protocols that contain methotrexate, cyclophosphamide, 5-fluorouracil, or doxorubicin. Of these medications, cyclophosphamide is most notorious. The risk of premature ovarian failure depends on duration of treatment, age, and cumulative dose.[31] Gonadotropin-releasing hormone (GnRH) analogs used to induce ovarian failure in premenopausal women can lead to a decrease in bone density of the spine seen 6 months after initiation of treatment.[32] Tamoxifen, which acts as an estrogen antagonist, is also known to cause loss in bone density in the spine and hip of premenopausal women, but it may preserve bone density in postmenopausal women.[33, 34]

Other treatment strategies in breast cancer involve the use of aromatase inhibitors, which also suppress estrogen levels; however, whether there is any increase in the risk of fractures from this therapy is unclear.

Recent studies comparing anastrozole to tamoxifen and letrozole to tamoxifen showed statistically significant difference in the rate of fractures, favoring tamoxifen over both aromatase inhibitors as causing less fractures.[35]

On the other hand, 5% of the men treated with GnRH analogs for prostate cancer were found to develop osteoporosis-related fractures.[36] Therefore, men with prostate cancer who get surgical or medical castration with anti-androgens should be considered at high risk for osteoporosis.

Finally, osteoporosis and osteomalacia can develop following gastrectomy in patients with early gastric cancer due to decreased absorption of vitamin D and calcium.

Most forms of osteoporosis induced by the treatment of malignancies can be prevented. For example, timely hormone replacement in the hypogonadism associated with nonhormone-dependent tumors prevents the expected bone loss in this group of patients. Bisphosphonates may be useful in patients with hormone-dependent tumors, in which hormone therapy is problematic or contraindicated. In such circumstances, the bisphosphonates are almost equivalent to the sex hormones with regard to their effects on bone metabolism.

Unless there is a clear contraindication (e.g., hypercalcemia), all patients with documented osteopenia or osteoporosis, or who are on chronic steroid therapy should be considered for basic therapy with calcium and vitamin D_3.

RHEUMATIC DISEASES AND MALIGNANCY

The association between malignancy and musculoskeletal or rheumatic disease is complex. The musculoskeletal system may be either directly or indirectly associated with cancer (e.g., dermatomyositis, systemic sclerosis, and RA), or paraneoplastic syndrome and malignancy may arise in preexisting rheumatic disease (e.g., hypertrophic osteoarthropathy, myasthenia gravis, amyloidosis, lymphoma). In addition, treatment of rheumatic disease with immunosuppressants may result in malignancy, and, conversely, chemotherapeutic treatment of the malignancy may result in rheumatic syndromes. Investigation of the intricate relationships among these diseases may enhance our understanding of their etiologies and therefore lead to better control.

CONCLUSION

Due to recent therapeutic advances, in many cases cancer has become a chronic disease rather than a fatal one. Many acute and chronic rheumatic manifestations develop in cancer survivors as side effects of the disease itself or from treatment regimens. These disorders are generally self-limiting, and their treatment may improve patient morbidity and well-being.

REFERENCES

1. Loprinzi CL, Duffy J, Ingle JN. Postchemotherapy rheumatism. *J Clin Oncol.* 1993;11:768–770.
2. Raderer M, Scheithauer W. Postchemotherapy rheumatism following adjuvant therapy for ovarian cancer. *Scand J Rheumatol.* 1994;23:291–292.
3. Warner E, Keshavjee al-N, Shupak R, et al. Rheumatic symptoms following adjuvant therapy for breast cancer. *Am J Clin Oncol.* 1997;20:322–326.
4. Siegel JE. Postchemotherapy rheumatism: is this a menopausal symptom? *J Clin Oncol.* 1993;11:2051(letter).
5. Michl I, Zielinski CC. More postchemotherapy rheumatism. *J Clin Oncol.* 1993;11:2051–2052(letter).
6. Smith DE. Additional cases of postchemotherapy rheumatism. *J Clin Oncol.* 1993;11:1625–1626.
7. Creamer P, Lim K, George E, et al. Acute inflammatory polyarthritis in association with tamoxifen. *Br J Rheumatol.* 1994,33:583–585.
8. Vogelzang NJ, Bosl GJ, Johnson K, et al. Raynaud's phenomenon: a common toxicity after combination therapy for testicular cancer. *Ann Intern Med.* 1981;95:288–295.
9. Papamichael D, Amft N, Slevin ML, et al. 5-Fluorouracil-induced Raynaud's phenomenon. *Eur J Cancer.* 1998;34:1983.
10. Janusch M, Fischer M, Marsch WCh, et al. The hand-foot syndrome—a frequent secondary manifestation in antineoplastic chemotherapy. *Eur J Dermatol.* 2006;16(5):494–499.
11. Kerr LD, Spiera H. Scleroderma in association with the use of bleomycin: a report of 3 cases. *J Rheumatol.* 1992;19:294–296.
12. Behrens S, Reuther T, von Kobyletzki G, et al. Bleomycin-induced PSS-like pseudoscleroderma. Case report and review of the literature. *Hautarzt.* 1998;49:725–729.
13. Yamamoto T, Takagawa S, Katayama I, et al. Animal model of sclerotic skin. I: Local injections of bleomycin induce sclerotic skin mimicking scleroderma. *J Invest Dermatol.* 1999;112:456–462.

14. Casciola-Rosen L, Wigley F, Rosen A. Scleroderma autoantigens are uniquely fragmented by metal-catalyzed oxidation reactions: implications for pathogenesis. *J Exp Med.* 1997;185:71.
15. D'Cruz D. Autoimmune diseases associated with drugs, chemicals and environmental factors. *Toxicol Lett.* 2000;112–113:421–432.
16. Samuels ML, Johnson DE, Holoye PY, et al. Large-dose bleomycin therapy and pulmonary toxicity: a possible role of prior radiotherapy. *JAMA.* 1976;235:1117–1120.
17. Yagoda A, Mukherji B, Young C, et al. Bleomycin, an antitumor antibiotic: clinical experience in 274 patients. *Ann Intern Med.* 1972;77:961–970.
18. Garrison JA, McCune JS, Livingston RB, et al. Myalgias and arthralgias associated with paclitaxel. *Oncology (Huntingt).* 2003;17:271.
19. Akerley W III. Paclitaxel in advanced non-small cell lung cancer: an alternative high-dose weekly schedule. *Chest.* 2000;117:152S.
20. van Deventer H, Bernard S. Use of gabapentin to treat taxane-induced myalgias. *J Clin Oncol.* 1999;17:434.
21. Schiller JH, Storer B, Tutsch K, et al. A phase I trial of 3-hour infusions of paclitaxel (Taxol) with or without granulocyte colony-stimulating factor. *Semin Oncol.* 1994;21(suppl 8):9–14.
22. Tsukadaira A, Okubo Y, Takashi S, et al. Repeated arthralgia associated with granulocyte colony stimulating factor administration. *Ann Rheum Dis.* 2002;61(9):849–850.
23. Ostensen M, Aune B, Husby G. Effects of pregnancy and hormonal changes on the activity of rheumatoid arthritis. *Scand J Rheumatol.* 1983;12:69–72.
24. Wandl UB, Nagel-Hiemke M, May D, et al. Lupus-like autoimmune disease induced by interferon therapy for myeloproliferative disorders. *Clin Immunol Immunopathol.* 1992;65:70–74.
25. Ronnblom LE, Alm GV, Oberg KE. Autoimmunity after alpha-interferon therapy for malignant carcinoid. *Ann Intern Med.* 1991;115:178–183.
26. Passos de Souza E, Evangelista Segundo PT, José FF, et al. Rheumatoid arthritis unduced by alpha-interferon therapy. *Clin Rheumatol.* 2001;20: 297–299.
27. Wang EP, Kaban LB, Strewler GJ, et al. Incidence of osteonecrosis of the jaw in patients with multiple myeloma and breast or prostate cancer on intravenous bisphosphonate therapy. *J Oral Maxillofac Surg.* 2007;65(7): 1328–1331.
28. Tauchmanova L, De Rosa G, Serio B, et al. Avascular necrosis in long-term survivors after allogeneic or autologous stem cell transplantation: a single center experience and a review. *Cancer.* 2003;97(10):2453–2461.

29. Schulte CM, Beelen DW. Avascular osteonecrosis after allogeneic hematopoietic stem-cell transplantation: diagnosis and gender matter. *Transplantation.* 2004;78(7):1055–1063.

30. Mendenhall WM. Mandibular osteoradionecrosis. *J Clin Oncol.* 2004;22: 4867.

31. Reichmann BS, Green KB. Breast cancer in young women: effect of chemotherapy on ovarian function, fertility, and birth defects. *J Natl Cancer Inst Monogr.* 1994;16:125–129.

32. Johansen J, Riis B, Hassager C, et al. The effect of gonadotropin-releasing hormone agonist analog (nafarelin) on bone metabolism. *J Clin Endocrinol Metab.* 1988;67:701–706.

33. Powles TJ, Hickish T, Kanis JA, et al. Effect of tamoxifen on bone mineral density measured by dual-energy x-ray absorptiometry in healthy pre-menopausal, and postmenopausal women. *J Clin Oncol.* 1996;14:78–84.

34. Ramaswamy B, Shapiro CL. Osteopenia and osteoporosis in women with breast cancer. *Semin Oncol.* 2003;30(6):763–775.

35. Ryan PD, Goss PE. Adjuvant hormonal therapy in peri- and post-menopausal breast cancer. *Oncologist.* 2006;11:718–731.

36. Townsend MF, Sanders WH, Northway RO, et al. Bone fractures associated with luteinizing hormone-releasing hormone agonists used in the treatment of prostate carcinoma. *Cancer.* 1997;79:545–550.

28

Cognitive Dysfunction— "Chemobrain" or "Chemofog"

Cara Miller, BS

In the Words of Cancer Survivors . . .

My mental stamina is limited, and if I do too much I feel exhausted and need to rest. I used to be good at multitasking, but now I need to focus all of my energies on doing one task at a time. At its worst, I would describe the feeling I have as "shredded cardboard" in my brain.

—Barbara, a 65-year-old breast cancer survivor who received chemotherapy

The problem is the inability to remember names and sometimes common words. It's not a problem when I write because I can take my time to remember the word in question, but sometimes it is embarrassing when I can't remember ordinary words like "appetizer" or "washing machine" in a conversation, and I feel the other person staring at me. I even had to put a post-it note on my microwave with the word "fennel" written in bold since I kept forgetting this word again and again. Interestingly, it's mostly ordinary words of objects and not abstract words like "truth," "ambivalence," or "conflict" when I draw a blank; I clearly see the object in my mind but simply can't remember what the object is called.

—Clarissa, a 70-year-old breast cancer survivor who received both chemotherapy and radiation therapy

ABSTRACT

Cognitive dysfunction (also known as "chemobrain" or "chemofog") has been reported in over 20% of patients following treatment with chemotherapy. Affected patients common complain of impairment of attention span, concentration, psychomoter speed, and information processing which often, but not always, improve following treatment. The pathophysiology of cognitive dysfunction are the topic on ongoing study as are possible pharmacologic interventions to treat these symptoms. Learning behavioral strategies to cope with cognitive dysfunction and rehabilitative services may be helpful to patients.

INTRODUCTION

Cognitive changes associated with chemotherapy are not uncommon. In fact, a reported 20% to 30% of cancer patients report symptoms of chemotherapy-induced neurocognitive impairment—"chemobrain" or "chemofog," as it is sometimes colloquially termed.[1] Estimates of female breast cancer patients who experience this condition are 15% and 16% to 40%.

Symptoms of cognitive changes induced by chemotherapy were first reported by female breast cancer patients complaining of problems with word finding, memory, multitasking, learning, processing speed, attention, concentration, language, and judging spaces and layout (Figure 28.1). Previously, doctors assumed that cognitive changes were the byproduct of other chemotherapy side effects such as anemia, fatigue, and depression. This assumption, coupled with the fact that cognitive impairment may manifest differently in many cancer patients, has frequently resulted in underreporting of cognitive changes. For some, cognitive changes are a temporary "mild annoyance," while for others, the long-lasting debilitating condition may prevent return to work and return to normal functioning (Table 28.1).

It is difficult to predict which patients will be affected by neurocognitive changes, and furthermore, such changes can be subtle and difficult to measure. Neuropsychological tests that measure memory and speed are typically developed to assess patients with fairly severe brain pathologies, not those with subtle changes, as may be seen in chemotherapy-induced neurocognitive impairment. Thus, not only

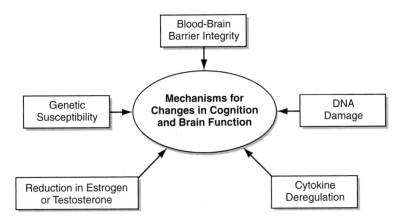

FIGURE 28.1 Mechanisms for changes in cognition and brain function.

Source: Ahles TA, Saykin AJ. Candidate mechanisms for chemotherapy-induced cognitive changes. *Nat Rev Cancer.* 2007;7(3):192–201.

may it be difficult to differentiate the neurologic complications of chemotherapy from other neurologic complications of cancer, but assessment results of cancer patients with cognitive impairments may still be within normal limits. Despite these "normal" scores, the patient's cognitive functioning may be significantly diminished compared to results that would have been otherwise obtained prior to treatment. As Dr. Barbara Collins states, "The brightest and the best and those most likely to have a high cognitive demand in their lives may be the most likely to complain that there is something wrong."[2]

TABLE 28.1 Domains of Cognitive Function

• Attention	• Language
• Concentration	• Psychomotor Speed
• Executive Function	• Visuospatial Skill
• Information Processing Speed	• Visual Memory
• Verbal Memory	• Intelligence
	• Verbal Fluency

BACKGROUND

Research on chemotherapy-induced neurocognitive impairment has been increasing in the past decade. In 1990, Appleton, Farrell, Zaide, and Rogers studied child leukemia survivors who were 2 years into remission. All had received chemotherapy. Of the children observed, half had apparent "decline in head circumference centile," and of those with reduced head growth, "performance was significantly impaired in neuropsychological tests designed to assess concentration and short term memory."[3] These children also demonstrated clinically significant "learning difficulties in the classroom," as well as "minor neurological dysfunction."[3]

In 1998, van Dam and colleagues compared cognitive deficits in patients with high-risk breast cancer.[4] In van Dam's study, patients were randomly assigned to receive either high-dose or standard-dose chemotherapy. Both groups of patients, in addition to a control group that had not received chemotherapy, were given a battery of neuropsychological tests as well as interviews related to cognitive problems and assessments of patients' reported quality of life and feelings of anxiety and depression. The study concluded that cognitive impairment was found in 32% of patients treated with high-dose chemotherapy, compared to 17% of patients treated with standard doses of chemotherapy. Only 9% of control patients, those who had cancer without chemotherapy treatments, reported any resulting cognitive changes.[4]

Also in 1998, Schagen and colleagues examined breast cancer patients treated with chemotherapy and compared this group with a control group of breast cancer patients who had been treated with surgery and radiation therapy.[5] The chemotherapy patients reported significantly more problems than control patients in regard to concentration (31% vs 6%) and memory (21% vs 3%). However, no relationship was found between patients' reported complaints of cognitive impairment and their results on neuropsychological tests. Instead, tests indicated that 28% of chemotherapy patients displayed symptoms of cognitive functioning compared to 12% of the control patient group. The cognitive impairments seen by Schagen and colleagues were evident in impaired attention, mental flexibility, visual functioning, motor functioning, and speed of information processing. Study results concluded that the differences in the chemotherapy and control groups were not accounted for by hormonal therapy, anxiety, depression, fatigue, time since treatment, or self-reported complaints of cognitive dysfunction.[5]

Ahles and Saykin found that cancer patients treated with chemotherapy scored significantly lower on standardized tests measuring mental and psychological functions than those who had only local therapy. Their scores were lower on average whether or not patients reported having depression, anxiety, or fatigue, indicating that the lower scores resulted from cognitive impairment due to chemotherapy.[6]

Tannock and colleagues did a study on female breast cancer patients who were undergoing or who had had chemotherapy 2 years earlier. The study concluded that those patients performed worse on "certain cognitive tests," which were not elaborated upon, than did a control group of women without cancer. Furthermore, the difference in results could not be explained by the women's age, education, mood, or menopausal status.[7]

Ahles and Saykin later compared men and women who had had chemotherapy for breast cancer or lymphoma with other cancer patients who were treated with only surgery and localized radiation. All subjects were still in remission 5 years post-treatment. The subjects who were treated with chemotherapy were found to perform worse on "pen-and-paper" tests of cognitive functioning.[6]

In 2006, Silverman compared positron emission tomography (PET) scans evaluating chemotherapy patients' brain function to PET scans from breast-cancer patients who only underwent surgery as well as control subjects who did not have breast cancer or chemotherapy. The participants in the study did short-term memory exercises while their resting brain metabolism and blood flow were measured. Silverman and his colleagues found a link between neurocognitive symptoms from chemotherapy and lower brain metabolism. Specifically, the lower a patient's resting brain metabolism rate was, the more difficulty she had with memory tests. The researchers concluded that the observed spike in blood flow to the areas of the frontal cortex, cerebellum, and basal ganglia suggested that those chemotherapy subjects "worked harder than control subjects to recall the same information."[8]

Other studies have examined the cognitive impact of chemotherapy on survivors of childhood cancer. Kadan-Lottick found a spectrum of structural changes, ranging from leukoencephalopathy and impaired gray matter growth to impaired glucose metabolism in the hippocampus.[9] Clinical findings after chemotherapy included seizures and acute problems with behavior and attention, as well as decreases in full scale and verbal IQ, mathematics achievement, reading, spelling, and executive functioning. Academically, these children had difficulties with math multiplication and division as well as recall and comprehension when reading. They also had problems with visual memory, processing speed, and visual-motor integration. These children were at greater risk of needing special education and not completing high school.[9]

PATHOPHYSIOLOGY

A current pilot study at Yale University is testing a hypothetical association between impairment in attention and memory with changes in white matter of basal ganglia and frontal cortex in child cancer survivors.

Other studies have looked at cognitive changes in animals that were administered chemotherapy drugs. Dietrich exposed and compared mice brain cells and human neural cells that were given the chemotherapy drugs cisplatin, carmustine, and cytarabine.[10] These drugs were found to have destroyed both neural stem cells and oligodendrocytes in mice; oligodendrocytes are neural cells that produce myelin and affect speed and efficacy of neurotransmission. Even 6 weeks after receiving the chemotherapy drugs, the mice's brain cells continued dying. In human subjects, the chemotherapy drugs destroyed only 40% to 80% of cancer cells, but approximately 70% to 100% of human brain cells.[10]

Currently, four main theories have been proposed to account for chemotherapy-induced neurocognitive impairment. The first is that chemotherapy drugs cross the blood-brain barrier and thus cause direct neurotoxicity. It should be noted that previously, chemotherapy drugs were thought to be too large to transverse the blood-brain barrier. This theory proposes that the neurotoxic chemicals found in chemotherapy drugs pass through the barrier and thus enter the blood supply to the brain.

The second theory proposes degeneration of DNA. Specifically, telomeres, which are the ends of chromosomes, may be shortened as a result of chemotherapy, and thus reduce the stability of the DNA.

The third theory suggests that cognitive changes are the results of cytokines that are suppressed when patients receive chemotherapy. Normally, cytokines, which are substances produced by our immune system, are important to normal neurocognitive functioning. During chemotherapy treatment, the quantity and nature of the cytokine milieu may change and result in neurocognitive consequences.

Finally, the fourth hypothesis is that receiving chemotherapy may reduce hormone levels, which then leads to relevant cognitive declines. Decreases in circulating estrogen and testosterone may affect those hormones' normal impact on neurocognitive functioning.

ONGOING AND FUTURE RESEARCH

Although previous research has established a probable link between chemotherapy and cognitive changes, many prior studies have been limited by both controllable and unforeseeable methodological limitations. These include limited sample sizes, lack of baseline assessment of patients' cognitive functioning, and lack of controls for potential confounding factors.[11] The Hurricane Voices Breast Cancer Foundation outlined five priorities for future research in the area of neurocognitive impairment related to chemotherapy, as follows[12]:

1. *Large-scale clinical studies using a longitudinal design with concurrent evaluation of cancer patients who do not receive chemotherapy. Address probability and magnitude of cognitive deficits, factors that predict them, and underlying mechanisms.* Studies of this sort will be important to look at covariables that can contribute or count for cognitive changes of and by themselves.

2. *Exploration of discrepancies between subjective reports of cognitive dysfunction and objective results of cognitive testing.* Of note, "objective testing" perhaps is not sensitive enough to measure true changes that occur and are perceived by an individual.

3. *Studies of cognitive function in patients receiving treatment for diseases other than breast cancer, in both men and women, to address the hypothesis that underlying mechanisms relate to changes in serum levels of sex hormones and/or to chemotherapy-induced menopause.* Although breast cancer is extremely common, the

largest majority of newly diagnosed patients have other types of cancers.

4. *Development of interventions to alleviate chemotherapy-induced cognitive dysfunction.* Characterizing cognitive deficits is certainly of value, but remediating them is the next important step.

5. *Development of animal models and imaging techniques to address mechanisms that might cause cognitive impairment associated with chemotherapy.* An improved understanding of the underlying physiologic and structural mechanisms may improve the efficacy of therapeutic interventions.

COGNITIVE REHABILITATION AND TREATMENT

Some pharmacologic approaches can be suggested, but primarily a behavioral approach has been suggested as a first form of remediation. For many patients, the neurocognitive changes gradually improve over time, and so strategies to compensate for the temporary deficits can be helpful. As suggested by the Mayo Clinic, these include[1]:

▷ Decrease workload
▷ Avoid multiple tasks
▷ "Prepare for tomorrow today"
▷ Make lists
▷ Increase sleep
▷ Use mnemonics and wordplay
▷ Use electronic calendars to record appointments
▷ Use key chains that beep when pressed
▷ Color-code and label items
▷ Track memory problems in small diaries
▷ Play crossword puzzles and Sudoku squares
▷ Try systematic computer training (e.g., MindFit)

There is very limited information on pharmacologic interventions. Treatments for attention deficit hyperactivity disorder and other neurodegenerative diseases have been seen to have some protective factors. Similarly, at least preliminary data suggest that erythropoietin may have "neuroprotective abilities."[13]

In summary, neurocognitive changes associated with chemotherapy may be subtle but can be observed consistently, may be durable, and can be disabling in many individuals. While current underlying mechanisms responsible for such cognitive deficits are unknown, preliminary studies have suggested genetic predispositions as a possible factor. Currently, cognitive impairments may be accompanied by changes in the brain that are detectable by neuroimaging as well as by self-reports from individuals and their families.

The number of cancer survivors, fortunately, continues to grow. As McDonald states[14]:

> As cancer patients are treated more aggressively, receive more chemotherapy, and live longer, and as new chemotherapeutic agents are developed and existing agents are used more intensively or in novel ways, neurologic complications of cancer chemotherapy will become more common, serious, and complex. The recognition and treatment of chemotherapy-induced neurotoxicity will become a frequent and important clinical problem.

The challenges to clinicians include attempting to minimize neurocognitive side effects of treatment without sacrificing efficacy, better understanding the pathogenesis of neurocognitive changes, and providing rehabilitative services to optimize quality of life.

REFERENCES

1. Chemobrain. MayoClinic.com Web site. http://mayoclinic.com/health/cancer-treatment/CA00044. Published October 11, 2008. Accessed December 17, 2008.
2. Hoag H. The foggy world of chemobrain. *The Star.* http://www.thestar.com/article/273121. Published November 3, 2007. Accessed December 17, 2008.
3. Appleton RE, Farrell K, Zaide J, Rogers P. Decline in head growth and cognitive impairment in survivors of acute lymphoblastic leukaemia. *Arch Dis Child.* 1990;65:530–534.
4. van Dam FS, Schagen SB, Muller MJ, et al. Impairment of cognitive function in women receiving adjuvant treatment for high-risk breast cancer: high-dose versus standard-dose chemotherapy. *J Natl Cancer Inst.* 1998; 90(3):210.
5. Schagen SB, Frits SAM, van Dam FS, et al. Cognitive deficits after postoperative adjuvant chemotherapy for breast carcinoma. *Cancer.* 1999;85: 640–650.

6. Ahles TA, Saykin AJ. Candidate mechanisms for chemotherapy-induced cognitive changes. *Nat Rev Cancer.* 2007;7(3):192–201.

7. Tannock IF, Brezden CB, Abdolell M, Bunston T. Cognitive function in breast cancer patients receiving adjuvant chemotherapy. *J Clin Oncol.* 2000;18(14):2695–2701.

8. Silverman DHS. Altered frontocortical, cerebellar, and basal ganglia activity in adjuvant-treated breast cancer survivors 5–10 years after chemotherapy. *Breast Cancer Res Treatment.* 2007;103(3):303–311.

9. Kaydan-Lottick N. Late effects in survivors of childhood cancer. Presentation to Department of Pediatrics, Yale University School of Medicine; 2007.

10. Dietrich J, Han R, Yang Y, Mayer-Proschel M, Noble M. CNS progenitor cells and oligodendrocytes are targets of chemotherapeutic agents in vitro and in vivo. *J Biol.* 2006;5(22).

11. Minisni A, Atalay G, Bottomley A, Puglisi F, Piccart M, Bignaozoli L. What is the effect of systematic anticancer treatment on cognitive function? *Lancet Oncol.* 2004 May;5(5):273–282.

12. Cognitive changes related to breast cancer treatment. Hurricane Voices Web site. http://www.hurricanevoices.org. Accessed December 17, 2008.

13. Staat K, Segatore M. The phenomenon of chemo brain. *Clin J Oncol Nurs.* 2005;9(6):713–721.

14. MacDonald DR. Neurologic complications of chemotherapy. *Neurol Clin.* 1991;9(4):955–967.

FURTHER READING

Brain MRI result. Greg's Place Web site. http://hewletts.org:8080/archives/000263.html#000263. Published February 4, 2004. Accessed December 17, 2008.

Cancer fast stats. National Center for Health Statistics Web site. http://www.cdc.gov/nchs/fastats/cancer.htm. Updated and accessed December 17, 2008.

Cancer statistics. National Cancer Institute Web site. http://www.cancer.gov/statistics/. Accessed December 17, 2008.

Chemotherapy: what it is, how it works. American Cancer Society Web site. http://www.cancer.org/docroot/ETO/content/ETO_1_2X_Chemotherapy_What_It_Is_How_It_Helps.asp. Updated April 4, 2008. Accessed December 17, 2008.

Fauber J. Lost in cancer's fog: "chemobrain" impairs thinking, memory after chemotherapy; anecdotal brain effects are just starting to get serious study. JSOnline. http://www.jsonline.com/story/index.aspx?id=655669. Published September 2, 2007. Accessed December 17, 2008.

Ferguson RJ, Ahles TA, Saykin AJ, McDonald BC. Cognitive-behavioral management of chemotherapy-related cognitive change. *Psycho-Oncol.* 2007; 16(8):772.

Losing the cancer war. Cancer Prevention Coalition Web site. http://www.preventcancer.com/losing/nci/manipulates.htm. Accessed December 17, 2008.

Smyth S. Chemo brain. Abreast in the World Web site. http://abreastintheworld.blogspot.com/2007/10/chemo-brain.html. Published October 8, 2007. Accessed December 17, 2008.

Tannock IF, Ahles TA, Ganz PA, van Dam FS. Cognitive impairment associated with chemotherapy for cancer: report of a workshop. *J Clin Oncol.* 2004;22(11):2233–2239.

Fertility Preservation in Cancer Survivors

Jason G. Bromer, MD

&

Emre Seli, MD

ABSTRACT

Seventy-five percent of cancer survivors report wanting to have children in the future. However, many common cancer therapies are toxic to the ovaries and testes. For this reason, a number of fertility preservation strategies have been developed, including gamete and embryo cryopreservation, ovarian tissue cryopreservation, and gonadotropin-releasing hormone agonist (GnRHa) cotreatment.

INTRODUCTION

Cancer is not uncommon among younger women. In the United States, approximately 600 000 women are diagnosed with cancer every year, and 10% of these women are under 40 years of age.[1] Of teenage girls and young women diagnosed with cancer, 90% will survive,[2] and it is estimated that by 2010, 1 in 250 adults will be a cancer survivor.[3]

The treatment required for most of the common cancer types occurring in younger women may involve removal of the reproductive organs and/or cytotoxic treatment that could partially or definitively affect reproductive function (Table 29.1). Therefore, women diagnosed with cancer prior to or during their reproductive period often have to deal not only with the uncertainty of long-term survival but also with the partial or total loss of fertility as a result of cancer treatment. In fact, there is ample evidence that women with cancer are highly interested in the topic of fertility preservation in their treatment regimens. In recent surveys, 75% of patients with cancer reported wanting children in the future, 80% felt their cancer experience would make them better parents, 67% wanted a child even if they were to die young, and less than 10% stated they would choose adoption due to the possible increased risk their treatment could pose for a biological child.[4,5]

Nonetheless, there remains a sharp divide between patient interest and caregiver education on the topic of fertility preservation. Only 60% of survivors diagnosed with cancer in young adulthood recall discussing cancer-related infertility. Furthermore, in a survey of 162 oncologists in two major cancer centers, 90% agreed that all men whose fertility could be impaired should be offered sperm banking; however, 50% stated they never or rarely addressed this topic with eligible patients.[4,5] In a survey of 697 women diagnosed with breast cancer before the age of 40, 72% of respondents stated they had discussed infertility with their physician, 17% had consulted an infertility specialist, but only 55% were satisfied that their concerns about childbearing were addressed.[6]

TABLE 29.1 ∽   Alkylating Agents and Gonadotoxicity

- Alkylating agents, particularly cyclophosphamide, are used in the treatment of cancer, as well as a number of rheumatic and renal disorders.
- All alkylating agents are toxic to both ovaries and testes.
- The incidence of gonadal dysfunction is dependent upon age, gender, and total dose. For example, Boumpas et al. (Ann Intern Med, 1993) and Huong et al. (J Rheumatol, 1993) found that IV cyclophosphamide administered to menstruating women for the treatment of rheumatologic disorders (SLE, Wegener's granuomatosis) results in ovarian failure in 0–12% of women < 25 years old, and 60% of women > 35 years old.

In this chapter, we will describe both the established and experimental strategies for fertility preservation in women with malignancies. Most available options may also be applicable to women who face gonadotoxic treatment due to other nonmalignant disorders (such as systemic lupus erythematosus).

ESTABLISHED TREATMENT OPTIONS

Embryo Cryopreservation

Currently, the only widely available option for fertility preservation in female patients who need chemo- and/or radiotherapy is the cryopreservation of fertilized oocytes and embryos. Cryopreservation of embryos involves an initial exposure to cryoprotectants, cooling to subzero temperatures, and storage. The embryos then may be thawed on demand, with a return to physiological conditions.

The methods involved in embryo cryopreservation and their success rates have been well-established. Reported survival rates per thawed embryo range between 35% and 90%, with implantation rates between 8% and 30%.[7–12] In the United States, approximately 16,000 assisted reproductive technology (ART) cycles using frozen nondonor embryos are performed yearly with a pregnancy rate of 25% per transfer, compared to a 35% pregnancy rate in cycles using fresh nondonor embryos.[13] It is noteworthy that the effects of different types of malignancies upon reproductive potential is not yet known, and these statistics may not predict the outcome in women undergoing embryo cryopreservation for fertility preservation due to malignancy.

Despite well-defined success rates, embryo cryopreservation has a few critical pitfalls. First, it requires that the patient has a male partner or uses donor sperm to fertilize retrieved eggs. Second, ovarian stimulation precedes oocyte retrieval for in vitro fertilization (IVF), necessitating a delay in initiating chemo- or radiotherapy that may not be acceptable. Third, the high serum estrogen concentrations associated with ovarian stimulation may be contraindicated in women with estrogen-sensitive malignancies. However, given the success of ovarian-stimulation protocols, including letrozole, in leading to successful term birth,[14,15] their combination with embryo cryopreservation is also likely to be successful.

ALTERNATIVE STRATEGIES FOR OVARIAN STIMULATION IN WOMEN WITH ESTROGEN-SENSITIVE MALIGNANCIES

Ovarian stimulation protocols lead to an expansion of the pool of growing follicles and thus an increase in serum estrogen. Recently, new strategies for ovarian stimulation prior to IVF have been investigated for women with breast cancer, with the aim of retrieving more oocytes than would be available in a natural cycle but without causing a significant increase in serum estrogen. Women with breast cancer constitute a special group due to the 6-week hiatus between surgery and chemotherapy in most treatment protocols; this break typically allows sufficient time for ovarian stimulation and egg retrieval.

Oktay and colleagues first used tamoxifen to stimulate follicle growth for IVF in 12 women with breast cancer.[16] Using a dose of 40 mg to 60 mg daily, beginning on day 2 or 3 of the menstrual cycle, they obtained a higher number of oocytes and embryos per cycle compared to a retrospective control group consisting of breast cancer patients attempting natural-cycle (unstimulated) IVF.[16] However, mean peak estradiol level in the tamoxifen group was significantly higher than in natural-cycle IVF patients. Following this initial study, Oktay and colleagues reported better stimulation and embryo development using a combination of follicle-stimulating hormone (FSH) with tamoxifen or the aromatase inhibitor letrozole.[17] While they obtained a similar number of mature oocytes and embryos per cycle in both groups, the mean peak estradiol was significantly lower in the letrozole group. In the most recent study to date, Oktay et al. determined that combination of an aromatase inhibitor with gonadotropin treatment in breast cancer patients produces comparable results to standard in vitro fertilization. Compared to age matched retrospective controls, letrozole and FSH stimulation resulted in significantly lower peak estradiol levels and 44% reduction in gonadotropin requirement; however, the length of stimulation, number of embryos obtained, and fertilization rates were similar.

EXPERIMENTAL STRATEGIES

Oocyte Cryopreservation

The cryopreservation of oocytes avoids the need for sperm and thus is applicable to a larger group of patients compared to embryo cryopreservation. In addition, oocyte cryopreservation may circumvent ethical or legal considerations associated with embryo freezing. Moreover, it also has considerable advantages compared to ovarian tissue cryopreservation, at least in the short term. However, although the first human live birth from cryopreserved oocytes was reported more than 20 years ago,[19] success rates in ARTs using frozen oocytes have lagged behind those using frozen embryos, most likely as a result of the biochemical and physical properties of the oocyte.

Due to the low efficiency of oocyte maturation in vitro, mature Metaphase II (MII) oocytes are most commonly used for cryopreservation. These oocytes are among the largest cells in the human body and contain the very delicate meiotic spindle. Because their cytoplasm contains a high proportion of water in comparison to other cells, damage due to ice crystal formation was an initial hurdle to oocyte viability after frozen storage. Recent protocols that include dehydration of the oocytes before or during the cooling procedure have reduced ice crystal formation and have led to much-improved clinical outcomes.

Cryopreservation of mature oocytes has also been shown to cause hardening of the zona pellucida, resulting in adverse effects on fertilization.[20] Significant improvement in the fertilization of cryopreserved oocytes has been achieved with the use of intracytoplasmic sperm injection,[21,22] likely due to avoiding the effects of zona hardening.

The two most common freezing protocols used are *slow cooling* and *vitrification*. In the last 2 years, each protocol has shown increasing promise, and as a result, oocyte cryopreservation is becoming more routine and less experimental.

SLOW COOLING PROCEDURE

The first protocol used to freeze oocytes was based on a slow cooling and rapid thawing method that had already been applied successfully for the cryopreservation of embryos. Since then, much progress has been made, mostly in the optimization of cryoprotectant concentration and exposure time. Recent pooled reports on outcomes with this protocol have suggested a 47% oocyte survival rate, with a subsequent 52% fertilization rate, leading to an overall pregnancy rate of 1.9% per thawed oocyte.[23]

VITRIFICATION

Vitrification may be defined as a physical process in which a highly concentrated solution of cryoprotectants solidifies during cooling without the formation of ice crystals.[24] Vitrification has certain advantages over freezing because it avoids the damage caused by intracellular ice formation and the osmotic effects caused by extracellular ice formation. Pregnancy outcomes to date have been similar to those seen with the slow cooling protocol, with a 68.4% survival rate per oocyte, a 48.5% fertilization rate, and a 2.0% pregnancy rate per vitrified oocyte.[23]

Ovarian Tissue Cryopreservation

Cryopreservation of primordial follicles within ovarian tissue has several potential advantages over both embryo and oocyte freezing. Hundreds of primordial follicles containing immature oocytes may be cryopreserved without the necessity for ovarian stimulation and delay in initiating cancer treatment. Moreover, primordial follicles are significantly less susceptible to cryo-injury compared to both mature and immature oocytes due to their smaller size, slower metabolic rates, and the absence of zona pellucida. Two approaches to ovarian tissue cryopreservation are currently being investigated: cryopreservation of ovarian cortical strips and cryopreservation of whole ovaries.

CRYOPRESERVATION OF OVARIAN CORTICAL STRIPS

The outer cortical layer of the ovary contains most of the primordial follicles. Therefore, it is conceivable to cryopreserve pieces of ovarian cortical tissue. The ovarian cortex is removed via laparoscopy or laparotomy and cut into strips of tissue 1 mm to 3 mm in thickness and less than or equal to 1 cm^2 in total area in order to ensure adequate penetration of cryoprotectants.[25] It is necessary to analyze a piece of the cortical tissue to confirm the presence of follicles and the absence of malignant metastasis.[12,26] Once the ovarian tissue is cryopreserved, future options include transplantation of the tissue back to the donor (autotransplantation), transplantation to nude mice (xenotransplantation), or culture of the follicles in vitro.

Autotransplantation studies using animal models have resulted in the return of ovarian function as well as pregnancies and live births.[27–29]

Two different surgical approaches have been used in humans for transplantation: orthotopic (pelvic) or heterotopic. Orthotopic transplantation places ovarian tissue at close proximity of the infundibulo-pelvic ligament with the hope that natural pregnancy may occur. Two live births have been reported to date with this method. Heterotopic transplantation is an alternative approach in which cryopreserved ovarian tissue is transplanted to a site outside of the pelvis. Transplantation to a heterotopic site such as the forearm[25,30] or abdomen[31] is technically easier and imposes fewer surgery-associated risks compared to orthotopic transplantation. In vitro fertilization and embryo transfer is absolutely necessary in order to achieve pregnancy.

In 2001, Oktay and colleagues were first to report return of ovarian endocrine function with the development of a dominant follicle and resumption of menstrual cycles in two women using this approach.[31] In one case, after stimulation with human menopausal gonadotropin, they performed percutaneous oocyte retrieval from the forearm; however, fertilization was not achieved.[31] More recently, Oktay and colleagues were able to restore ovarian function in a woman previously treated for breast cancer by transplanting the cryopreserved ovarian tissue beneath the abdominal skin. They performed eight cycles of controlled ovarian stimulation using a combination of recombinant FSH and human menopausal gonadotropins for stimulation. A total of 20 oocytes were retrieved, of which one fertilized normally, but pregnancy did not occur.[31]

A significant source of concern associated with autotransplantation is the risk of transmission of metastatic cancer cells. Xenotransplantation of cryopreserved ovarian tissue into nude mice eliminates the possibility of cancer cell transmission and relapse, because the oocytes are retrieved from the host animal. Another advantage is the possible application in women in whom hormonal stimulation is contraindicated. However, possible transmission of zoonoses to humans is a serious concern, and this method is unlikely to be clinically available in the near future.

CRYOPRESERVATION OF WHOLE OVARIES

Animal studies suggest that fresh whole ovaries can be successfully transplanted. Although the duration of subsequent ovarian function has initially been limited, mostly due to ischemia resulting from thrombosis,[32] the use of microsurgical techniques has led to improvements in graft survival.[32–36] In addition, careful dissection of ovarian vessels during ovariectomy and perfusion of ovary with cryoprotectants through these vessels improved tissue survival and led to similar rates of follicular viability and apoptosis compared to ovarian cortical strips.[34]

Bedaiwy and colleagues investigated the immediate post-thawing injury to the ovary that was cryopreserved as a whole with its vascular pedicle or as cortical strips.[37] Bilateral oophorectomy was performed in two women (46 and 44 years old) undergoing hysterectomy. In both patients, one of the harvested ovaries was sectioned and cryopreserved as ovarian cortical strips. The other ovary was cryopreserved intact with its vascular pedicle. After thawing 7 days later, the overall viability of the primordial follicles was 75% to 78% in intact cryopreserved-thawed ovaries and 81% to 83% in ovarian cortical strips. Comparable primordial follicle counts and absence of features of necrosis or apoptotic markers led them to conclude that cryopreservation injury is not associated with significant follicular damage.

While these results are encouraging, definitive restoration of fertility resulting from the transplantation of a cryopreserved-thawed whole human ovary remains to be demonstrated. This technique does carry potentially increased risk of returning metastatic disease to the patient, compared to the handling of oocytes or even cortical strips.

Ovarian Transposition

Transposition of the ovaries (oophoropexy) outside of the pelvis to protect them from pelvic radiation was initially described in 1958.[38] The procedure is indicated in patients diagnosed with malignancies that require pelvic radiation, but not removal of the ovaries, as part of their treatment. The most common indications are Hodgkin disease, cervical and vaginal cancer, and pelvic sarcomas. Initially, the procedure was performed through a laparotomy incision. More recently, oophoropexy has been described laparoscopically.[39] During the last 4 decades, several reports have documented different degrees of ovarian function and ability to conceive a pregnancy after radiation treatment. The procedure has been successful in 16% to 90% of the reported cases.[12,40,41] The variations are likely due to the inability to calculate and prevent scatter radiation, different doses of radiation utilized, and concomitant use of chemotherapy.[12]

Gonadotropin-Releasing Hormone Agonist Cotreatment

Based on the postulated role of gonadal suppression in the preservation of testicular function in men receiving chemotherapy and the belief that the fertility of prepubertal girls is not affected by gonadotoxic treatment, the effect of GnRHa treatment in preserving fertility by creating a prepubertal hormonal environment has been investigated.[12] Animal studies have shown a protective role for GnRHa treatment against chemotherapy-induced gonadal damage.[42,43] Ataya and colleagues demonstrated that loss of primordial follicles in response to cyclophosphamide chemotherapy was significantly less in Rhesus monkeys receiving GnRHa cotreatment compared to those receiving chemotherapy alone.[44] Interestingly, they did not find GnRHa cotreatment to be effective in protecting against radiotherapy-induced gonadal damage.[45]

Following encouraging findings in animal models, nonrandomized studies with short-term follow-up have suggested a protective role for GnRHa cotreatment.[46–50] However, these studies have been criticized for their lack of randomization and the use of ovarian failure as an endpoint that may not reflect the decrease in primordial follicle count in response to chemotherapy in young women.[12] Presently, despite encouraging reports, the benefits and long-term effects of GnRHa cotreatment are unclear, and a consensus regarding the effectiveness of ovarian suppression is lacking.

SUMMARY

Fertility preservation in females diagnosed with cancer has become an important area of investigation due to increasing cancer survival rates combined with delayed childbearing. Alternative treatment strategies for early stage gynecologic cancers have recently been studied with promising results for both survival and fertility preservation. In addition to embryo cryopreservation, encouraging findings have recently been reported using oocyte cryopreservation, ovarian cryopreservation, and GnRHa cotreatment with chemotherapy. In addition to the possibilities for surgical management, female patients today have a wide range of options for fertility preservation that should be discussed prior to undergoing gonadotoxic therapy.

REFERENCES

1. Cancer Facts & Figures, 2001. American Cancer Society Web site. http://www.cancer.org/downloads/STT/F&F2001.pdf. Accessed December 17, 2008.

2. Ries LAG, Percy CL, Bunin GR. Introduction. In: Ries LAG, Smith MA, Gurney JG, eds. *Cancer Incidence and Survival Among Children and Adolescents: United States SEER Program, 1975–1995*. National Cancer Institute: Bethesda, MD; 1999.

3. Bleyer WA. The impact of childhood cancer on the United States and the world. *Cancer*. 1990;40:355–367.

4. Schover LR, Brey K, Lichtin A, Lipshultz LI, Jeha S. Knowledge and experience regarding cancer, infertility, and sperm banking in younger male survivors. *J Clin Oncol*. 2002;20(7):1880–1889.

5. Schover LR, Rybicki LA, Martin BA, Bringelsen KA. Having children after cancer. A pilot survey of survivors' attitudes and experiences. *Cancer*. 1999;86(4):697–709.

6. Partridge AH, Gelber S, Peppercorn J, et al. Web-based survey of fertility issues in young women with breast cancer. *J Clin Oncol*. 2004;22(20): 4174–4183.

7. Son WY, Yoon SH, Yoon HJ, Lee SM, Lim JH. Pregnancy outcome following transfer of human blastocysts vitrified on electron microscopy grids after induced collapse of the blastocoele. *Hum Reprod*. 2003;18(1):137–139.

8. Wang JX, Yap YY, Matthews CD. Frozen-thawed embryo transfer: influence of clinical factors on implantation rate and risk of multiple conception. *Hum Reprod*. 2001;16(11):2316–2319.

9. Senn A, Vozzi C, Chanson A, De Grandi P, Germond M. Prospective randomized study of two cryopreservation policies avoiding embryo selection: the pronucleate stage leads to a higher cumulative delivery rate than the early cleavage stage. *Fertil Steril*. 2000;74(5):946–952.

10. Frederick JL, Ord T, Kettel LM, Stone SC, Balmaceda JP, Asch RH. Successful pregnancy outcome after cryopreservation of all fresh embryos with subsequent transfer into an unstimulated cycle. *Fertil Steril*. 1995; 64(5):987–990.

11. Selick CE, Hofmann GE, Albano C, et al. Embryo quality and pregnancy potential of fresh compared with frozen embryos—is freezing detrimental to high quality embryos? *Hum Reprod*. 1995;10(2):392–395.

12. Sonmezer M, Oktay K. Fertility preservation in female patients. *Hum Reprod*. 2004;10(3):251–266(update).

13. Society for Assisted Reproductive Technology (SART). Assisted reproductive technology success rates. National summary and fertility clinic reports. Centers for Disease Control: USA; 2002.

14. Baysoy A, Serdaroglu H, Jamal H, Karatekeli E, Ozornek H, Attar E. Letrozole versus human menopausal gonadotrophin in women undergoing intrauterine insemination. *Reprod Biomed Online.* 2006;13:208–212.
15. Bedaiwy MA, Forman R, Mousa NA, Al Inany HG, Casper RF. Cost-effectiveness of aromatase inhibitor co-treatment for controlled ovarian stimulation. *Hum Reprod.* 2006;21:2838–2844.
16. Oktay K, Buyuk E, Davis O, Yermakova I, Veeck L, Rosenwaks Z. Fertility preservation in breast cancer patients: IVF and embryo cryopreservation after ovarian stimulation with tamoxifen. *Hum Reprod.* 2003;18(1): 90–95.
17. Oktay K, Buyuk E, Libertella N, Akar M, Rosenwaks Z. Fertility preservation in breast cancer patients: a prospective controlled comparison of ovarian stimulation with tamoxifen and letrozole for embryo cryopreservation. *J Clin Oncol.* 2005;23(19):4259–4261.
18. Oktay K, Hourvitz A, Sahin G, et al. Letrozole reduces estrogen and gonadotropin exposure in women with breast cancer undergoing ovarian stimulation before chemotherapy. *J Clin Endocrinal Metab.* 2006;91: 3885–3890.
19. Chen C. Pregnancy after human oocyte cryopreservation. *Lancet.* 1986;1: 884–886.
20. Matson PL, Graefling J, Junk SM, Yovich JL, Edirisinghe WR. Cryopreservation of oocytes and embryos: use of a mouse model to investigate effects upon zona hardness and formulate treatment strategies in an in-vitro fertilization programme. *Hum Reprod.*1997;12(7):1550–1553.
21. Porcu E, Fabbri R, Seracchioli R, et al. Birth of a healthy female after intracytoplasmic sperm injection of cryopreserved human oocytes. *Fertil Steril.* 1997;68:724–726.
22. Polak de Fried E, Notrica J, Rubinstein M, Marazzi A, Gómez Gonzalez M. Pregnancy after human donor oocyte cryopreservation and thawing in association with intracytoplasmic sperm injection in a patient with ovarian failure. *Fertil Steril.* 1998;69:555–557.
23. Oktay K, Cil PA, Bang H. Efficiency of oocyte cryopreservation: a meta-analysis. *Fertil Steril.* 2006;86:70–80.
24. Mazur P. Equilibrium, quasi-equilibrium, and nonequilibrium freezing of mammalian embryos. *Cell Biophysiol.* 1990;17:53.
25. Oktay K, Buyuk E, Rosenwaks Z, Rucinski J. A technique for transplantation of ovarian cortical strips to the forearm. *Fertil Steril.* 2003;80(1): 193–198.
26. Blumenfeld Z. Gynaecologic concerns for young women exposed to gonadotoxic chemotherapy. *Curr Opin Obstet Gynecol.* 2003;15(5): 359–370.

27. Gosden RG, Baird DT, Wade JC, Webb R. Restoration of fertility to oophorectomised sheep by ovarian autografts stored at −196 degrees C. *Hum Reprod.* 1994;9:597–603.

28. Salle B, Demirci B, Franck M, Rudigoz RC, Guerin JF, Lornage J. Normal pregnancies and live births after autograft of frozen-thawed hemi-ovaries into ewes. *Fertil Steril.* 2002;77:403–408.

29. Sztein J, Sweet H, Farley J, Mobraaten L. Cryopreservation and orthotopic transplantation of mouse ovaries: new approach in gamete banking. *Biol Reprod.* 1998;58(4):1071–1074.

30. Oktay K, Economos K, Kan M, Rucinski J, Veeck L, Rosenwaks Z. Endocrine function and oocyte retrieval after autologous transplantation of ovarian cortical strips to the forearm. *JAMA.* 2001;286(12):1490–1493 (comment).

31. Oktay K, Buyuk E, Veeck L, et al. Embryo development after heterotopic transplantation of cryopreserved ovarian tissue. *Lancet.* 2004;363(9412): 837–840(comment).

32. Yin H, Wang X, Kim SS, Chen H, Tan SL, Gosden RG. Transplantation of intact rat gonads using vascular anastomosis: effects of cryopreservation, ischaemia and genotype. *Hum Reprod.* 2003;18(6):1165–1172.

33. Jeremias E, Bedaiwy MA, Nelson D, Biscotti CV, Falcone T. Assessment of tissue injury in cryopreserved ovarian tissue. *Fertil Steril.* 2003;79(3): 651–653.

34. Bedaiwy MA, Jeremias E, Gurunluoglu R, et al. Restoration of ovarian function after autotransplantation of intact frozen-thawed sheep ovaries with microvascular anastomosis. *Fertil Steril.* 2003;79(3): 594–602.

35. Jeremias E, Bedaiwy MA, Gurunluoglu R, Biscotti CV, Siemionow M, Falcone T. Heterotopic autotransplantation of the ovary with microvascular anastomosis: a novel surgical technique. *Fertil Steril.* 2002;77(6): 1278–1282.

36. Wang X, Chen H, Win H, et al. Fertility after intact ovary transplantation. *Nature.* 2002;415(6870):385.

37. Bedaiwy MA, Hussein MR, Biscotti C, Falcone T. Cryopreservation of intact human ovary with its vascular pedicle. *Hum Reprod.* 2006;21: 3258–3269.

38. McCall ML, Keaty EC, Thompson JD. Conservation of ovarian tissue in the treatment of carcinoma of the cervix with radical surgery. *Am J Obstet Gynecol.* 1958;75:590–600.

39. Morice P, Castaigne D, Haie-Meder C, et al. Laparoscopic ovarian transposition for pelvic malignancies: indications and functional outcomes. *Fertil Steril.* 1998;70:956–960.

40. Bisharah M, Tulandi T. Laparoscopic preservation of ovarian function: an underused procedure. *Am J Obstet Gynecol.* 2003;188:367–370.

41. Morice P, Thiam-Ba R, Castaigne D, et al. Fertility results after ovarian transposition for pelvic malignancies treated by external irradiation or brachytherapy. *Hum Reprod.* 1998;13:660–663.

42. Glode LM, Robinson J, Gould SF. Protection from cyclophosphamide-induced testicular damage with an analogue of gonadotropin-releasing hormone. *Lancet.* 1981;1:1132–1134.

43. Ataya K, Moghissi K. Chemotherapy-induced premature ovarian failure: mechanisms and prevention. *Steroids.* 1989;54(6):607–626.

44. Ataya K, Rao LV, Lawrence E, Kimmel R. Luteinizing hormone-releasing hormone agonist inhibits cyclophosphamide-induced ovarian follicular depletion in rhesus monkeys. *Biol Reprod.* 1995;52(2):365–372.

45. Ataya K, Pydyn E, Ramahi-Ataya A, Orton CG. Is radiation-induced ovarian failure in rhesus monkeys preventable by luteinizing hormone-releasing hormone agonists? Preliminary observations. *J Clin Endocrinol Metab.* 1995;80(3):790–795.

46. Blumenfeld Z, Avivi I, Linn S, Epelbaum R, Ben-Shahar M, Haim N. Prevention of irreversible chemotherapy-induced ovarian damage in young women with lymphoma by a gonadotrophin-releasing hormone agonist in parallel to chemotherapy. *Hum Reprod.* 1996;11(8):1620–1626.

47. Blumenfeld Z, Avivi I, Ritter M, Rowe JM. Preservation of fertility and ovarian function and minimizing chemotherapy-induced gonadotoxicity in young women. *J Soc Gynecol Invest.* 1999;6(5):229–239.

48. Blumenfeld Z, Shapiro D, Shteinberg M, Avivi I, Nahir M. Preservation of fertility and ovarian function and minimizing gonadotoxicity in young women with systemic lupus erythematosus treated by chemotherapy. *Lupus.* 2000;9(6):401–405.

49. Blumenfeld Z, Dann E, Avivi I, et al. Fertility after treatment for Hodgkin's disease. *Ann Oncol.* 2002;13(suppl 1):138–147(comment).

50. Recchia F, Sica G, De Filippis S, Saggio G, Rosselli M, Rea S. Goserelin as ovarian protection in the adjuvant treatment of premenopausal breast cancer: a phase II pilot study. *Anticancer Drugs.* 2002;13:417–424.

FURTHER READING

Lee SJ, Schover LR, Partridge AH, et al. American Society of Clinical Oncology recommendations on fertility preservation in cancer patients. *J Clin Oncol.* 2006;24(18):2917–2931.

chapter

30

Postoperative Lymphedema: Evaluation and Treatment

Dalliah Black, MD, FACS

ABSTRACT

Lymphedema can develop any time after surgical or radiation treatment for cancer. Most patients with lymphedema experience mild, reversible swelling; however, few patients have marked edema causing moderate to severe limitation in daily functions. This chapter will review the assessment, prevention, treatment, and current research in lymphedema management.

THE LYMPHATIC SYSTEM AND CANCER TREATMENT

Cancer staging comprises tumor size, regional lymph node involvement, and the presence of distant metastasis. Lymph nodes are often removed during an operation for melanoma, breast cancer, and gynecologic cancer to assess whether or not a cancer has spread locally. Lymph nodes normally filter about 2 liters of protein-rich lymph fluid throughout the human body a day. They also limit and fight infections. Tumor cells can spread by way of the lymphatic system and lodge in nearby lymph nodes.

427

Surgical removal of lymph nodes and disruption of lymphatic channels predisposes a patient to develop lymphedema (swelling due to abnormal buildup of lymph fluid). Sentinel lymph node biopsy (SLNB) has
become an accepted method for checking lymph nodes for tumor metastasis, particularly in breast cancer and melanoma cases. During an SLNB,
an average of one to three lymph nodes are removed from the regional
nodal basin (axilla, inguinal, popliteal fossa). If metastasis is found, usually the remainder of the lymph nodes in that basin are removed, which
may number between 10 and 25 nodes. The likelihood of lymphedema
increases as more lymph nodes are removed. For breast cancer surgery,
SLNB has a 4% to 7% chance of arm lymphedema, and complete lymph
node dissection has a 15% to 20% chance of lymphedema.[1]

Radiation therapy, often given to prevent local tumor recurrence,
can also damage lymphatic channels by scarring down these channels
and thereby causing lymphedema. The chance of lymphedema after surgical lymph node removal is increased with the addition of postsurgical
radiation therapy.[2]

DEFINITION AND TYPES OF SECONDARY LYMPHEDEMA

Primary lymphedema results from underdevelopment or an inadequate
number of lymphatic channels. This swelling usually presents at birth
or later in early life. Secondary lymphedema is tissue swelling caused by
an accumulation of lymph fluid after the removal of lymph nodes or
lymphatic channel disruption, most commonly after surgery or radiation
treatment.[3] Secondary lymphedema can occur within 1 year of treatment
or more than 20 years after treatment. Lymphedema can occur anywhere
in the body because lymph nodes are throughout the body. Most commonly, lymphedema presents as swelling of the arm, leg, trunk, or neck,
depending on where the treatment was given. There are three types of
secondary lymphedema: (1) spontaneously reducible, (2) not spontaneously reducible, and (3) elephantitis. This chapter will discuss secondary lymphedema and how it is related to cancer treatment.

SECONDARY LYMPHEDEMA EVALUATION AND
DIFFERENTIAL DIAGNOSIS

Secondary lymphedema can occur at any time after surgery or radiation treatment. Many healthcare providers and patients think that if

lymphedema has not happened within a year or 2 years after surgery there is no chance of developing it. It is difficult to tell which patient will get lymphedema after treatment; however, there are risk factors that can increase a patient's chance. These risk factors include surgical removal of lymph nodes for cancer staging or surgical scars that disrupt lymphatic channels and lymphatic drainage. Lymphedema can occur after any type of surgery but is commonly seen in breast lumpectomy, which result in breast or arm swelling, plastic surgery, and heart or lung surgery, which can result in chest swelling. Melanoma excision and removal of its draining lymph nodes can cause extremity lymphedema. Patients can have genital or bilateral lower extremity swelling after excision of a gynecologic or urologic tumor and its pelvic lymph nodes. Radiation therapy is a risk factor of developing lymphedema, because the radiation damages lymphatic channels while killing tumor cells. These damaged lymphatic channels may then scar down and no longer drain the lymph fluid, causing swelling in the irradiated area. There are data to suggest that chemotherapy also has a damaging effect on lymphatic channels and increases the chance of lymphedema. Obese patients and infections at the surgical site also increase the chance of lymphedema.[4] The more risk factors a patient has, the higher the chance of lymphedema (Table 30.1).

The occurrence of secondary lymphedema varies and treatment is often delayed because healthcare providers oftentimes do not recognize the symptoms and signs of lymphedema. Early treatment begins with taking a good history and performing a physical exam. There are numerous symptoms a patient may experience. Patients may describe skin tightness, shooting pain, asymmetry, uncomfortable fit of clothing on one side, or a deep, achy heaviness in the affected area. Some patients

TABLE 30.1 Risk Factors for Secondary Lymphedema

• Lymph node removal
• Breast cancer, melanoma, gynecologic cancer cases
• Plastic surgery cases, cardiac and lung cases
• Radiated areas
• Obese patients
• Postoperative wound infection
• Some evidence for patients receiving chemotherapy

may not remember having a surgical procedure that may explain their newly acquired lymphedema until the healthcare provider notices the scar. Measuring the affected side is helpful in diagnosing mild lymphedema that may be difficult to appreciate on physical exam alone. A simple way to measure an extremity in the clinic is with a tape measure at every 10 centimeters compared to the contralateral side. A difference of 5% to 10% is considered mild lymphedema. Healthcare providers such as physical therapists may employ calipers or a water displacement technique to diagnose lymphedema.[5] New studies to more accurately measure lymphedema use laser capture pictures for computer-generated measurements.[6]

Not every patient with swelling has lymphedema. A common cause of unilateral extremity swelling is venous insufficiency. Another cause is a blood clot in the vein, also known as deep venous thrombosis. Lymphangitis, infection in the lymphatic channels, or a tumor that is obstructing lymphatic flow can also cause unilateral swelling.[7] Inflammatory or rheumatologic disorders can present as swelling in one extremity or joint. Congestive heart failure and renal insufficiency more often present as generalized swelling and are usually not limited to one extremity. A venous duplex ultrasound can evaluate for blood clot in the vein. A chest x-ray, echocardiogram, and bloodwork may help to evaluate for congestive heart failure, renal failure, or inflammatory disorders.

∿ Case Example 30.1

Edna, a 68-year-old female, presented with a 6.5 centimeter right breast cancer in 1997. She received chemotherapy before having a modified radical mastectomy, which showed a residual 3 centimeter tumor, and 5 out of 11 axillary lymph nodes had tumor. Postoperatively, she received radiation to the chest wall and axilla as well as additional chemotherapy. In 2002 she noticed right arm swelling. She did not have signs of heart or kidney insufficiency. The differential diagnosis included lymphedema, tumor recurrence in the axilla causing lymphatic obstruction, or venous obstruction from a blood clot.

On physical exam, the right arm was soft and almost twice the size of the left arm. There was a strong radial pulse, and the arm had no signs of ischemia. There was no axillary lymphadenopathy or palpable chest wall mass. Arm duplex ultrasound showed no venous clot.

She was referred to physical therapy for evaluation and treatment of lymphedema. She underwent manual drainage and wore an arm sleeve with good result. However, 1 year later she stopped all treatment and the swelling reoccurred.

TREATMENT OF SECONDARY LYMPHEDEMA

There is no cure for lymphedema, only treatment. The best treatment is prevention and, failing this, early recognition and treatment. A physical therapist or occupational therapist specializing in lymphedema therapy is the major component of treatment.[8] During physical therapy, manual lymphatic drainage is performed with light massage to redirect drainage of lymphatic fluid from the area of swelling to another unaffected area of lymph nodes. Initially, this treatment is done two to five times a week, depending on the degree of lymphedema. If a surgical scar is in the route of redirecting lymphatic fluid, then the therapist may try to break down scar formation with devices such as ultrasound. Compression bandaging such as arm sleeves, truncal bras, or ACE wraps are useful in minimizing reaccumulation of fluid, but oftentimes they must be used in combination with manual lymphatic drainage. Massage pumps should be used under the direction of a therapist with at least weekly clinical follow-up. Massage pumps are used by the patient to apply pressure to continue redirecting the lymphatic flow recently established by the therapist. Weight management and thorough skin care are also essential to lymphedema treatment. Diuretics and low-protein diets are not effective in treating lymphedema.[5]

PREVENTION OF SECONDARY LYMPHEDEMA

Patients at high risk for lymphedema should be aware of preventative measures. Table 30.2 provides a list of simple steps one can take after surgery or radiation treatment.

CURRENT RESEARCH IN SECONDARY LYMPHEDEMA

Ongoing research in secondary lymphedema focuses on developing more accurate ways to measure, prevent, and treat lymphedema. As

TABLE 30.2 ∾ Post-treatment Preventative Measures for Lymphedema

I. Protect your skin from infection.
   a. Use an antibacterial soap.
   b. Keep arm hydrated with moisturizing lotion.
   c. Use an electric shaver or wax for hair removal. If using a razor, do so carefully in a mirror to avoid breaks in the skin.
   d. Avoid pet scratches and insect bites.
   e. Wear gloves when gardening or taking out the trash.
   f. Avoid cutting cuticles during a manicure.
   g. If you get a cut or burn, wash the area with an antibacterial soap, apply an antibacterial ointment, and cover with a bandage. Immediately call your doctor because you may need to start antibiotics by mouth.

II. Avoid constricting movements.
   a. Do not have IVs, blood pressures taken, or blood draws in the extremity if a complete axillary dissection was done.
   b. Do not wear tight sleeves or jewelry.

III. Avoid exposure to excessive heat and burns.
   a. Wear sunscreen.
   b. Avoid saunas or hot tubs.

IV. Gradually return to normal activity.
   a. Immediately after surgery, avoid repetitive vigorous arm movement such as vacuuming.
   b. Avoid lifting anything greater than 10 pounds.
   c. Carry heavy items on your other arm.

mentioned previously, one group has found laser capture scanning to be an alternate method for extremity measurement in the evaluation of lymphedema.[6]

Axillary sentinel lymph node biopsy is a surgical technique that minimizes the risk of lymphedema and is performed by injecting the breast with a tracer that travels to the axillary sentinel lymph node. These nodes are then identified by the surgeon and removed while leaving the rest of the lymph nodes in the axilla. Thompson and colleagues reported a technique of injecting blue dye into the arm and a radioactive tracer into the breast so that the lymph nodes draining the arm can be differentiated from lymph nodes that drain the breast. By specifically removing nodes that drain only the breast, arm swelling was less likely to occur, and the technique was accurate in identifying breast cancer lymph node metastasis.[9]

Surgeons in Italy have also reported techniques of reimplanting benign lymph nodes into the venous and lymphatic channels of the affected extremity by microvascular anastomosis with some success.[10] This surgery is tedious, and its long-term benefit is not known. Therefore, it has not been met with interest as a routine treatment option for lymphedema in the United States.

Lymphedema is not an uncommon side effect of surgery and cancer treatment. If it occurs, it commonly presents as mild swelling. Currently, assessing cancer spread to nearby lymph nodes usually requires surgical excision. The benefits this information provides in accurately staging a cancer help tailor treatment options to provide patients with the best outcome in the future and outweigh the potential risk of lymphedema. Preventing lymphedema by maintaining a healthy weight, avoiding infections, gradually returning to full activity and early recognition and intervention are ways patients can minimize swelling risks.

REFERENCES

1. Langer I, Guller U, Berclaz G, et al. Morbidity of sentinel lymph node biopsy (SLN) alone versus SLN and completion axillary lymph node dissection after breast cancer surgery: a prospective Swiss multicenter study on 659 patients. *Ann Surg.* 2007;245(3):452–461.

2. Aitken RJ, Gaze MN, Rodger A, et al. Arm morbidity within a trial of mastectomy and either nodal sample with selective radiotherapy or axillary clearance. *Br J Surg.* 1989;76(6):568–571.

3. Moseley AL, Carati CJ, Piller NB. A systematic review of common conservative therapies for arm lymphedema secondary to breast cancer treatment. *Ann Oncol.* 2007;18(4):639–646.

4. Soran A, D'Angelo G, Begovic M, et al. Breast cancer-related lymphedema—what are the significant predictors and how they affect the severity of lymphedema? *Breast J.* 2006;12(6):536–543.

5. Harris J, Lippman M, Morrow M, et al. *Diseases of the Breast.* 3rd ed. Philadelphia: Lippincott Williams & Wilkins; 2004:1453–1463.

6. McKinnon J, Wong V, Temple WJ, et al. Measurement of limb volume: laser scanning versus volume displacement. *J Surg Oncol.* 2007;96(5): 381–388.

7. Zakaria S, Johnson R, Pockaj BA, Degnim AC. Breast cancer presenting as unilateral arm edema. *J Gen Intern Med.* 2007;22(5):675–676.
8. Hamner JB, Fleming MD. Lymphedema therapy reduces the volume of edema and pain in patients with breast cancer. *Ann Surg Oncol.* 2007; 14(6):1904–1908.
9. Thompson M, Korourian S, Henry-Tillman R, et al. Axillary reverse mapping (ARM): a new concept to identify and enhance lymphatic preservation. *Ann Surg Oncol.* 2007;14(6):1890–1895.
10. Campisi C, Eretta C, Pertile D, et al. Microsurgery for treatment of peripheral lymphedema: long-term outcome and future perspectives. *Microsurgery.* 2007;27(4):333–338.

chapter

31

Conclusion

Kenneth D. Miller, MD

When President Nixon signed the Cancer Act in 1971, it is estimated there were approximately 3 million cancer survivors; today that number is close to 12 million.[1] By the year 2020, this number will be about 20 million men, women, and children.[2]

One cancer survivor, Dr. Fitzhugh Mullan, described his own journey as a cancer survivor in the article "Seasons of Survival: Reflections of a Physician with Cancer." In it, Dr. Mullan wrote:[3]

> Survival was not one condition but many. It was desperate days of nausea and depression. It was the elation at the birth of a daughter in the midst of treatment. It was the anxiety of my monthly chest x-rays. . . . It was survival, an absolutely predictable but ill-defined condition that all cancer patients pass through as they struggle with their illness.

Dr. Mullan defined three seasons of survival. The first was *Acute Survival*—a medical stage including the time of diagnosis and then the initial therapy. The second was *Extended Survival*—a time of watchful waiting with celebration, uncertainty, and transition. Finally, the third was *Permanent Survival*—a time when a gradual sense of confidence develops when the risk of recurrence is low and the chance of long-term survival is great. (See Figure 31.1.)

Today, there is a large and growing number of cancer survivors, and many short- and long-term sequelae of treatment have been identified. The medical impact of cancer on an individual is related to many factors, including the cancer survivor's age and comorbidities, the

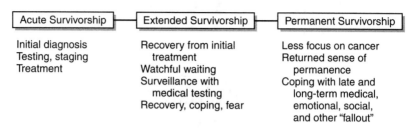

FIGURE 31.1 Seasons of survivorship proposed by Fitzhugh Mullan, MD, in 1985.[3]

specific diagnosis, location of the tumor, type of treatment (surgery, radiation, or chemotherapy), the intensity of the treatment, and the effect of time and age after cancer treatment. The risk of a second or subsequent malignancy is also becoming more relevant because of the side effects of high-dose therapy and because cancer survivors are living longer. (See Chapter 15 of this text.)

There is a growing understanding of the psychosocial impact of the diagnosis of cancer and its treatment on cancer survivors. Understandably, fear of recurrence is common for cancer survivors, and anxiety and depression are problems for others. Sexual problems are observed in at least 50% of survivors of breast cancer and gynecological cancer, as well as up to 90% of men treated for prostate cancer.[4] As a result, survivors frequently report that life after diagnosis is characterized by new emotional depth and personal growth. Cancer survivors talk about "stopping to smell the roses."

Cancer survivors are a growing group with increasing heterogeneity. Increasing numbers of cancer survivors have moved beyond cancer and are healthy. On the other hand, others are cancer-free but "not free of cancer," because consequences of cancer continue to affect their health, sexuality, career, and insurability; moreover, some reenter the system years later with a second cancer that may or may not be related to their previous cancer and its treatment. Other growing populations of cancer survivors include those living with advanced cancer for long periods of time and those who are in a remission that is dependent upon the use of a targeted agent such as imatinib (for patients with chronic myelogenous leukemia).

Recognition of the heterogeneity of cancer survivorship results in a modified model of the "Seasons of Survivorship," incorporating what has been learned about cancer survivorship during the past 20 years. (See Figure 31.2.)

It is essential to note that survivorship for individual cancer survivors is quite variable, largely because they are a large group of people with tremendous diversity in sex, age, culture, socioeconomic status, religion, family, education, and multiple other factors that influence and define them.[5] Cancer survivors share some of the common experiences of acute survivorship, when the diagnosis is made and treatment follows. Some cancer survivors do not live long beyond acute survivorship, but the growing majority do and enter a season known as transitional survivorship, which is the beginning of watchful waiting or of ongoing therapy after the initial diagnosis and the most intense treatment. The next season is extended survivorship, during which a diverse group of patients are in a stable complete remission with a good prognosis, are in remission because of ongoing therapy, or are living with active cancer and its sequelae. Finally, there is a growing group of permanent survivors that includes those who are medically and emotionally cancer-free, those who have ongoing "fallout" from the cancer experience, and those who reenter the system with second or with secondary cancers.[6]

Improving our understanding of the "seasons of survivorship" is important because it may improve the clinical care we offer. Late and long-term medical complications of cancer treatment may be amenable to early and ongoing intervention and may improve the long-term health of our patients. The roots of post-traumatic stress syndrome probably arise in acute survivorship, and specific interventions during that time may improve long-term adjustment and coping. In long-term cancer survivorship, emphasizing comprehensive cancer screening and

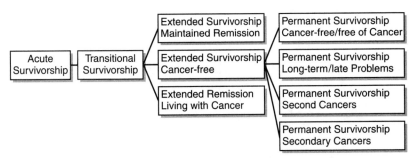

FIGURE 31.2 Proposed model for the "Seasons of Survivorship."[3]

healthy cancer survivorship practices, including ongoing exercise and a prudent diet, might reduce the morbidity and mortality of second and secondary cancers.

Over 22 years have passed since the founding of the National Coalition for Cancer Survivorship, the new definition that cancer survivorship starts from the moment of diagnosis, and the landmark article by Dr. Mullans. The chance of living beyond acute cancer survivorship has increased, as has the total number of "permanent survivors." Because cancer survivors are living more years after their diagnosis, it is an important goal to help them enjoy the best possible quality of life during those years.

REFERENCES

1. National Coalition for Cancer Survivorship (NCCS): NCCS Charter. Silver Spring, MD: National Coalition for Cancer Survivorship; 1986.
2. SEER Cancer Statistics Review, 1975–2005. National Cancer Institute Web site. http://seer.cancer.gov/csr/1975_2005/index.html. Accessed January 27, 2009.
3. Miller K, Merry B, Miller J. Seasons of survivorship revisited. *Cancer J.* 2008 Nov–Dec; 14(6):369–374.
4. Schover LR. Sexuality and fertility after cancer. *Hematol Am Soc Hematol Educ Program.* 2005:523–527.
5. Foley KL, Farmer DF, Petronis VM, et al. A qualitative exploration of the cancer experience among long-term survivors: comparisons by cancer type, ethnicity, gender, and age. *Psycho-Oncol.* 2006;15:248–258.
7. Miller KD. The cancer journal. The journal of principles & practice of oncology. From the guest editor. *Cancer J.* 2008;14(6):358–360.

Index

Italicized pages indicate a photo/figure; tables are noted with a t.